READER'S DIGEST
HEALTH SECRETS

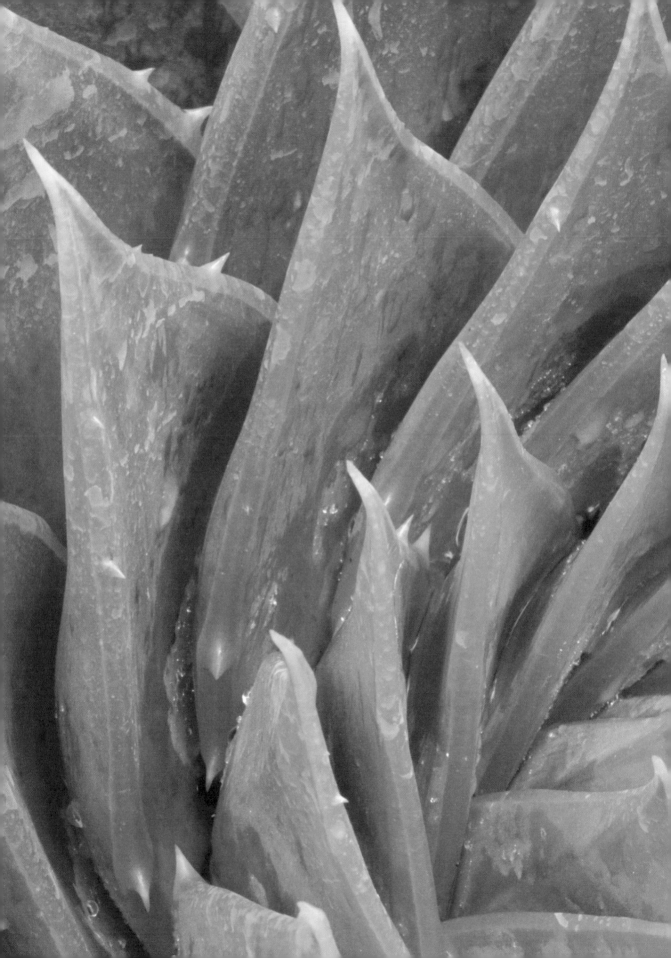

READER'S DIGEST
HEALTH
SECRETS

Reader's
digest

The Reader's Digest Association, Inc.

New York, NY / Montreal

CONTENTS

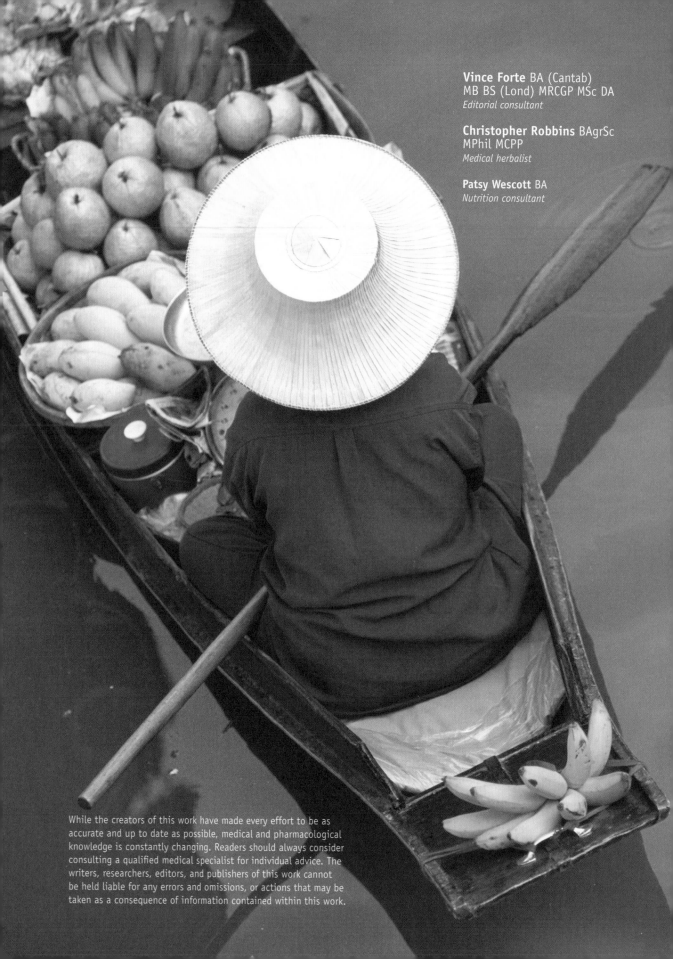

Vince Forte BA (Cantab)
MB BS (Lond) MRCGP MSc DA
Editorial consultant

Christopher Robbins BAgrSc
MPhil MCPP
Medical herbalist

Patsy Wescott BA
Nutrition consultant

Why you need
THESE HEALTH SECRETS

As a family doctor, I am only too aware that every patient who comes through my office door is an individual. Everyone has a unique set of genes, family background, upbringing, temperament, and physical constitution, all of which impact on their health—as do age, gender, and ethnicity.

Equally, I recognize that there is no one answer to any health problem, which is what makes *Reader's Digest Health Secrets* such an exciting and useful new book. With information drawn from worldwide sources, it contains a huge variety of dependable hints and tips for so many ailments and conditions, enabling you to pick and choose what is most helpful to you and your family.

While the media is awash with health advice and news stories announcing the benefits of the latest "cure," often the difficulty is sorting out the strategies that really work from the merely speculative. This is why this book is so helpful. It will give you the sound information you need to take charge of your own and your family's health and well-being. And much of it is the sort of lifestyle guidance, touching on diet, exercise, or simple home treatments that a busy doctor may not have time to impart.

For example, did you know that eating red foods such as tomatoes, peppers, and pomegranates can help protect against sunburn and prematurely aged skin, that turning on the radio could bring instant relief from tinnitus, and that the ingredients in chicken soup could help to bring down blood pressure levels? These are just three of the hundreds of health secrets you are about to discover as you leaf through the following pages. Many will be new to you, some familiar, while others that were previously dismissed as old wives' tales have now gained the stamp of scientific approval.

I don't always have the time to share the latest research with my patients or discuss the range of self-help strategies they could use. I hope this book will enlighten and empower you to take charge of your own and your family's health and lead to better communication between you and your doctor for the sake of your health and well-being and that of your family.

Dr. Vince Forte
Practicing GP

About
THIS BOOK

You will discover a whole new approach to managing your health in this ground-breaking new family reference book from Reader's Digest. Every page outlines useful and often surprising advice about how good health can be enhanced and illness prevented and treated in simple ways that are accessible to all. You'll learn how simple and often unexpected changes or additions to your diet, exercise habits, and daily routine boost your physical and mental health at every stage of life from childhood to old age.

From homespun remedies to cutting-edge science

Reader's Digest has gathered wide-ranging health tips from around the globe and chosen the best to include in this book. Many have been validated by cutting-edge research but others reflect popular usage, recognizing that conventional medical science does not hold all the answers to our health, and alternative therapies can be equally, or in some instances, more effective. The result is a volume that encompasses everything from special diets to prescription drugs and herbal medicine. It draws on the wisdom of tribal societies as well as top academic institutions to present hard-hitting information on subjects ranging from superfoods to the latest surgical techniques.

By reading this book, you will reap the benefits of the latest scientific thinking and its practical applications. For instance, research has disproved the notion (often suggested by orthopedic specialists) that a hard mattress can ease an aching back. In fact, it can actually exacerbate the pain; a medium to firm mattress with plenty of support is more helpful. And you'll gain some other intriguing insights as researchers examine traditional remedies and put them to the test. For example, if your mother ever warned you that eating cheese late at night might give you nightmares, she was right. Studies have revealed that cheese contains tyramine, a compound that raises blood pressure, a stress symptom often associated with bad dreams. Wherever possible, the science behind the secret is revealed to help you understand why or how it works.

Simple, practical, and new

An added benefit of this book's secrets is that many of them are so simple. Did you know, for instance, that brushing your teeth can help prevent a heart attack or that chewing gum has been shown to improve memory? Others, such as putting a bar of soap in your bed to prevent night cramps, might seem a little quirky but are worthy of inclusion because so many people claim they work.

And that's not all. The information about more complex health problems that may affect you and your family from cancer to dementia, from arthritis to heart disease is largely new and different. Rather than giving you well-worn advice on causes and treatments that you can find elsewhere, here is something of more immediate value, such as the lesser-known but typical signs of a heart attack (nausea, sweating, and in women, back pain and light-headedness)—information that could be invaluable in an emergency.

Above all, the book provides a holistic view of health, embracing the indisputable truth that symptoms cannot be treated in isolation and effective treatments may have physical, mental, even spiritual dimensions. From proof that acupuncture can alleviate backache or that beta blockers, ordinarily used to lower blood pressure, may also inhibit the spread of cancer cells, the book includes a wealth of insights from a wide range of authoritative sources.

The result is a mix of ancient lore, home remedies, and new scientific discoveries that will entertain, inform and, above all, help you and your family stay fit and healthy—for life.

Mind and body

Reader's Digest Health Secrets recognizes the crucial interaction between body and mind, with tips that benefit both physical and mental health, arranged system by system in two main sections.

Section one, **Body Health Secrets,** includes chapters on key aspects of physical health such as the heart, circulation, bones and muscles, breathing, nutrition, weight control, hormones, reproduction, teeth, skin and hair health, as well as the aging process.

The second section, **Mind Health Secrets,** focuses on the brain and nervous system, including ways to keep them healthy, how to boost mood, improve memory, and keep your senses sharp. There is also advice on improving sleep, and how to combat fears, phobias, and addictions as well as advice on coping with the symptoms of illnesses such as Alzheimer's and Parkinson's disease.

Throughout the book special panels highlight the effects of physical processes on psychological health and well-being, and vice versa. In Body Health Secrets, "Mind Power" boxes illustrate how certain thought processes affect physical health. For instance, researchers have now discovered that women who suffer from depression have lower bone density and higher levels of blood cortisol, a hormone related to bone loss.

By contrast, other studies show that a positive approach to life boosts health and can even help you live longer. Similarly, in Mind Health Secrets, "Body Power" boxes explain how certain physical actions help to boost your mood and keep your brain firing on all cylinders.

Within each chapter you will also find colorful features that investigate fascinating topics in greater depth. Many of these focus on the wide geographical and often ancient origins of treatments scientists are studying today.

For example, you'll discover why the older people of the Japanese islands of Okinawa live so long; the secret lies in their traditional diet. Or that aloe vera, much used today for its healing and antiseptic properties, was valued by the ancient Egyptians and grown by King Solomon. Other features take a different perspective, providing insights into new medical research that may pave the way for the treatments of the future.

PROTECTING YOUR HEART
BLOOD AND CIRCULATION
BREATH OF LIFE
BUILDING STRONG BONES AND MUSCLES

Body Health Secrets

NUTRITION AND WEIGHT CONTROL
IMPROVING YOUR DIGESTION
URINARY HEALTH
HEALTHY HORMONES
THE CYCLE OF LIFE
FIGHTING INVADERS
GLEAMING TEETH, HEALTHY MOUTH
PROTECT YOUR SKIN
SHINING HAIR, STRONG NAILS
AGING WELL

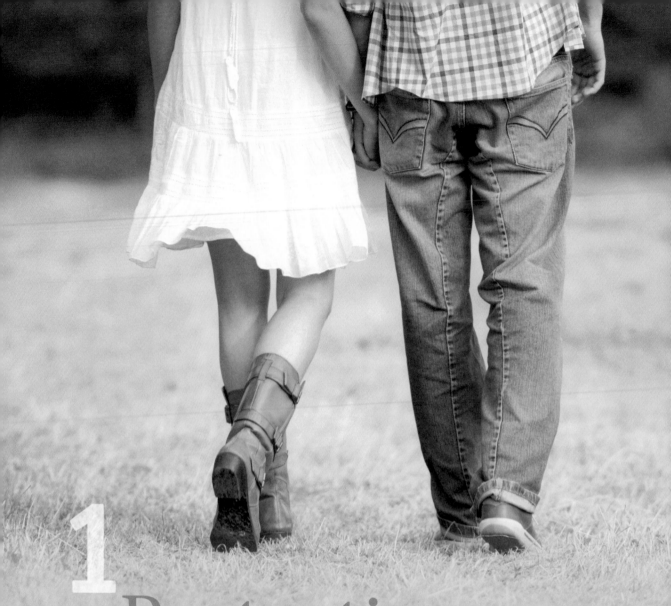

1 Protecting
YOUR HEART

Your amazing heart pumps blood around a vast 60,000-mile (96,560-km) network to feed your body's thousands of billions of cells. Read on to discover what it loves and hates—advice that your doctor may never have passed on—and the simple steps you can take to improve and preserve your heart health for all the years to come.

Everyday LIVING

Studies from around the world show that heart health is linked more closely to lifestyle than anything else—so there is plenty you can do to prevent damage to this vital organ. On the following pages, you'll find suggestions for small changes that can make a big difference.

● **Check your neck size** According to recent studies, the thickness of your neck may provide more clues to your risk of heart disease than the size of your waist. American researchers have found that the greater the circumference, the higher the risk of heart disease. The average neck circumference for an American woman is 13½in (34.2cm), and 16in (40.5cm) for a man. A fat neck may be a sign of heart-unfriendly visceral fat deposits around the liver and heart.

● **Aim for 10,000 steps a day** That's what US experts advise for healthy adults to maintain heart well-being. It's a great incentive to buy a pedometer—and one for a friend—and see how many steps you can fit into your day. Most of us walk no more than 4,000 steps a day— too little to give the heart the exercise it needs. Medical experts say that, along with diet, inactivity is a major contributor to heart problems.

● **Watch TV standing up** Every 2 hours spent sitting in front of the tube raises heart disease risk by 15 percent, say American researchers. So stand up or better still, turn it off and get moving. Doing something active could prevent two in every 1,000 people from developing heart problems. The risk of heart disease and early death from any cause doubles in people who spend more than 4 hours a day in front of a computer or television screen. Limit your own and your children's viewing. If you work with a computer, make sure you walk away and take active breaks every 30 minutes.

● **Do the math** Researchers at the University of Glasgow have identified your BMI (body mass index) as the clearest indicator of your heart's present and future health. Calculate your BMI using the formulas at the Centers for Disease Control's website: www.cdc.gov/healthyweight/assessing/bmi/adult_bmi/index.html. Then refer to the "Know Your BMI" chart on page 80 for an estimate of the risk to your heart

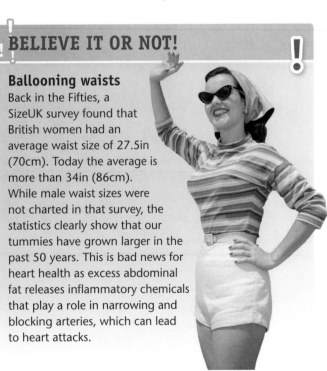

BELIEVE IT OR NOT!

Ballooning waists

Back in the Fifties, a SizeUK survey found that British women had an average waist size of 27.5in (70cm). Today the average is more than 34in (86cm). While male waist sizes were not charted in that survey, the statistics clearly show that our tummies have grown larger in the past 50 years. This is bad news for heart health as excess abdominal fat releases inflammatory chemicals that play a role in narrowing and blocking arteries, which can lead to heart attacks.

health. For adults, a BMI between 18.5 and 24.9 is normal, 25–29.9 is overweight, and above 30 is considered to be obese (unless you are heavily muscled).

● **Don't sleep for too long** Too much sleep is bad for your heart, according to a 2010 study from the West Virginia University School of Medicine. The research into more than 30,000 adults showed that those who regularly slept more than nine hours a night were over one and a half times more likely to develop heart disease. Getting seven hours a night was best, while getting less than five was worst; sleep-deprived adults were twice as likely to suffer heart problems.

For further tips on improving your sleep, see Chapter 20, *A Better Night's Sleep*

A potted plant can be your secret weapon against heart-damaging pollutants.

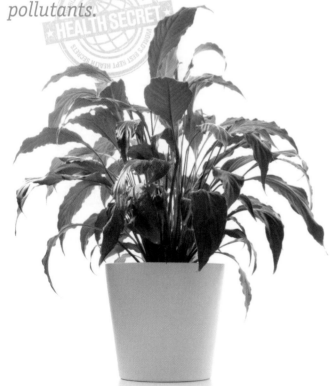

● **Get some gum** For the sake of your heart, make the decision to quit smoking now and ask your doctor for the help you need—such as nicotine patches or gum—to kick the habit. Within as little as 8 hours of quitting smoking, your oxygen levels increase and your circulation improves, and within a year, your risk of heart disease is reduced by up to 50 percent. And just five years after giving up tobacco, your risk of dying prematurely from heart disease is about the same as that of someone who has never smoked.

● **Avoid polluted air** Heavy traffic fumes, smoke, and dust all raise heart attack risk but can be hard to escape if you work or live in a town or city. Just being aware is the first step. If possible, try not to travel during rush hour. Escape to a park or riverside at lunchtime and, whenever possible, get out into the country. And try the air-purifying benefits of certain houseplants. The right kind of potted plant in your home or office, such as a rubber plant or peace lily, will help remove pollutants and could do your heart good.

● **Make your glass half full** Optimists have a lower risk of heart attack and death from cardiovascular disease than those with a more negative outlook on life. In one study that followed the fortunes of 122 men who had suffered a heart attack, eight years after the attack, 21 of the pessimists had died compared with just six of the optimists. Looking on the bright side can bring health as well as happiness.

● **Throw a pebble** Visitors to the Scottish isle of Iona like to follow a potent ancient tradition. They throw a pebble from the beach into the sea to get rid of the bad things in their lives and pick up a new one to represent the future. It's a strategy that works for worries, too. Brooding over problems can raise levels of the stress hormone cortisol which is linked to inflammation and heart disorders.

Externalizing them, throwing them away, or writing them down, then sorting them out is a much more positive response. But be sure to see your doctor if you find it hard to deal with stress or if you suffer from ongoing depression or anxiety. Depression can make you twice as vulnerable to a heart attack.

● **Shut down your computer** to help make your home a special place in which you can relax and get away from the heart-damaging stresses in your life. Here are some tips to help you create a tranquil refuge from the day's worries:
★ **Get rid of** clutter.
★ **Choose** restful colors.

And when you're ready to relax:
★ **Switch off** your phone.
★ **Play** music you enjoy.

Letting a pebble symbolize the bad things in your life, then throwing it away, is liberating.

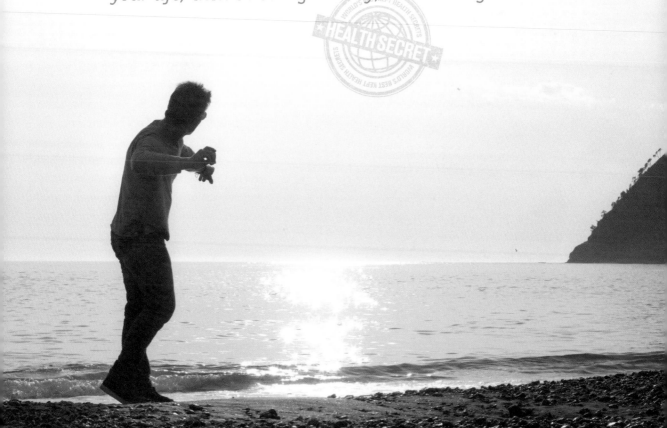

● **Train your brain** Controlling your thoughts can help to keep a heart problem in check, according to a study from the British Heart Foundation. When scientists studied the health of people who had just been diagnosed with heart disease, they found that those who took part in a cognitive behavioral therapy (CBT) course—which teaches you to think more constructively—reduced their risk of having a heart attack by 41 percent. It is not known exactly how CBT might reduce heart attack risk but the researchers think it teaches you to acknowledge and deal with negative areas in your life, reducing high stress levels. Talk to your doctor about the availability of CBT and the possibility of a referral.

For further tips on coping with depression, see *Chapter 16, Managing Your Mood*

● **Get help, if necessary** Your heart suffers when you are depressed. Scientists suggest that people who suffer from a mood disorder such as depression are twice as likely to have a heart attack. By contrast, a five-year study of older people shows that those who feel happiest are less likely to smoke and more likely to exercise —factors, together with a healthy diet that are known to benefit heart health. So don't live with low spirits, get expert help.

A toothbrush can help reduce your risk of heart disease.

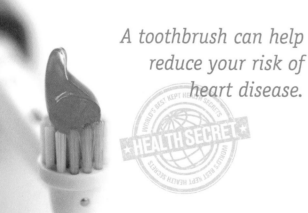

SECRETS OF SUCCESS

Why laughter works wonders
Researchers suggest that a good laugh benefits your heart because the tissue that forms the inner lining of our blood vessels expands when we chuckle, which helps to increase blood flow by around 25 percent. That's equivalent to the impact of a stroll in the park or even being on cholesterol-lowering drugs. It's so good for you that experts advise 15 minutes of laughter a day. So watch a funny movie or go to a stand-up comedy show. Anything that makes you giggle will lift your heart, too.

● **Avoid the news** The constant barrage of news headlines—often concerned with disasters or frightening events—can create a potent and damaging cocktail of worry and feelings of powerlessness. Give your heart a break by giving the news a vacation for a few days. You'll be surprised how much better you feel.

● **Get brushing** Your mouth may seem a long way from your heart, but if you neglect your teeth, you could be putting your heart and your life at peril. Poor oral hygiene is a major cause of gum disease. It produces low-grade inflammation, which in turn is a high risk factor for heart disease. Studies show people with infected gums are nearly twice as likely to have heart attacks as those with healthy gums. To reduce heart-damaging gum inflammation:
★ **Brush** (preferably with an electric toothbrush) for at least 2 minutes and floss or use interdental brushes twice a day.
★ **Replace** your toothbrush every two to three months.
★ **Visit** the dental hygienist regularly.

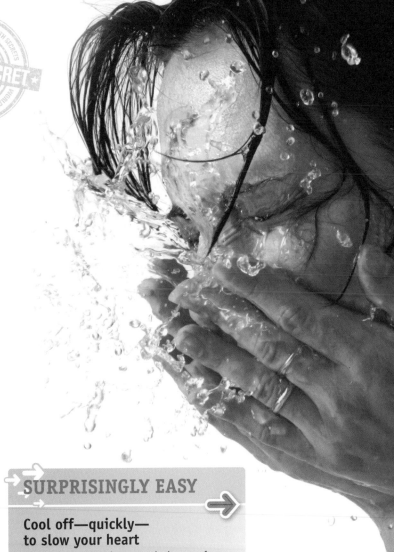

Splashing cold water on your face can slow a racing heart.

● **Listen to your heart** Is your heartbeat frequently fast and irregular? That's one symptom of atrial fibrillation (AFib), a common heart rhythm disturbance and a major risk factor for stroke. In a survey by the British Stroke Association of more than 1,000 people and 1,000 family doctors, a staggering 66 percent were unaware of the signs. According to the charity, earlier treatment of AFib could prevent around 4,500 people having a devastating stroke each year. Check your heart rate and rhythm by feeling your pulse in your neck or wrist. Consult your doctor if your heartbeat is irregular or fast (over 140 beats a minute at rest), or if you have other symptoms such as palpitations, shortness of breath, lightheadedness, or faintness.

● **Get a winter flu shot** to reduce your chance of suffering a heart attack by almost a fifth. Heart attacks are more common in winter and studies show there is a link between having an infection such as flu a week or two earlier. The risk is even higher for those who already have a heart condition. People in this category are up to four times more likely to suffer an attack following an infection.

● **Time it right** A UK study has suggested that getting a flu vaccination in late autumn or early winter is more effective than one given later in the year. It therefore makes sense to schedule your appointment for a flu shot with this in mind.

SURPRISINGLY EASY

Cool off—quickly— to slow your heart

To slow a racing heart, splash your face with cold water or cover your face with a cold, wet washcloth for a few minutes. A natural reaction to cold water can cause the heart to slow down.

You could also try the following:

● Take a deep breath—inhaling as much as possible until you can't take in any more air—and then exhale as fast as you can.

● Repeat until you feel your heart slowing down.

● Take a very deep breath to help get oxygen to your brain and restore your breathing rhythm to normal. Ordinary deep breathing won't do the trick.

Heart
HEALTHY EATING

Making sensible food choices can really help your heart. It's well known that reducing levels of harmful fats and salt is a must for heart health, but the trick is knowing how to do this without making mealtimes a misery. Here are some practical—and delicious—tips.

● **Eat six meals a day** Small, frequent meals can help keep cholesterol levels low suggests a 2001 study published in the *British Medical Journal*. Researchers found that people who ate six small meals a day had a 5 percent lower average cholesterol level and also lower levels of artery-clogging "bad" low-density lipoprotein (LDL) cholesterol than those who ate just one or two large meals. This reduction is enough to shrink your risk of heart disease by 10 to 20 percent. It seems that grazing during the day may balance metabolism and prevent the dramatic rises and falls in blood glucose that are linked to increased cholesterol production. So snacking can be good for you—as long as you choose healthy nibbles.

● **Go brown** Whole-grain brown rice, with its mild nutty flavor, offers heart benefits for carnivores and vegetarians alike.

Researchers suggest that an extract in brown rice may work against a protein called angiotensin—a known trigger of high blood pressure and hardening of the arteries, key risk factors for heart disease. Brown rice is also a good source of fiber, and for most of us makes a healthy addition to a balanced diet. So choose brown over white whenever you can.

● **Try acai berries** Acai berries from the Brazilian rainforest are on course to become a favorite "super food." American research has revealed that these berries are rich in anti-inflammatory substances, which may help to protect against hardening of the arteries—a major risk factor for heart disease. Another study suggests that the berries can also help to lower high cholesterol levels as well as reduce the risk of type 2 diabetes, both of which predispose you to heart disease. Scientists think that acai juice helps

Acai berries from the rainforest can help lower your cholesterol levels.

HEALTH SECRET

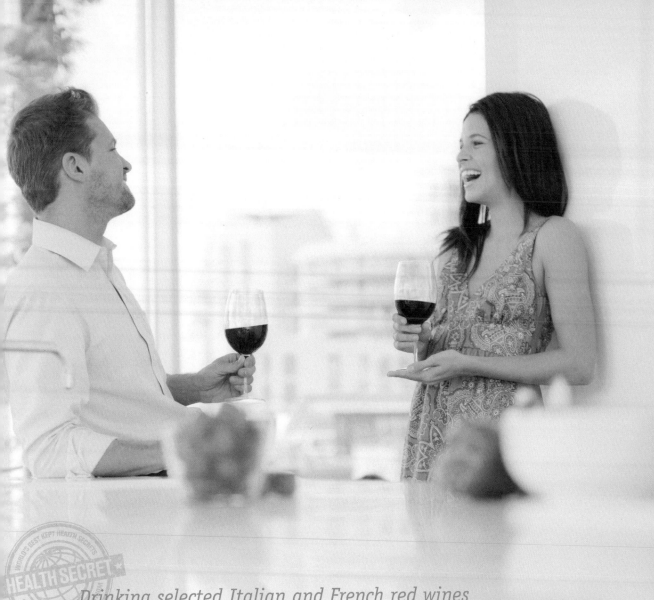

Drinking selected Italian and French red wines could give your heart health an extra boost.

to block the production of inflammatory chemicals that increase the risk of narrowed arteries. Look for acai juice, freeze-dried berries, or acai extract capsules in health food stores.

● **Choose the right red wine** Some red wines may offer extra special heart benefits, suggests a new study from the University of London. Scientists have known for a while that resveratrol—a plant chemical in red wine—has a heart-protective effect. Now

other potentially protective chemicals— procyandins—are also receiving credit. Red wines from Sardinia and southwest France are thought to have especially high levels of these helpful compounds. But moderation is key—the benefits are easily outweighed by the risks of excessive alcohol consumption.

● **Say "no" to sugary drinks** Pay heed if you love sugary canned or bottled drinks. Research from the Harvard School of Public Health shows that having just one sugar-

Eggs are low in heart-damaging fats

They may be rich in cholesterol, but when it comes to heart disease, it is not the amount of cholesterol in the food that matters but the amount of saturated fat—and eggs are low in saturated fat. What's more, eggs are one of the few dietary sources of vitamin D, which now also appears to benefit heart

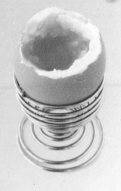

health, and they supply good amounts of vitamins A, B, and E and essential minerals. Unless you have been advised by your doctor or dietitian not to eat them, you can include eggs in your balanced and varied diet.

sweetened drink a day (1¼ cups/350ml) can increase your risk of heart disease by at least 20 percent. And studies suggest that people who consume sugary drinks are more likely to accumulate harmful belly fat, also linked to heart disease. While sugar-sweetened beverages are not necessarily a direct cause of heart disease, high sugar intake does contribute to certain risk factors for heart problems. So it makes sense to keep your consumption of all sugar-ladened foods to a minimum.

● **Have more bananas** Potassium-rich bananas can help to keep a check on heart-damaging high blood pressure. Slice them into fruit salads or blend them in shakes and smoothies. But a word of warning: Check with your doctor if you are taking diuretics. Some of these medicines may cause a build-up of potassium in the body.

● **Get more than five** We are used to hearing that we should eat five portions of fruit and vegetables a day for good health.

Now the British Heart Foundation is emphasizing that this should be the minimum. Our heart health would benefit even more if we adapted our diet to include as many as eight portions of fruit and veggies every day.

● **Go for tangerines** These tasty fruits are not just a rich source of vitamin C and fiber. Researchers at Canada's University of Western Ontario have recently discovered that tangerines also contain a flavonoid called nobiletin that may help prevent obesity and protect against atherosclerosis (hardening of the arteries), which can lead to heart disease.

● **Add flavor to reduce risk** Instead of salt, which contributes to high blood pressure, a risk factor for heart disease, use spices and fresh herbs to flavor food. Try to include the three below, which are reputed to have additional special benefits for heart health.

★ **Garlic** Research suggests that allicin is the key ingredient that makes eating garlic so good for you. In the body, allicin is broken down into compounds that react with red blood cells to produce hydrogen sulphide, which relaxes blood vessels and helps blood flow more easily.

★ **Ginger** In a study published in the *Journal of Nutrition*, extract of ginger was shown to reduce overall blood cholesterol levels as well as inhibiting LDL oxidation. This suggests it could help protect against hardening of the arteries and heart disease.

★ **Turmeric** Japanese research suggests that curcumin—a plant compound that gives the turmeric its yellow color—may prevent heart failure. Further research is needed to confirm this effect, but it is possible that curcumin could form the basis of new treatments for this condition.

● **Get the avocado habit** Studies show that eating one avocado a day as part of a healthy diet can lower heart-clogging LDL ("bad") cholesterol by as much as 17 percent while raising levels of HDL ("good") cholesterol. Try some guacamole and combine the health benefits of avocado and garlic.

● **Whip up a super smoothie** French researchers from the University of Strasbourg have come up with a smoothie recipe specially designed to boost heart health. The tasty drink is a blend of apples, blueberries, grapes, strawberries, acerola cherries, lingonberries, and chokeberries.

● **Have a heart-healthy stir-fry** Yes, you can enjoy fried food without risk to your health— if you use the right kind of oil. This good news, in a study published in the *British Medical Journal*, found that heart risk factors linked to eating fried foods do not apply when foods are fried in olive and sunflower oils. Olive oil is a source of heart-friendly monounsaturated fatty acids, while sunflower oil contains omega-6 fatty acids. But be careful to use fresh oil each time you fry. Overheating or reheating oil causes chemical changes, turning healthy fats into heart-damaging trans fats.

A delicious blend of grapes, apples, blueberries, strawberries, and other berries can boost your heart's health.

SURPRISINGLY EASY

Low-fat frying
Reduce the amount of oil you use when frying by using an oil-water spray. Simply fill a spray bottle with seven-eighths water and one-eighth heart-healthy canola or olive oil, and spray the mixture onto your griddle or roasting pan before cooking.

● **Enjoy milk and cheese** Researchers who examined the records of 3,630 middle-aged Costa Rican men and women found no significant link between heart attack risk and eating dairy foods. They suggest that the saturated fat in dairy foods may be offset by protective calcium and a "good" fat called conjugated linoleic acid.

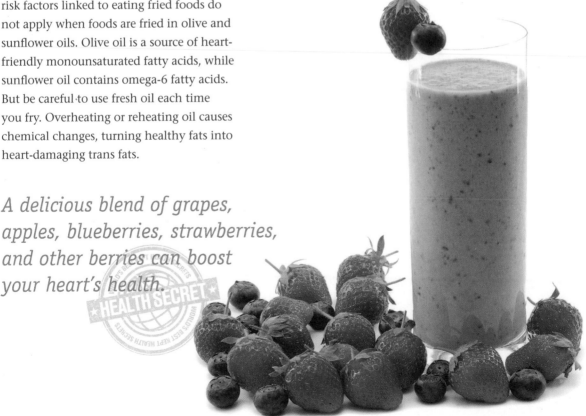

Secrets of a HEART-HEALTHY DIET

While heart disease has reached epidemic proportions in many Western countries, scientists have discovered some societies—from South America to the Pacific and the Arctic—where it is much less widespread. Their research has identified important factors that these populations share.

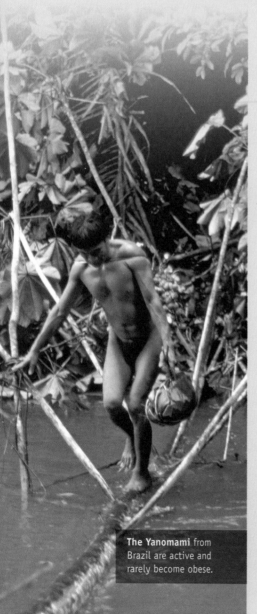

The Yanomami from Brazil are active and rarely become obese.

A few decades ago when the first global studies showed huge disparities in heart disease around the world, scientists wanted to know why. What they discovered in heart-healthy communities, such as the three populations below, has provided vital clues and is helping health experts to advise and educate much wealthier nations.

The Yanomami Indians

In a study of 52 populations across four continents, the Yanomami Indians of Brazil were shown to have the lowest blood pressure levels. The figures from the INTERSALT study were dramatic—the Yanomami average was 95/61 compared to 120/80–140/90 for people in the UK. Researchers concluded that their secret is a diet that contains virtually no salt or alcohol, and their active lifestyle. The men hunt and fish and the women cultivate vegetables, which accounts for around 80 percent of what they eat.

The people of Okinawa

People in the Okinawan islands of Japan traditionally eat a diet low in saturated fats and high in essential minerals, antioxidants, and phytonutrients—compounds that give fruit and vegetables their hue. The Okinawan Centenarian Study, launched in 1975, ascribed the astonishingly low rates of heart disease in large part to this diet. That many younger Okinawans have abandoned their traditional diet and are falling prey to heart disease underlines the value of this way of eating.

The Inuit

Two Danish researchers Hans Olaf Bang and Jorn Dyerberg, working in the 1970s, became intrigued by the fact that, despite eating huge amounts of fat and protein with little fruit and vegetables, the Greenland Inuit were almost free of heart disease. They concluded that the explanation for the heart health of the Inuits was that their diet was rich in omega-3 fatty acids, which lower cholesterol and reduce inflammation.

Share the health benefits

Populations in which heart disease is very rare have a diet low in saturated fats, high in monounsaturated and polyunsaturated fats, and rich in the vitamins, minerals and other compounds that promote a healthy heart. You can share the health benefits of the diets of these cultures by adapting their menus (described here). You'll need to substitute some of the foods—for example, venison for moose, sardines for seal, and seafood for frogs and grubs.

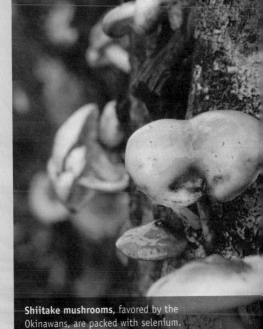

Shiitake mushrooms, favored by the Okinawans, are packed with selenium.

Yanomami foods

- **Fruit and vegetables**
Potassium-rich bananas, carotene-rich mangoes, sweet potatoes, papaya, and the starchy cassava or manioc, rich in the antioxidant mineral manganese and vitamin C.
- **Frogs, land crabs, caterpillars, and other grubs**—high in protein and healthy omega-3 fatty acids, vitamins B12 and C, folate, and essential minerals such as magnesium, calcium, copper, zinc, phosphorus, and iron.
- **Nuts**, rich in unsaturated fats.
- **Honey**, which contains vitamins and minerals plus high levels of friendly bacteria.

Okinawan foods

- **Shiitake mushrooms**, for selenium and vitamin D.
- **Kombu** (kelp), rich in iodine.
- **Vegetables** such as Chinese okra and green papaya, rich in vitamins, minerals, and phytonutrients.
- **Sweet potato**, the main starchy food rather than rice. It's rich in beta-carotene and has a low glycemic index score.
- **Soy products** such as tofu and miso, which lower levels of blood cholesterol, raise those of good cholesterol (HDL), and reduce harmful triglycerides.
- **Fish and lean meat** in small quantities.

- **Turmeric**, a spice that is high in anti-inflammatory, cholesterol-lowering curcumin.
- **Daikon** (Japanese radish), which has high levels of enzymes that aid the absorption of fats and carbohydrates, vitamin C, and phytonutrients.

Inuit foods

- **Sea mammals** such as whale and seal, which are high in monounsaturated fats and omega-3 fatty acids, and rich in selenium and vitamins A, D, and E.
- **Oily fish** such as salmon and Arctic char.
- **Raw fish,** such as frozen raw whitefish, thinly sliced.
- **Fermented foods,** rich in probiotic bacteria that promote a healthy gut. Prized delicacies include fermented seal flipper.
- **Wild gamebirds and meats,** such as moose, which are low in saturated fats, high in healthy unsaturated fats, and rich in vitamins B, C, and E.

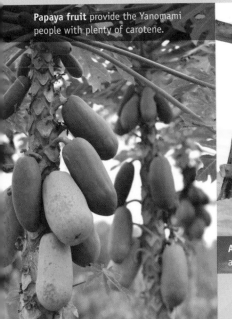

Papaya fruit provide the Yanomami people with plenty of carotene.

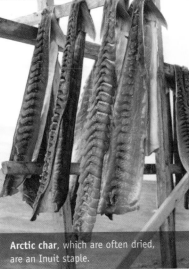

Arctic char, which are often dried, are an Inuit staple.

Keep it
MOVING

Physical activity is key to heart health. Even a moderate level of exercise strengthens the muscles of your heart by making it pump faster. There are many effective ways to get fit that can be easily worked into a hectic day. Just get moving.

● **Take small steps** Anything that gets your heart beating faster is good for heart health. Exercising for 15 minutes a day or 90 minutes a week is enough; initially the pace is unimportant. Something is always better than nothing. But the more exercise you do and the more vigorous it is, the more your heart will benefit. Start out modestly but aim to build up to at least 30 minutes of moderate physical activity most days of the week by doing aerobic exercise—any activity that gets your heart beating faster and leaves you feeling warm and a little out of breath.

● **Leave the car at home** There are plenty of ways you can build exercise into your daily life. Leave the car at home and walk briskly to the store, get off the bus a stop early and walk the rest, mow the lawn, put on your favorite music and dance around the living room, or take the family for a bike ride. You don't have to do 30 minutes at a time; break it down into 10-minute slots through the day if that's easier for you to achieve.

Here are some more—perhaps surprising—ways to increase your daily exercise with very little effort:

★ **Cook dinner** rather than calling for takeout—standing and cooking burns more calories than sitting and waiting for the delivery to arrive.

★ **Unload** the washing machine, stack the dishwasher, or do another household chore during the commercial breaks on television instead of sitting in front of the screen and having a snack.

★ **Park** as far away as you can from the grocery store or mall to get the longest possible walk to your destination.

★ **Stand up** to answer the phone and don't sit down until you have finished the call. Walk around the house, garden, or office to add extra steps.

★ **Plan a weekend walk** with someone who is faster and fitter than you—it will push you that little bit more.

★ **Think on your feet**—stand up when you write notes or lists, whether at home or in the office. That way you will stretch your legs more regularly.

Lifting weights can lower your blood pressure.

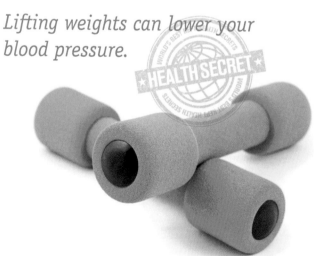

● **Get strong** Strength-training exercise such as lifting weights is not just good for increasing muscle power. Research reported in the *Journal of Strength and Conditioning* shows that it can be as good for your heart as aerobic exercise. It improves blood flow and triggers a long lasting drop in blood pressure. For maximum effect, aim for two sessions a week, each at least 30 minutes, in addition to your regular aerobic workouts. If you have a heart condition, ask your doctor before starting such training.

● **Help your child's heart** One of the best things you can do for your children's future heart health is to keep them moving. A study carried out in Sweden on a group of 11-year-olds showed that the less active among them were at a higher risk of later heart problems. Aim to get your kids active for at least 60 minutes a day. Games of tag,

cycling, and soccer are all good choices. Research suggests that youngsters with plenty of friends tend to get more exercise, so invite other children to join in.

● **Work out to music** Let your favorite sounds boost the cardiovascular benefits of training. Research suggests that running to your favorite beat increases stamina by up to 20 percent.

● **Walk your way to recovery** Many people are afraid to exercise after a heart attack for fear of triggering another attack, but the evidence suggests that doing aerobic exercise helps to speed recovery. Working your large muscles hard will also strengthen your heart muscle. Good choices include brisk walking, swimming, or gardening. Check with your cardiologist or doctor before you start and build up gradually.

Children need at least an hour's activity a day to guard against future heart problems.

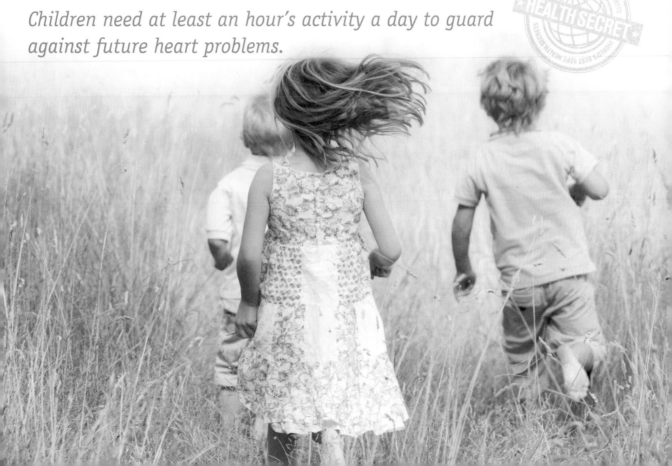

On the MEDICAL FRONT

While scientists cannot change the way we live, medical research can help us identify risks, pinpoint problems, and rescue hearts in danger. On these pages, you'll discover some of the ways new knowledge can help you look after your heart.

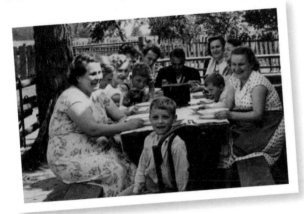

Your family's genes may hold the key to your heart attack risk.

● **Know all the symptoms** Severe and crushing chest pain is the heart attack symptom most of us are aware of. Another classic sign is an aching discomfort in the chest, similar to indigestion. But there are several other more vague and less dramatic symptoms that can indicate the onset of a heart attack. And there is some evidence that women are less likely to feel chest pain and often suffer these less common, non-specific warnings of heart trouble. They include the following:

★ **Jaw, shoulder, or arm pain**
★ **Tiredness, weakness, or feeling generally unwell**
★ **Dizziness or lightheadedness**
★ **Nausea or vomiting**

If you are experiencing any symptoms that make you suspect you have a heart problem, consult your doctor as soon as possible. Seek emergency medical help if you think you may be having a heart attack.

● **Check out your family history** Your genetic inheritance could have a huge impact on your risk of heart disease. A British Heart Foundation study has found that one in five men have a variation of the male-only Y chromosome, which could increase their heart disease risk and could

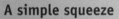

SECRETS OF SUCCESS

A simple squeeze

Squeezing the upper arm tightly using a normal blood pressure measuring cuff could limit heart damage following a heart attack. This new technique, called conditioning, which is being investigated by scientists, could reduce injury after a heart attack by as much as one-quarter. It could also help reduce the risk of heart failure, a major cause of illness and death, later in life.

The theory is that temporarily cutting off the blood supply to a muscle makes it resistant to further damage. Intriguingly, protection from one muscle can be transferred through the bloodstream to another muscle. If this theory proves to be right, squeezing an arm for a few minutes could protect the heart during the recovery period.

explain why several men from the same family may all have heart attacks at a young age. Researchers hope this discovery leads to new tests and treatments for men. If early heart problems run in your family, discuss preventive treatment with your doctor.

● **Keep up your estrogen levels** For women after menopause, boosting levels of the female sex hormone estrogen may benefit heart health. Studies have shown that estrogen acts on white blood cells—part of your body's natural defense system—preventing them from sticking to the insides of your blood vessels, which can damage arteries, veins, and capillaries and lead to heart disease. Hormone replacement therapy (HRT) can restore estrogen levels, which decline naturally after menopause, but it's not suitable for everyone. Ask your doctor whether it's right for you.

● **Seek help for erection problems** Erectile dysfunction (ED) can be an early sign of clogged arteries. Men with ED are 1.6 times more likely to suffer from a serious cardiovascular problem such as a heart attack or stroke, according to a study in the *Journal of the American Heart Association*. The arteries supplying the penis are narrow, so erection problems could be an early sign of clogging and narrowing in other blood vessels. If you are experiencing this problem, seeing your doctor is a vital precaution, as well as the best way to get help for your ED.

● **Get the best view** Magnetic resonance imaging (MRI) may offer the most accurate diagnosis of your heart problems. Research has shown that an MRI is better than the most commonly used alternative—a single photon emission computed tomography (SPECT) scan, which uses radioactive material to track blood flow to tissues and organs. An MRI scan does not use radiation. If your doctor suggests a scan, ask if this option is available.

● **Time it right** Research suggests that ACE inhibitors (often given to those with high blood pressure, after a heart attack, or to treat heart failure) may work better if taken at bedtime rather than first thing in the morning as is usually advised. They work by reducing levels of a hormone (angiotensin-converting enzyme), which tend to rise at night. So targeting the highest levels, may be more effective. Discuss the timing of your dose with your doctor.

● **Don't pocket your headphones** The tiny magnets found inside headphones can interfere with the operation of your pacemaker, according to US researchers. In a recent study, 20 percent of pacemakers reacted when headphones were placed directly over them. If you have an implanted pacemaker, don't carry your headphones in your breast pocket or let them dangle unused on your chest.

BELIEVE IT OR NOT!

"Staying Alive" can keep you alive

Many people are reluctant to give mouth-to-mouth resuscitation, fearing close contact with a stranger or doing it incorrectly. But the latest advice from the British Heart Foundation (BHF) for carrying out cardiopulmonary resuscitation (CPR) is to forget mouth-to-mouth and concentrate on chest compressions. To get the tempo right, work to the tune of the Bee Gees' hit "Staying Alive." Hands-only CPR should give you the confidence to step in and help when somebody is in cardiac arrest, says the BHF. You need to press hard and fast in the center of the chest at a depth of 2 to 3in (5 to 6cm), at a rate of 100 to 120 compressions a minute.

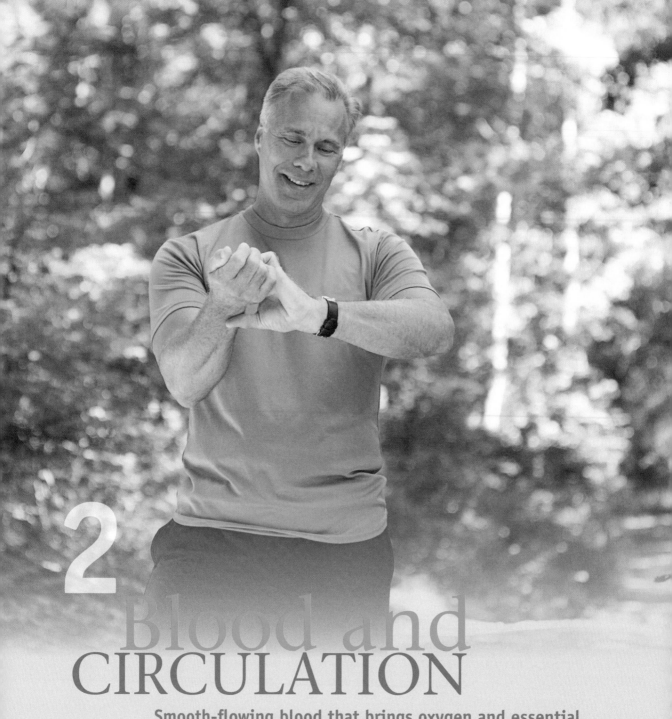

2
Blood and
CIRCULATION

Smooth-flowing blood that brings oxygen and essential nutrients to every cell in the body is vital for health and well-being. To improve your circulation and reduce your risk of disease, you need a healthy level of fats and other blood constituents as well as optimum blood pressure. Find out how to achieve this in effective and sometimes surprising ways.

Better BLOOD

There's plenty you can do to keep your blood healthy and able to supply your body with the nutrients it needs. Your diet and the amount you exercise can influence the composition of your blood. Genetics and environmental factors also have a role to play.

● **Have beans with your steak** Iron is the key component of hemoglobin, the oxygen-carrying substance in red blood cells. To maximize your absorption of this valuable mineral, eat vegetable, meat, or fish sources of iron in the same meal. Iron-rich foods include meat, poultry, fish, dark green vegetables, dried beans, and dried fruits. The adult body contains around 4g of iron, half of which is found in our red blood cells. If iron levels fall too low, anemia (low levels of red blood cells) can result.

● **Drink orange juice with your muesli** Did you know that some foods can actually block the absorption of iron from our diet? Notable iron-blocking foods include fiber-rich whole-grain cereals, dairy products, such as milk and cheese, and drinks such as tea, coffee, and chocolate. It's not possible—or advisable—to avoid many of these foods, but you can counteract their effect on iron absorption by drinking beverages between rather than with meals and by having foods or drinks that are rich in vitamin C, which boosts iron uptake. Citrus fruit, such as oranges, are particularly high in vitamin C.

● **Sprinkle nuts on your salad** Seeds, nuts, oats, barley, and soy products actively lower your blood levels of cholesterol. One study found that including a portfolio of foods that actively lower cholesterol may be

SURPRISINGLY EASY

Get more garlic
A review from New York Medical College suggested this pungent bulb may help your blood fats stay within the healthy zone. The results showed that a group of people with a total cholesterol of over 193 (5mmol/L) who were given garlic had a significant reduction in blood fats. Half to one clove a day is enough to make a difference. Add garlic to salads, soups, and stews for a tasty circulation-boosting lift.

more effective, especially for lowering heart-damaging LDL cholesterol, than a low saturated fat diet alone. Try adding cholesterol-lowering foods to your low-fat regimen to maximize the benefits.

● **Drink green tea** to improve your balance of "good" to "bad" cholesterol. Chinese researchers have found that green tea helps lower blood levels of "bad" low-density lipoprotein (LDL) cholesterol without affecting "good" high-density lipoprotein (HDL) cholesterol. So while using other cholesterol-fighting tactics such as avoiding fatty foods, enjoy green tea as often as you like.

● **Watch the label** For blood vessel health, the most important ingredients to avoid are trans fats, which appear on ingredient labels as "hydrogenated" or

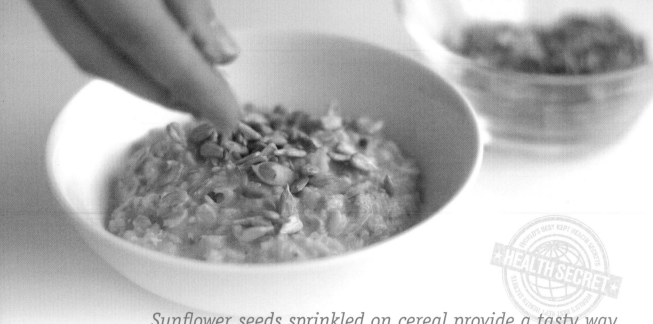

Sunflower seeds sprinkled on cereal provide a tasty way to benefit from circulation-friendly phytosterols.

"partially hydrogenated fats." They are often present in processed foods, such as cookies and cakes. Dutch scientists claim that cutting trans fats from the diet would reduce deaths from heart disease by 20 percent.

● **Snack on sunflower seeds** to lower your blood levels of cholesterol. They are one of the richest sources of phytosterols, plant compounds that help lower cholesterol and keep your blood flowing smoothly. Snack on these seeds or sprinkle a few over breakfast cereal or salads.

● **Take your tea black** Holding the milk in your tea could help to improve your blood fat profile. In one study from Mauritius, having three cups of black tea a day over three months improved the ratio of good to bad cholesterol and reduced levels of blood sugar and triglycerides (a damaging type of blood fat). Milk reduces these effects so have a slice of lemon in your tea instead.

● **Resist fried fast food** It may seem like a treat, but takeout fried fish or chicken could be especially bad for your arteries. The food has often been refried in oil that has been heated several times—which raises levels of trans fats, perhaps the most harmful type of fat for your arteries.

● **Move it** Combining exercise with a slimming diet not only boosts weight loss but also benefits the blood and circulation. Research has revealed that a mixture of exercise and a low-calorie diet raised levels of HDL cholesterol, lowered levels of damaging blood fats called triglycerides, and reduced blood pressure. Walking, jogging, and cycling are all good choices. Aim to exercise for 30 minutes on most days.

● **Get tested (if necessary)** Blood composition is a powerful indicator of numerous health conditions—particularly heart problems—and holds the key to effective treatment. One useful gauge is not only the overall level of cholesterol in the blood, but also the ratio between total cholesterol and that of "good" high-density lipoprotein (HDL) cholesterol. A high level of LDL, or "bad" cholesterol, increases your risk of heart disease, while a high level of

KNOW YOUR LEVELS

This chart shows the optimum levels of the different types of blood fats, including cholesterol and triglycerides, for people at high and low risk of heart disease.

	People at low risk of heart disease	People at high risk of heart disease
Total cholesterol (TC)	193mg/dl (5mmol/l) or less	155mg/dl (4mmol/l) or less
HDL cholesterol	Men: above 39mg/dl (1.0mmol/l) Women: above 46mg/dl (1.2mmol/l)	Men: above 39mg/dl (1.0mmol/l) Women: above 46mg/dl (1.2mmol/l)
LDL cholesterol	116mg/dl (3mmol/l) or less	77mg/dl (2mmol/l) or less
TC/HDL ratio	4.5 or less	3.5 or less
Triglycerides	66mg/dl (1.7mmol/l) or less	50mg/dL (1.3mmol/l) or less

HDL, or "good" cholesterol, helps protect your heart. You should have your levels tested if you:

★ **Have been diagnosed** with coronary heart disease, stroke or mini-stroke (TIA), or peripheral arterial disease
★ **Are over 40**
★ **Have a family history** of early heart disease or inherited high cholesterol
★ **Are overweight** or obese
★ **Have high blood pressure** or diabetes.

● **Don't rely on pills** If your doctor has prescribed medication to reduce your cholesterol levels, you must still make healthy lifestyle choices. The best results are achieved by a mix of diet, exercise, weight loss, and medication. Keep away from high-calorie, fat-laden foods and make sure you exercise regularly.

● **Take the stairs** Walking up and down stairs is an excellent way to lower cholesterol and blood pressure. As part of a study, over a period of 12 weeks, a group of hospital employees used the stairs rather than the elevator and increased the flights of stairs they walked up. As the number of flights rose, their blood pressure, cholesterol, weight, and waist circumference went down.

● **Walk, don't snooze** after a heavy meal to reduce your triglyceride levels. Experts now believe these fats are just as responsible as cholesterol, if not more so, for clogged arteries. Triglyceride levels, which rise after eating, gradually diminish over the following few hours. Exercise speeds up this process, so if you want to keep your triglyceride levels down, don't slump in the chair or go to bed just after a meal; get moving instead.

● **Steer clear of too much beer** Beer can be a cause of raised triglyceride levels. It not only reduces the breakdown of triglycerides but also encourages the liver to make even more of these damaging substances. So if you're a beer drinker, consider choosing a different beverage.

Secrets of
DVT AVOIDANCE

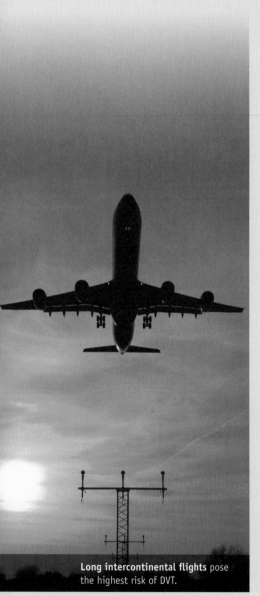

Although we have known about flight-related deep vein thrombosis (DVT)—in which a clot forms in a deep vein while flying—since the 1950s, there has been a lack of conclusive research into this potentially life-threatening condition. As medical science continues to provide insights, there are some practical measures you can take to protect yourself.

Flight-related DVT was first reported in 1954 when US surgeon John Homas diagnosed the condition in a man who had flown for 14 hours. In fact, a 1940 study of the sixfold rise in sudden death associated with DVT among Londoners had already uncovered its underlying cause—prolonged immobility, in this case in air raid shelters. Most recently, so-called e-thrombosis has been diagnosed in people sitting in front of a computer for 12 hours or more. DVT becomes life-threatening if the thrombosis, or clot, becomes dislodged, because it may travel to the lungs and block—potentially fatally—the supply of oxygen. This is known as a pulmonary embolism (PE).

The condition began to receive huge publicity in 2000 after a 28-year-old British woman died of a PE following a flight from Sydney to London. In 2001, the World Health Organization (WHO) set up the WHO Research into Global Hazards of Travel (WRIGHT) Project. Phase I of the study, published in 2007, found that:

● Air travel longer than 4 hours increases the risk of DVT/PE twofold.
● Other risk factors include obesity, using an oral contraceptive, being very short or tall, and blood abnormalities related to the clotting mechanism.

Further studies have established that pregnancy, old age, recent surgery, heart failure, recent stroke, and the use of hormone replacement therapy also increase the risk. Surprisingly, endurance athletes may also be susceptible, according to many academics. Their fitness gives them a low resting heart rate, which when combined with factors such as inactivity due to travel or injury, makes clot formation more likely.

While there is no clear evidence about the incidence of DVT among those who fly frequently, especially flight crews, flight attendants tend to be active while the plane is airborne, minimizing their risk. And pilots undergo frequent medical checkups that identify any predisposing health problems, which is likely to offer a degree of extra protection. For healthy people, it's worth remembering that the overall incidence of DVT/PE is actually quite low—one event in 6,000 flights of 4 hours or more.

Long intercontinental flights pose the highest risk of DVT.

Flight check

However, as a sensible precaution, it's worth considering where you will sit and what you will do during a flight. If possible, choose an aisle seat to make it easier to move around. A 2009 Dutch study of more than 11,000 people on flights of longer than 4 hours found that window seat passengers doubled their risk of DVT, especially if they were overweight. Those who slept had 1.5 times the risk. Anxious passengers were found to have 2.5 times the risk.

Medical experts suggest the following protective measures:

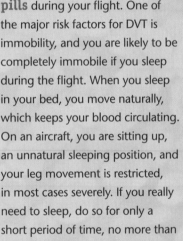

Move around the cabin and stretch to boost circulation during a long flight.

Consult your doctor before you take a flight longer than a few hours if you have any of the previously described risk factors.

Choose loose, comfortable clothing for your trip.

Buy some flight socks or compression stockings to wear during the flight. Wear only below-knee stockings, which exert a gentle pressure around the ankle to stimulate blood flow. It is vital that the stockings are measured and worn correctly, as ill-fitting stockings could increase the risk of DVT developing. Ask a pharmacist or health professional about obtaining the correct size and fitting.

Choose a low-risk seat You'll be more likely to move about if you sit next to the aisle. And ideally opt for a bulkhead seat, which is roomier.

Store luggage overhead so that your ability to move your legs is not unnecessarily restricted.

Be careful with drink If you must take advantage of in-flight alcoholic drinks, have no more than one. Drink plenty of water. There's no proof that water directly protects against DVT, but it can certainly help prevent dehydration, which may be a risk factor.

Avoid sleep and sleeping pills during your flight. One of the major risk factors for DVT is immobility, and you are likely to be completely immobile if you sleep during the flight. When you sleep in your bed, you move naturally, which keeps your blood circulating. On an aircraft, you are sitting up, an unnatural sleeping position, and your leg movement is restricted, in most cases severely. If you really need to sleep, do so for only a short period of time, no more than 30 minutes. Set an alarm to make sure you wake up and do anti-DVT exercises (see below).

Take a stroll around the cabin whenever you can.

Do anti-DVT exercises at least every half hour. Raise your heels, keeping your toes on the floor, then bring them down. Do this 10 times. Now raise and lower your toes 10 times.

Stay calm If you're afraid of flying, doing some deep breathing exercises will help to keep you calm. You could also put some lavender oil on a handkerchief, to inhale during the flight.

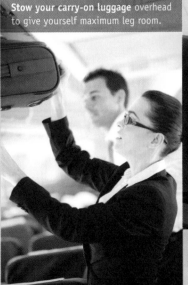

Stow your carry-on luggage overhead to give yourself maximum leg room.

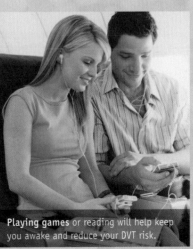

Playing games or reading will help keep you awake and reduce your DVT risk.

Controlling BLOOD PRESSURE

Known as the "silent killer" because there are usually no symptoms, dangerously high blood pressure may be revealed only after a checkup or, more seriously, after a stroke or heart attack. These essential tips will help you keep your blood pressure in check.

● **Go purple—with potatoes** Swapping your usual white potatoes for purple varieties could help reduce your blood pressure by around 4 percent. To prevent weight gain, microwave the potatoes and serve them plain, say Scottish researchers. The purple pigments in these potatoes contain high levels of antioxidant plant chemicals called anthocyanins and carotenoids, which reduce inflammation and help keep blood vessels healthy. This small drop in blood pressure may be enough to reduce your risk of heart disease.

● **Have some chicken soup** The popular cure-all, chicken soup, could help in your fight against high blood pressure. Researchers in Japan have found that chicken legs and breasts contain chemicals that act in a similar way to ACE inhibitors—

UNDERSTANDING YOUR BLOOD PRESSURE READING

A blood pressure reading of 120/80mmHg or lower is ideal according to the American Heart Association. The top number (systolic), refers to the pressure as your heart pumps; the bottom number (diastolic) is the measure of the pressure when your heart is at rest between beats.

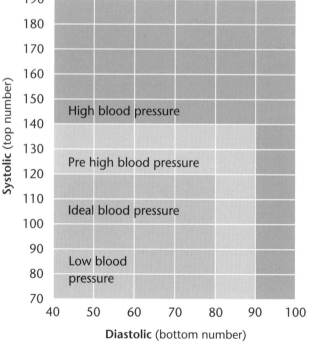

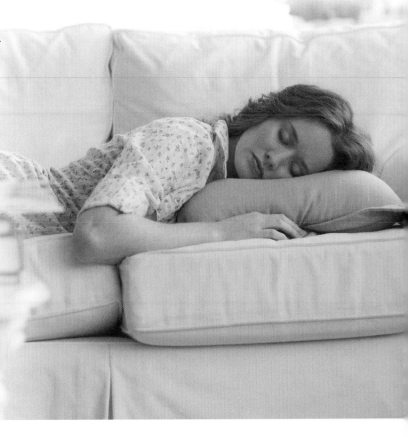

BELIEVE IT OR NOT!

Reduce blood pressure—fast

In as little as two weeks, you can reduce your blood pressure just by watching what you eat. The DASH (Dietary Approaches to Stop Hypertension) diet recommends reducing salt intake and eating increased amounts of fruit and vegetables, whole grains, lean proteins, and low-fat dairy foods. In a US trial of 459 healthy people with blood pressure just above normal (average 131/85mmHg), the DASH diet was successful at lowering blood pressure and cholesterol. It also reduced the participants' risk of developing heart disease in the following 10 years.

● **Take a siesta** If stress is causing your blood pressure to soar, a 45-minute nap could help keep it on a more even keel, according to a US study. The researchers found that a daytime sleep seemed to have a restorative effect on the heart, especially in people who slept badly at night. While this might not be a practical solution if you work full time away from home, you can adopt the rule on weekends and even try napping when you get home from work.

● **Beware of fast foods** Processed foods are a prime source of salt in our diet, and excessive salt intake is a leading cause of elevated blood pressure. Be extra vigilant

A daytime nap can lower your blood pressure.

a group of blood pressure-lowering drugs. They found that the systolic (top) blood pressure number of people who took a small daily dose of the ingredients in chicken soup dropped by an average of 11.8mmHg. If your blood pressure is on the high side, try dosing yourself with chicken soup, but keep taking any prescribed medication.

● **Know your numbers and save your health** Getting to know your blood pressure should be an essential part of your strategy to safeguard the health of your blood vessels and reduce your risk of heart attack and many other health problems. If you don't know your blood pressure reading, see your doctor or check it yourself at one of the many gyms and pharmacies that have blood pressure testing machines available. Be sure to sit down and rest for a few minutes before you test yourself. If your reading is above 120/80mmHg, make an appointment to see your doctor to discuss whether you need to take action to bring down your blood pressure.

when reading food labels—salt usually appears as sodium. The CDC recommended amount of sodium a day is 1,500mg, about a ¼ teaspoonful, with an upper limit of 2,300mg. For salt content, multiply the sodium figure by 2.5. Common salty culprits include savory snacks such as chips and crackers, canned fish and soup, ready-made meals, sauces, and packaged meals such as noodles and mixes. Many types of cheese are also high in salt, so consider eating low-salt varieties.

● **Try pomegranate juice** A daily glass of this juice may help to reduce your blood pressure, suggests a small study carried out at Queen Margaret University, Edinburgh. After a week, the blood pressure levels of healthy volunteers who drank 2 cups (500ml) of pomegranate juice daily had dropped. It's thought that pomegranate juice contains compounds that have a beneficial effect on elevated levels of cortisol, the stress hormone produced by your adrenal glands, which can contribute to high blood pressure. So enjoy a regular glass of tasty pomegranate juice as part of your blood pressure-lowering program.

● **Eat kiwi fruit** to lower blood pressure. In a small Norwegian study, a group of men and women with mildly elevated blood pressure who ate three kiwis a day for eight weeks had systolic blood pressure levels that were 3.6mmHg lower than those who snacked on an apple a day. Eat kiwis on their own, slice them into fruit salads, or blend them into a smoothie. But don't be tempted to swap them for your medication.

● **Take a dip to lower the pressure** Swim for 45 minutes three to four times a week to bring down high blood pressure, say US researchers. After 12 weeks of regular

swimming, in which the study participants gradually worked up to 45 minutes of swimming at each session, this group of over 60s had shaved an average of 9mmHg from their systolic blood pressure (the top figure in a blood pressure reading). Their arteries also became more flexible. The study suggests that this low-impact exercise could have a big impact on your health.

● **Tackle resistant blood pressure** If your blood pressure remains high in spite of efforts to improve your lifestyle, you may be among the 1 in 20 people in whom the problem is caused by an underlying medical problem called Conn's syndrome. Tiny benign growths in the adrenal glands interrupt the production of aldosterone, a hormone involved in regulating blood pressure. Although it is difficult to identify, new tests with a PET-CT scan can offer a more accurate diagnosis of the condition. If treatment has not lowered your blood pressure, ask your doctor about this test.

Clear
VESSELS

To have good circulation, you need blood vessels that are clear of fatty deposits and able to expand and contract to meet your body's needs. Regular exercise and a low-fat diet are at the core of a circulation-friendly lifestyle. Here are some extra tips to help you get it right.

● **Choose an aisle seat** It's good to be able to look out, but opting for the window seat on a long-haul flight could raise your risk of deep vein thrombosis (DVT), a condition in which blood clots form in the legs (see page 32). These clots can travel through the bloodstream to block blood flow to the lungs—a life-threatening pulmonary embolism. A window seat limits your mobility, one of the key risk factors for DVT. New guidelines from the American College of Chest Physicians advise anyone at risk of DVT on a flight of 6 hours or more to sit in an aisle seat.

BELIEVE IT OR NOT!

One a day is enough ...
Inhaling secondhand smoke from as little as one cigarette a day is enough to speed up the development of dangerous clogging and narrowing of the arteries (atherosclerosis) says the American Heart Association. The message is clear: If someone lights a cigarette, cigar, or pipe near you, move away fast, and make sure your house and car are kept as smoke-free zones.

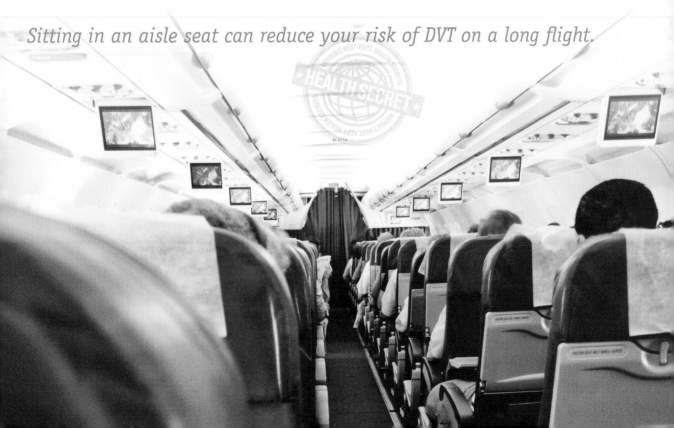

Sitting in an aisle seat can reduce your risk of DVT on a long flight.

● **Don't jog in traffic** Activity is good for your heart and blood vessels, but where and when you exercise can be just as important. Pollutants from traffic fumes, factories, and even wood-burning stoves can damage the inner lining of your arteries and curb the smooth flow of your circulation. Amazingly, the damaging effects can be seen within hours of exposure. When exercising, avoid rush hour if you can and try not to jog or cycle along busy roads. The air is fresher and better for your arteries in parks or in the country.

● **Get some herbal help** The following herbal remedies may help to keep your blood vessels in top condition—but take only one herbal remedy at a time:

★ **Garlic** To prevent hardening of the arteries take one to three 300mg capsules a day or 900mg of fresh garlic.

★ **Ginkgo** 15 drops of tincture in water a day may help to prevent hardening of the arteries and keep your veins strong.

★ **Grapeseed and grape leaves** Take one 30mg capsule of grapeseed extract daily to strengthen your veins and to help prevent varicose veins and hemorrhoids (piles). Grapevine leaves have similar properties and can form a part of your regular diet.

● **Pick up a tropical treat** Exotic fruit such as persimmons and papayas are a good source of vitamin C, a powerful antioxidant that can boost blood flow and may even reverse the damage caused by clogged, narrowed arteries. In a US study of heart disease patients, vitamin C improved the ability of the arteries to widen, boosting blood flow. Eat vitamin C-rich fruit in fruit salads, with cereals, or simply enjoy them on their own. But don't worry if you can't find these exotic fruits in your local grocery store. Strawberries, oranges, black currants, broccoli, kale, red peppers, and many other fruit and vegetables provide high levels of vitamin C. Include a wide selection of vitamin C-rich foods in your daily diet to keep your blood vessels in top condition.

Dark chocolate could lower your risk of cardiovascular disease.

● **Try tomato extract** An extract from ripe tomatoes, marketed as Fruitflow, is believed to "smooth" blood platelets, preventing life-threatening blood clots. Its manufacturers claim that it is free from the side effects associated with conventional "blood thinning" medicines such as warfarin. If you think you may be at risk of deep vein thrombosis (DVT) or blood clots, it may be worth a try. But do check with your doctor first if you are currently receiving treatment.

● **Have a piece of chocolate** A square of chocolate after dinner may help reduce your risk of blood clots—and lower your blood pressure as a bonus—but only if it's plain and dark. Researchers suggest that eating just 6.7g of chocolate a day could lower the risk of cardiovascular disease by as much as 19 percent. Dark chocolate is rich in chemical compounds that can help stop the oxidation of LDL ("bad" cholesterol), one of the key processes in clogging of the arteries. Choose chocolate that is high in cocoa solids for this delicious daily health boost.

● **Ask about foam therapy** Foam injections for varicose veins can get you on your feet even faster than laser surgery. According to a study from Imperial College, London, people treated with foam therapy had less pain and were able to return to normal activities in just three days compared with eight days after laser treatment. If you're hoping to get rid of painful or unsightly veins, ask your doctor about foam treatment.

● **Pine for your veins** An extract from the bark of a French maritime pine—Pycnogenol—can significantly improve symptoms of chronic venous insufficiency (CVI), a condition that leads to swelling of the legs. In an Italian study of 40 patients, 30 took Pycnogenol and ten a placebo; those taking the supplement had less heaviness and swelling in the legs and less pressure in their veins. It is thought that Pycnogenol works by stabilizing the layer of cells just beneath the skin or by scavenging free radicals (rogue molecules that cause cell damage) or by a combination of the two. Pycnogenol is available in many pharmacies and health food stores. Check with your doctor before taking this product.

● **Don't be squeamish—maggots can help cure leg ulcers** Reviving a practice that has been known for centuries, doctors in many hospitals recommend the use of maggot debridement, in which living maggots (fly larvae) inside a dressing are used to clean infected varicose ulcers. The dressing is left on the wound for 24 to 36 hours, during which time the maggots eat damaged tissue. Although the thought of it may make your flesh creep, most people report that they don't feel a thing.

✳ MIND POWER

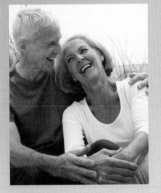

Laugh away leg ulcers

A good laugh—along with traditional nursing care—could heal leg ulcers more successfully than ultrasound therapy, suggests a recent study from Leeds University in the UK. Having a hearty chuckle can be beneficial because laughing gets the diaphragm working, which plays a vital part in moving blood around the body, helping the healing process. Have a giggle with a friend, watch a film comedy, or read a funny book. Anything that prompts a belly laugh should do the trick.

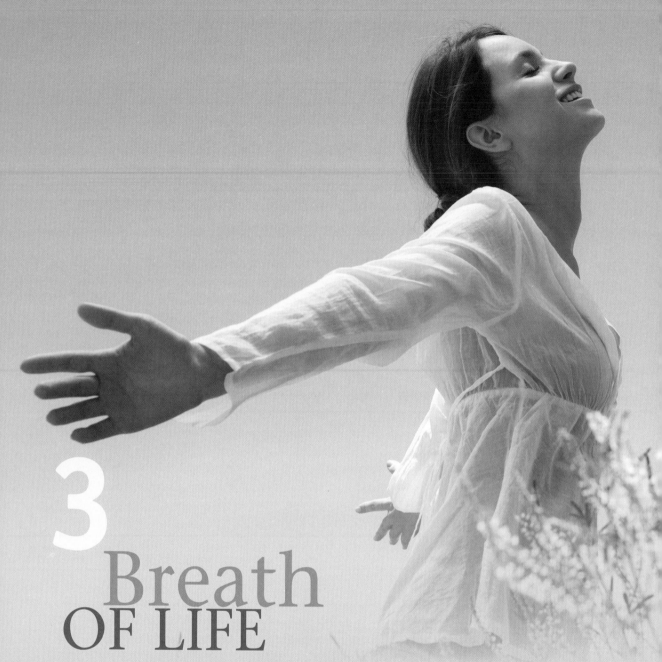

3 Breath
OF LIFE

The average person takes up to 30,000 breaths a day, inhaling as much as 318ft³ (9,000L) of air. This essential process supplies the body with the oxygen it needs for energy and life. In this chapter, you'll discover new and time-tested strategies to keep the hard-working organs that carry out this process—the respiratory system—in top condition.

Maximizing
LUNG HEALTH

Strong lungs are essential for enjoying your waking hours and for sleeping well at night. There is much you can do to keep your lungs healthy, including new exercises that won't just make them function better, but will also ease your stress.

BELIEVE IT OR NOT!

Wrinkles may indicate COPD

Most of us know that smoking causes wrinkles. Now scientists have shown that those who become most lined are very often the same people who go on to develop chronic obstructive pulmonary disease (COPD). Indeed, researchers have shown that middle-aged smokers with deep wrinkles are five times more likely to develop COPD than smokers who have fewer and less deep wrinkles. This is almost certainly because smoking damages lung elasticity in the same way it does that of the skin. Doctors are now being encouraged to look out for premature heavy wrinkling as a sign of COPD.

● **Learn yoga, qigong, or meditation** to develop a better breathing technique. Any one of the therapies can benefit your lungs by teaching you to:

★ **Be aware of** and increase the length of the in-breath and out-breath.

★ **Breathe** deeply down into the abdomen, then follow your out-breath up through the chest to the shoulders and head.

If you think a class could help you, ask your doctor for a recommendation. To find a yoga class in your area, try yogafinder.com.

● **Boost your breathing with color** To reduce wheezing and coughing, try eating a range of red, green, blue, yellow, and purple fruit and vegetables. A colorful diet that includes plenty of foods rich in antioxidants and vitamin C will help you to breathe better, according to Norwegian researchers.

A rainbow diet of fruit and vegetables could reduce breathing problems.

Breathing and movement in yoga

Combining deep breathing (pranayama) with fluid body movements makes yoga more than a mere physical workout. London yoga teacher Caron Ladkin says, "Yoga practiced well requires a great deal of concentration, with the mind and body working together. It's at these moments that people are able to change and find a level of inner calm. And the more you practice combining breathing with movement, the more it becomes part of normal everyday life."

● **Get deep inspiration** Breathing deeply and consciously can boost both mental and physical health. It can help to reduce stress and depression, lower blood pressure, improve asthma symptoms, sharpen brain function, and increase energy levels. A normal in-breath takes in about 0.018ft³ (500cm³) of air. You can increase this intake sixfold by breathing deeply, using both your abdomen and your lungs to achieve optimum expansion.

● **Keep surfaces clean**—especially if you have a smoker in the house. It's not just a question of being house proud. American research has revealed that nicotine can persist on indoor surfaces for several months. The resulting carcinogens can then be absorbed through the skin or ingested, and children are particularly at risk. Scientists believe this thirdhand smoke route explains how passive smoking causes cancer. The best advice is not to smoke or, if you must, to smoke outdoors. But if anyone does smoke in your house make sure that you wipe down all surfaces regularly.

● **Give your breathing muscles a workout** If you suffer from breathlessness, using a respiratory muscle trainer can improve your capacity for exercise. The device applies resistance as you breathe in through a valve, forcing the muscles to work harder. This is particularly beneficial for people who have weakened breathing muscles as a result of a lung condition such as asthma or chronic obstructive pulmonary disease (COPD). If you suffer from that or any similar disorder that causes you to feel breathless, ask your doctor if you can obtain a trainer with a prescription.

● **Breathe and relax** Try this abdominal breathing exercise to increase the supply of oxygen to the whole body, raising your energy levels and helping you to both relax and concentrate:

★ **Lie down** and put a lightweight book on your chest. Check that the book rises and falls as you breathe in and out. Practice this for a few minutes.

★ **Inhale slowly** through your nose, feeling the book on your chest rise.

★ **Push** your abdomen upward when the breath reaches your stomach, letting it rise slightly higher than the book as the diaphragm expands the capacity of your lungs.

★ **Hold** for one second and then reverse the process. Exhale slowly, letting the air out of your lungs through your nostrils, allowing your abdominal muscles to relax. Keep your jaw loose throughout. If you have time, continue to repeat the exercise until you feel fully relaxed.

Combat
COUGHS AND SNEEZES

Known medically as upper respiratory tract infections (or URTIs), coughs and colds are among the most common infections we experience. Protect against cold and flu viruses and treat the diseases they cause with these tips.

● **Adopt the French-style of greeting**
The French peck on both cheeks is less likely to pass on a cold than a regular handshake. The fingers of someone who has a cold are likely to be contaminated as a result of unconscious rubbing of the nose or eyes. It's riskier to shake hands with such a person than be close to a serial sniffer or even directly in the path of a giant sneeze—as long as any droplets stay away from your eyes and nose. Kissing on the cheeks is a much safer greeting.

● **Get out more ...** Vitamin D, which is generated in the body as a result of exposure to sunshine, helps to boost immunity and protects against colds and flu. But northern hemisphere sunshine is strong enough to produce sufficient levels of the vitamin only

A peck on both cheeks is less likely to pass on a cold than a handshake.

HEALTH SECRET

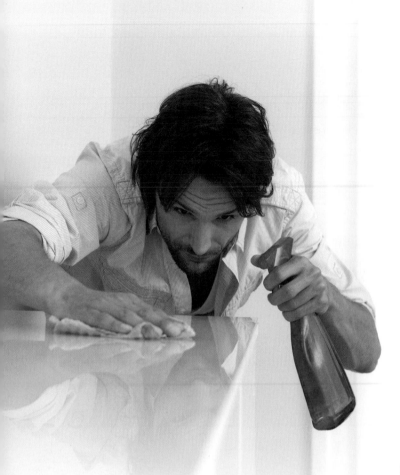

● Keep clean to beat winter bugs

Colds are more common in winter—but don't blame the weather. The only way to catch a cold is through direct contact with the cold virus itself. Colds spread more during winter because people spend more time indoors, increasing their chances of coming into close contact with someone who is infected or with something they have touched. Here are some tips for reducing the chance of having contact with the virus:

★ **Clean handles and surfaces** You are most likely to come into direct contact with a cold virus by touching a contaminated surface, such as a door handle, shared keyboard, faucet, or telephone handset. Young children at school or nursery are very likely to bring cold viruses home. The most effective way to prevent germs spreading is to regularly clean frequently touched surfaces in the home using a disinfectant

Using a disinfectant spray can reduce the virus count by up to 99.9 percent.

between April and September. To make up for this deficit, take a vitamin D supplement in winter and eat plenty of vitamin D-rich foods—especially oily fish—all year round.

● ... but keep warm

While you are out in winter weather, wear a hat and scarf to keep your head and neck warm. As well as its chill, wintry weather gives the cold virus an advantage—cold air causes blood vessels in the nose to constrict, compromising nasal defenses against infection. Protect yourself further with a healthy lifestyle and a balanced vitamin-rich diet, plenty of exercise, and hot drinks.

BELIEVE IT OR NOT!

Advantage of age

Medical scientists have been at a loss to explain why elderly people are less likely to succumb to swine flu than those in their 20s and 30s—unlike normal flu, in which those most severely affected are almost exclusively in older groups.

According to US researchers, anyone over the age of 50 is likely to have developed at least some immunity during the 1957 flu pandemic, which involved a virus that was similar to the H1N1 flu virus that causes swine flu. People with this type of protection, known as cell-mediated immunity, are as likely as anyone else to be infected with the swine flu virus. The difference is that they will almost always be only mildly ill and never develop the severe form of swine flu. It's even possible that this immunity can be inherited.

spray. This can reduce the virus count by 99.9 percent in just one minute.

★ **Wash your hands** Surfaces at work and on trains and buses are also likely to be contaminated, so wash your hands thoroughly and regularly during the day.

★ **Use a hand sanitizer** When soap and water are not available, use an alcohol-based antibacterial hand-cleaning product to keep the bugs at bay.

● **Exercise your lungs** US researchers found that sedentary, overweight, post-menopausal women who took brisk 45-minute walks five times a week reduced the number of colds they got a year by two-thirds. This benefit is likely to apply to anyone who starts to exercise in this way: Each bout of activity brings a small boost to the immune system—over time this translates into fewer days when you are laid low by the cold virus. Try establishing a routine that involves brisk walks several times a week and see if you get fewer colds.

● **Keep your teeth clean** The link between gum infections and chest infections is well established. It seems that bacteria that cause severe respiratory infections thrive in the warmth and wetness of the mouth. Swollen or bleeding gums are a significant cause of pneumonia: They can lead to the inhalation of fine droplets containing bacteria. Protect your chest and your teeth and gums with regular dental checkups and follow your dentist's advice.

● **Don't rely on vitamin C** It's an essential nutrient, but don't expect this vitamin to prevent the common cold, according to a review by the authoritative Cochrane Database of 30 trials. It concluded that for the vast majority of people, "regular ingestion of vitamin C has no effect on

Regular dental checks will protect your chest as well as your teeth and gums.

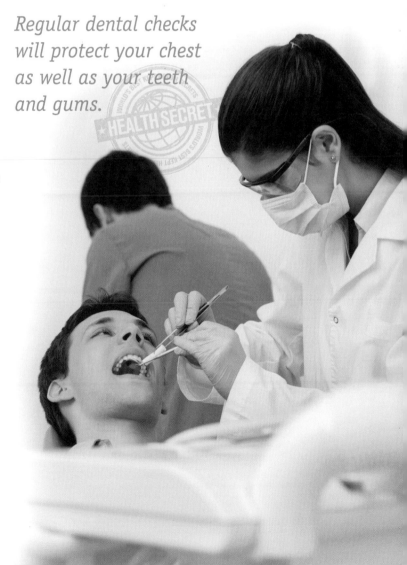

common cold incidence." That holds true even when large doses are taken. There might be an immune system benefit for people who take strenuous physical exercise, are exposed to extreme cold, or live in a very cold environment, but the advice for the rest of us is that regular intake of vitamin C as part of a balanced diet is all we need.

● Don't spread it—use a tissue

Sneezing protects you by ejecting viruses and other detritus from the body at 85 percent of the speed of sound. The expulsion of up to 40,000 droplets, however, inevitably spreads the virus. Many people make the situation worse by trying to contain their sneeze with a hand, which then becomes covered in germs that can be spread through shaking hands and touching surfaces. You can minimize the risk of spreading your cold virus by using tissues when you sneeze and making sure you wash your hands as soon as possible afterward.

● Take flu seriously

Don't play down the risk of flu or the value of a flu shot, especially if you have heart disease or are over 65. Flu, and the inflammatory response to the flu virus that causes it, raises the risk of heart attacks and strokes. Other groups at

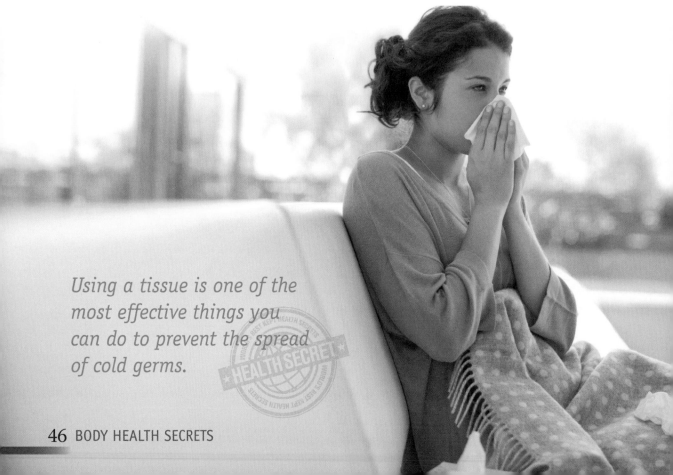

Using a tissue is one of the most effective things you can do to prevent the spread of cold germs.

high risk include people with a respiratory problem (including asthma), diabetes, serious kidney disease, or anyone who has had their spleen removed. So take whatever sensible precautions you can against flu.

● Use an old-fashioned cold remedy

When you get a cold and cough, shun the commercial remedy and sip a hot honey-and-lemon drink instead. Over-the-counter cough syrup is no more effective and a lot more expensive. A couple of teaspoons of honey at bedtime reduces nighttime coughing and improves sleep. Adding honey to a glass of hot water and lemon juice will provide a healthy shot of natural vitamin C as well as soothing your throat.

● Teatime for cough and cold

sufferers Infusions made from dried leaves, flowers, or roots of common plants are traditional remedies that have been used for centuries to help loosen phlegm and soothe sore throats and coughs—and have been found to be at least as effective as over-the-counter remedies. For a dry cough, try a traditional brew made from one of the following herbal helpers:
★ **Licorice**
★ **Mallow or marshmallow.**

Both are available as teabags or as loose herbs from health food stores. Just add to a cup of boiling water and allow to infuse for 10 minutes.

● Enjoy some medicinal chocolate

It's naughty and nice—and also rather good for you, according to researchers. An ingredient of chocolate, theobromine, is significantly more effective for stopping persistent coughs than leading over-the-counter cough syrups. The chemical suppresses the activity of the vagus nerve

SURPRISINGLY EASY

Clearing congestion
To clear nasal congestion in moments, many people find it helps to apply firm pressure with two fingers to the "dips" on either side of your nostrils and press ten times. It may also be beneficial to breathe deeply and visualize the congestion clearing.

that causes persistent coughing, particularly in those suffering from lung disease. Next time you have a cough, try a square or two of dark chocolate and see if it does the trick.

● Sweat it out

It may feel refreshing, but don't turn up the air conditioning if you're suffering from a cold or flu on a hot summer's day. Sweating helps to rid the body of toxins and is part of our infection-fighting mechanism. And even if you don't have a cold, beware of over-air conditioned environments, which can make you more susceptible to upper respiratory tract infections of all kinds, especially if you move frequently between the heat outside and the cold of an air conditioned office or store. Stay warm to stay well.

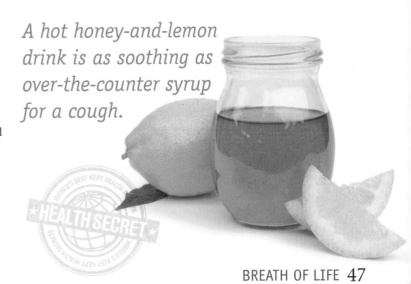

A hot honey-and-lemon drink is as soothing as over-the-counter syrup for a cough.

Secrets of fresh air
IN THE HOME

Noxious indoor air pollution kills as many as 2 million people a year—surprisingly, even more than outdoor air pollution, according to the World Health Organization. Among the pollutants, scientists have identified damaging chemicals in modern home materials—and discovered "green" ways to combat their effect.

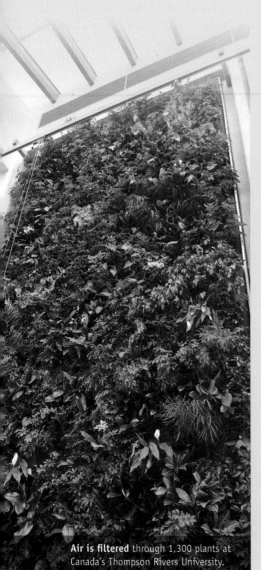

Air is filtered through 1,300 plants at Canada's Thompson Rivers University.

In the late 1960s, Dr. Bill Wolverton—an environmental scientist working with the US military to clean up toxins left behind by biological weapons research—revealed that swamp plants could eliminate the controversial herbicidal chemical known as Agent Orange from water. This success led to his employment by NASA to continue his research into the cleansing power of plants. During the 1973 *Skylab* space station mission, NASA scientists identified 107 health-damaging gases known as volatile organic compounds (VOCs) inside the spacecraft—they were being "off-gassed" by synthetic construction materials. If VOCs were present in *Skylab*, then they were also increasingly common in homes and public buildings as the use of synthetic materials spread.

In the 1980s, Dr. Wolverton's research continued with the NASA-developed BioHome—a small, airtight structure made entirely of synthetic materials. The BioHome caused a range of symptoms—irritated eyes and breathing difficulties—in anyone who entered. These symptoms were later characterized as "sick building syndrome." Dr. Wolverton found that VOCs in the BioHome were substantially reduced by the introduction of houseplants. The plants removed the VOCs through transpiration and photosynthesis, and the symptoms disappeared.

The rise of polluting buildings

The 1970s energy crisis spurred the construction industry to make buildings more energy efficient by sealing them more tightly, which also exacerbated the VOCs problem. Today, VOCs such as acetone, ammonia, benzene, formaldehyde, trichloroethylene, and xylene are given off by a huge variety of modern materials in homes, schools, workplaces, and public buildings including carpets, furnishings, paints, treated woods, glues, cleaning products, and air fresheners. Studies have linked them to many health problems, such as asthma, nasal congestion, headaches, eye irritation, and nausea and some have been linked with cancer. There is also evidence to suggest that they may contribute to liver, kidney, and central nervous system damage.

Reducing the risk

Newly decorated and furnished homes, which we tend to think of as being clean and healthy, may in fact have the highest levels of off-gassing. But you can now buy many paints and other products that are low risk or VOCfree. It is particularly important that babies' bedrooms—often specially decorated for a new arrival—are safe for young children as they may spend much of their early lives sleeping there. Whatever products you use, keep windows open for as long as possible after having your home repainted or recarpeted. And it may be worth considering the use of an indoor air purifier. These devices claim to remove a high proportion of pollutants. VOC testing kits are available from www.projectnesting.org.

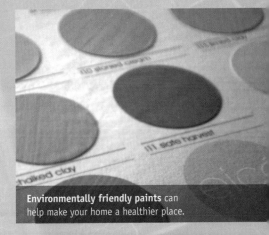

Environmentally friendly paints can help make your home a healthier place.

Houseplants that purify your air

You can easily put the fruits of NASA's research to use in your home. Naturally air-cleansing and decorative, plants are especially useful in modern houses and offices in which efficient insulation has reduced the natural ventilation provided by drafts. Dr. Wolverton identified many plants that are efficient at removing VOCs—here's a selection of the best:

Areca palm With cane-like stalks and feathery fronds, this plant excels at general toxin removal, is easy to care for and very attractive.

Bamboo palm This palm has slender canes and graceful fans, and is one of the best choices for removing benzene, formaldehyde, and trichloroethylene.

Boston fern This is one of the most effective plants for removing air pollutants in the home, especially formaldehyde but also xylene and benzene.

Dracaena "Janet Craig" Able to live for decades in dimly lit areas, this plant is easy to look after and scores well at toxin removal, especially trichloroethylene.

English ivy Very effective at removing formaldehyde, English ivy enjoys some time outdoors during spring or summer and benefits from cooler temperatures.

Peace lily With beautiful white spathes, this lily efficiently removes acetone, benzene, formaldehyde, and trichloroethylene.

Pot chrysanthemum Available all year round, this is one of the best flowering plants for removing ammonia, benzene, and formaldehyde from your home.

Rubber plant This tough plant with large, oval leaves tolerates dim light and is especially effective at removing formaldehyde. It requires very little care.

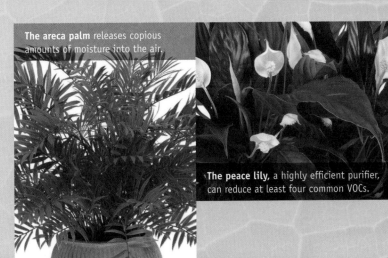

The areca palm releases copious amounts of moisture into the air.

The peace lily, a highly efficient purifier, can reduce at least four common VOCs.

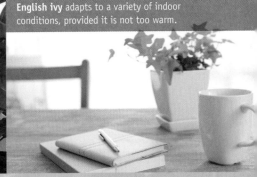

English ivy adapts to a variety of indoor conditions, provided it is not too warm.

Addressing
ALLERGIES

Allergic reactions affecting the respiratory system include the running nose and watering eyes of hay fever and the breathless attacks that characterize asthma. Today, a better understanding of the causes of allergic reactions and how to prevent and treat them has dramatically improved the well-being of those affected.

● **Irrigate your nose to cut allergy symptoms** The traditional Asian practice of nasal irrigation may provide relief for hay fever sufferers. Flushing out mucus and debris from the nose and sinuses may not sound appealing, but it has become accepted as a respectable technique for the prevention of this allergic condition. If you have hay fever, you may want to try this technique. But don't do it every day and don't do it if you have a current sinus infection. Here are some helpful pointers for carrying out nasal irrigation safely:

★ **Use a neti pot**, which looks like a tiny watering can, to pour saltwater into one nostril while letting it run through the other. Breathe through the mouth.

★ **Choose from** metal, glass, ceramic, or plastic neti pots. They are available cheaply on the Internet.

★ **Use only** an isotonic or hypertonic saltwater solution made with sachets of pharmaceutical grade salt; neti pot solutions can be bought from pharmacies or online.

★ **Never use** ordinary tap water as it can irritate the nasal membranes.

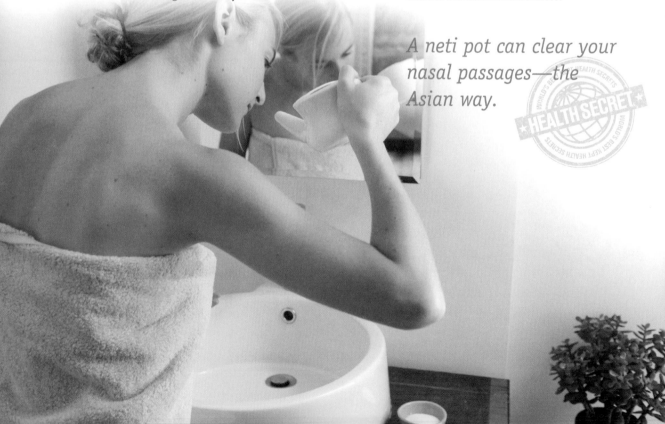

A neti pot can clear your nasal passages—the Asian way.

HEALTH SECRET

● **Try a pollen barrier** You may be able to reduce the frequency and severity of hay fever attacks by using a pollen barrier cream around your nostrils. The ointment traps enough pollen grains to significantly reduce the amount entering your nose and lungs and therefore minimizes symptoms. Ask about such products in your local pharmacy or health food store.

● **Got asthma? Rethink your home**
If anyone in your home suffers from asthma or if you have children, the following measures may help alleviate the condition and minimize the chance of this allergic condition developing:

★ **Swap carpets** for hard flooring.

★ **Vacuum** your sofa.

★ **Bag and freeze** the soft toys of a child with asthma for at least 6 hours every one to two weeks.

★ **Fit barrier coverings** on dust mites' favorite habitats, such as pillows and mattresses.

These measures will reduce exposure to asthma-provoking dust mites. There are about 19,000 of these tiny creatures in a gram of house dust. One in ten adults and up to eight in ten children are allergic to the droppings of these bugs, which live in the dust that builds up in carpets, bedding, and soft furnishings.

● **Cut down on fizzy drinks** Too many fizzy drinks can be bad for your breathing. An Australian study has shown that any consumption of these beverages increases the risk of developing asthma and chronic obstructive pulmonary disease (COPD). And the more you consume, the higher the risk. Carbonated drinks have no health benefits, so it makes sense to keep them as an occasional treat.

BELIEVE IT OR NOT!

Expose babies to dust mites?

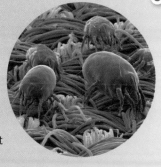

Parents are being invited to bring their babies into teaching hospitals in the Southampton area in the UK in order to swallow dust mites, the microscopic bugs that cause allergic conditions such as asthma, hay fever, and eczema. Scientists there believe that babies today are less likely to swallow dust mites as their mothers may not allow them to chew on soft toys and cushions. The infants are encouraged to swallow the dust mites to test the theory that exposure at a time when their immune systems are working out what is and isn't harmful "will allow us to teach their bodies to accept it and not become susceptible as they grow older," says Professor Graham Roberts, Southampton General Hospital's specialist in pediatric respiratory and allergy medicine.

If the studies show that babies who swallowed the dust mites suffer fewer allergies in later years, the researchers say that ingesting potential allergens could one day become a more widely used preventive measure.

● **Boost your breathing with Buteyko** If you have asthma, consider using the training program known as Buteyko breathing. Developed in Russia by Dr. K.P. Buteyko, this program focuses on "progressive breathlessness resilience" exercises that help people breath more deeply, more calmly, and less often. Buteyko training reduces the number of attacks and the intensity of symptoms experienced by asthma sufferers—with an average 300 percent increase in the capacity for physical activity and a reduced need for inhaled bronchodilator medication. If you have asthma, ask your doctor to recommend a Butekyo practitioner.

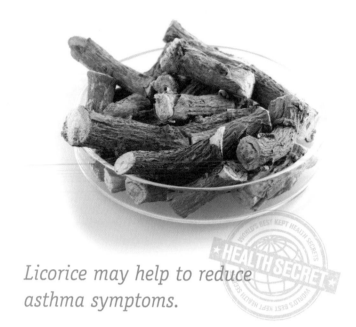

Licorice may help to reduce asthma symptoms.

● **Enjoy some licorice** This common confectionery ingredient is a core element in Tsumara saiboku-to, or TJ-96, a traditional Japanese herbal mix that is one of the most popular and best-studied anti-asthmatic herbal remedies. Researchers have found that TJ-96 helps reduce asthma symptoms, sometimes allowing medication to be reduced—but only under medical supervision. Discuss with your doctor whether this product is suitable for you.

● **Trim your weight** If you're overweight and have asthma, you may be able to improve your lung function simply by losing weight. Several studies have shown that asthma sufferers who slim down have fewer flare-ups and are able to control their condition successfully with reduced levels of medication. As well as making exercise easier, losing weight seems to prevent the airways in your lungs from closing too early on the out-breath.

● **Keep the air fresh, not fragranced** There is some evidence that products used to scent our homes can trigger attacks in those prone to asthma. A variety of chemicals that have the potential to irritate the lungs are commonly used in their manufacture, and even though they are present only in small amounts, can lead to breathing difficulties, especially in young children and those with pre-existing lung problems. Open a window or use natural fragrances, rather than squirting an aerosol to mask bad smells.

● **Get salty** Inhaling salty air may help to control asthma symptoms, according to Asthma UK. People in eastern Europe have been taking the air in salt caves for their lung health for 150 years. Now a Lithuanian study has confirmed that salt therapy for an hour a day improves breathing in nine out of ten people with asthma. The findings have led to the development of an inhaler that delivers minute salt particles into the lungs at the touch of a button, and salt "caves" have been opened in various places in the UK. Discuss the possible benefits of this therapy with your doctor.

● **Get the exercise you need** People with asthma often worry that exercise will provoke an attack of breathlessness. But if your medication is correct for you and if you take some sensible precautions, there is no need for you to deprive yourself of the

● **Check your medicines** If your asthma attacks have increased recently, check your prescription drugs with your doctor. Recent evidence suggests that cholesterol-lowering statin drugs may worsen asthma control. US researchers found that people with asthma who were taking statins had more airway inflammatory obstruction and increased symptoms. So far, studies have been too small to provide solid proof of a link. But if your asthma has worsened since starting a course of statins, talk to your doctor.

innumerable fitness benefits that exercise can bring. Here are some tips for safe exercise if you have asthma:

★ **Swimming** is good exercise for people with asthma, but the chlorine used in many swimming pools can trigger asthma in some people. Some pools don't use chlorine, so ask at your local pool what method is used to keep the water germ free.

★ **Don't forget your inhaler** when you exercise. You may need to use the reliever just before exercise or if you have an attack. As a precaution, be sure to ask your doctor for advice on controlling your asthma during exercise.

● **Avoid pollution** Asthma attacks can be triggered and worsened by the presence of pollutants in the air we breathe. Specific culprits include:

★ **Particulates** Tiny particles in poorly filtered diesel exhaust and from a variety of industrial processes.

★ **Ozone** An irritant chemical formed in the atmosphere by the action of sunlight.

MIND POWER

Asthma blues

If you have asthma, watch out for signs of depression, which is more common in people with this condition. Older people are especially at risk and asthma can appear for the first time in later life. Researchers have found substantial evidence that depression may reduce the ability of people with asthma to manage their health problems—and it may also lead to smoking, physical inactivity, and insufficient sleep. Health professionals and the friends and family of people with asthma are advised to look out for signs of depression to increase the chances of early diagnosis and treatment.

If you have asthma or a similar disorder, it may be worth trying to reduce your exposure to such pollutants, for example, by staying inside with the windows closed when ozone levels are high.

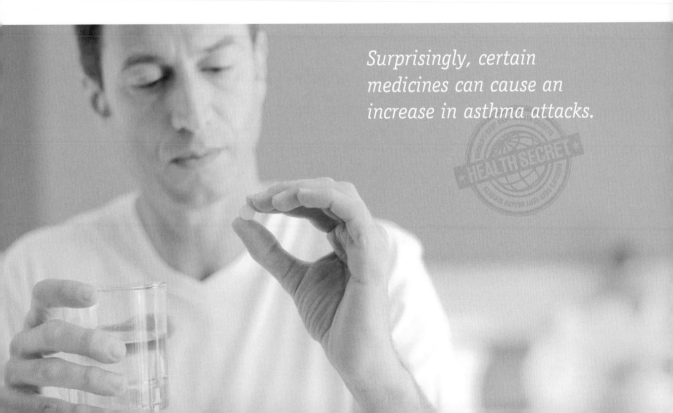

Surprisingly, certain medicines can cause an increase in asthma attacks.

HEALTH SECRET

4

Building strong
BONES AND
MUSCLES

Human beings are designed to move—bones, muscles, and joints support our bodies and enable us to perform myriad everyday activities. What we often overlook is our essential role in keeping them healthy and strong so they can keep us mobile all our lives.

Boosting
YOUR BONES

Like every other part of your body, your bones are a living structure designed to grow and to renew and repair itself. But as we age, bone density can be lost, resulting in osteoporosis. Eating foods that are key to bone health, getting enough exercise, and following the other tips below will all help keep your bones strong.

● **Have more of the sunshine vitamin** Vitamin D helps calcium absorption, and bone growth and repair. Without it, bones can become thin, brittle, or misshapen as you age. There is little vitamin D in most foods, so we have to get the amounts our bodies need from exposure to sunlight or from supplements. In the UK the recommended daily intake for adults is 10mcg, but in the USA the recommended intake is higher: up to 20mcg daily for those over 70. The vitamin D content of common foods is listed at http://ods.od.nih.gov/factsheets/VitaminD-HealthProfessional/.

● **Pick up a prune** In a US study of postmenopausal women, those who ate about 10 prunes a day had significantly higher bone-mineral density in the ulna—one of long bones in the forearm—and in the bones of the spine than a control group who ate dried apples. It is thought that ingredients in prunes suppress the breakdown of bone.

● **Know your needs** Our bodies contain around 2 lb (about 1kg) of calcium, 99 percent of which is carried in our bones. Adults need at least 700mg of calcium a day to maintain bone density and avoid the risk of osteoporosis. You can find the calcium content of common foods by visiting http://www.iofbonehealth.org/calcium-rich-foods.

SURPRISINGLY EASY

Bone up on sardines
Canned sardines and salmon can boost your calcium intake. The reason? The canning process softens the bones, making the calcium easier to absorb. So why not have one of those old favorites—sardines on toast or salmon and cucumber sandwiches—for a light lunch or afternoon snack?

● **Get calcium from non-dairy foods, too** While milk and dairy foods are excellent calcium sources, did you know that you can increase your intake from lots of other food sources as well? A 7oz (200ml) glass of milk, a 5oz (150ml) container of yogurt, and a small piece of cheese will meet your daily calcium requirements. Here's how some non-dairy calcium-rich foods can contribute to your calcium intake:

★ **Figs** Just one dried fig contains 130mg of calcium.

★ **Greens** Spring greens, savoy cabbage, broccoli, and kale are packed with calcium; one cup of cooked kale contains nearly 200mg of calcium—around a quarter of your daily requirement.

★ **Almonds** Just 1oz (26g) of almonds provides 60mg of calcium. Toast them and sprinkle them over salads, cereals, or fruit compote. You can add them to tagines and meatballs or use them in pesto, and a small handful of almonds is an ideal snack.

● **Major on magnesium** This mineral found in bone is essential for keeping our skeleton strong. Get plenty of green vegetables, beans, peas, nuts, and seeds and whole, unrefined grains. Whole-grain bread provides more magnesium than white because magnesium-rich wheat germ and bran are removed from flour as it is refined and processed. Eating a magnesium-rich diet is particularly important for older people because as we age, the risk of magnesium deficiency increases.

● **Eat seeds to slow bone breakdown** Make seeds and oils derived from seeds part of your bone health plan. Studies funded by the US space agency NASA suggest that omega-3 fatty acids may reduce the bone breakdown experienced by astronauts during spaceflight. Experts think they may help people with osteoporosis. Essential fatty acids seem to increase the amount of calcium the body absorbs, reduce the amount lost in urine, and improve bone strength and bone growth. To get omega-3

❄ MIND POWER

Depression is bad for bones
If you suffer from depression, it may be worth having your bone density checked. Women who are depressed are at greater risk of osteoporosis, according to research. The reason is probably that hormonal changes associated with depression also deplete bone mass. In one study, women with depression had much higher blood levels of an inflammatory protein made by the immune system and linked to bone loss than women without depression. The depressed women also had much lower levels of anti-inflammatory proteins.

Omega-3 fatty acids may reduce bone breakdown in astronauts—and could do the same for you.

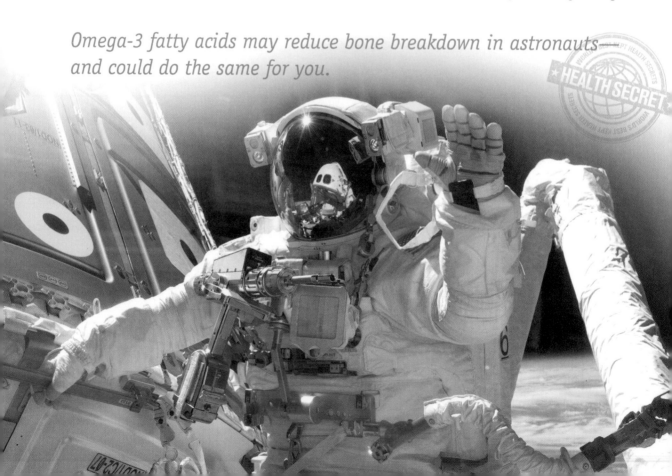

fatty acids into your diet, use canola and flaxseed (linseed) oil in cooking and food preparation; add chia seeds to salads; snack on walnuts; and include meals containing oily fish such as salmon, mackerel, sardines, and herring as part of your regular diet.

● **Eat your greens** Research suggests that vitamin K can reduce fracture rates in people affected by osteoporosis. We obtain most of our vitamin K from friendly bacteria in our gut, but you can give your intake a boost by eating plenty of leafy green vegetables such as kale, broccoli, sprouts, spinach, and watercress. Fermented soy (also known as natto) is another excellent source.

● **Savor some soy** Natto, a fermented soy breakfast food beloved by the Japanese, is the richest natural source (and one of only two natural sources) of vitamin K2, which has been linked to improved bone health. Legend has it that fermented soy was discovered by the 11th-century Samurai warrior Yoshiie Minamoto after he was forced to abandon his boiled soybeans during an attack. When he returned to eat the now fermented beans, he found he enjoyed them more than expected and told all his friends. Natto has since become part of the traditional Japanese diet. Its sticky texture and strong flavor may not appeal to all Western tastes, but you can buy it in supplement form in health food stores.

● **Watch your cola consumption**
While some foods help us to build strong bones, there are other foods and drinks that actively leach calcium from bones and prevent the absorption of new calcium. Research has shown that consumption of cola drinks, alcohol, caffeine, and salt can have this effect, so limit your intake to prevent avoidable loss of bone density. And

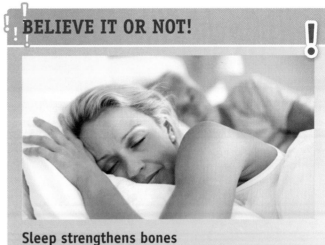

there is evidence to suggest that eating pasta too often can have the same effect. Every now and then, have potatoes instead.

● **Carry that load** Whatever your age, it's never too late to start bone-strengthening weight-bearing exercise. Although most of our bone mass is laid down by our mid-20s, you can still reduce your risk of osteoporosis by exercising later in life. Taking regular, weight-bearing exercise stimulates your bones to absorb calcium—this is as vital for older men as it is for women, and is healthy for people of all ages. Ask your doctor about safe weight-bearing workouts.

● **Get walking** A US study has found that post-menopausal women who walk about 7.5mi (12km)—a half-hour walk four days a week—retain bone density four to seven years longer than those who don't walk at all. Walking is also beneficial for men.

Muscle POWER

Skeletal muscles thrive on hard work; the more we use them the stronger they become. And strong muscles are key to avoiding injury, as well as enabling us to perform everyday activities with ease and enjoyment. Check out these tips for boosting your muscle power.

● **Be voracious with vegetables**
Eat plenty of fruit, legumes, and vegetables—especially the green leafy kinds—to get enough potassium, which regulates muscle and nerve function, and balances sodium levels in cells. Low levels of this mineral can cause muscle weakness and cramps.

● **Go nuts** Be sure to get plenty of muscle-conditioning magnesium in your diet to avoid cramps. You can obtain this key nutrient from Brazil, cashew, and pine nuts, sesame and sunflower seeds, and dark green leafy vegetables.

● **Have a ball** Using an exercise ball is an effective way to build up core muscle strength. Because you are in an unstable position on the ball, you automatically engage and exercise the muscles in your abdomen, back, and pelvis. These core muscles support your lower back and spine, help you maintain posture, and control your twisting, reaching, and bending movements.

● **Wield some weights** Join a gym and get some advice on a weight-bearing exercise program. In one landmark US study, 40 women aged 50 to 70 who took up twice-weekly weight-training built muscle, lost fat, and, bucking all expectation, became physically stronger than their daughters.

● **Watch your medication** If you're taking diuretics (often prescribed to treat high blood pressure), be aware that some

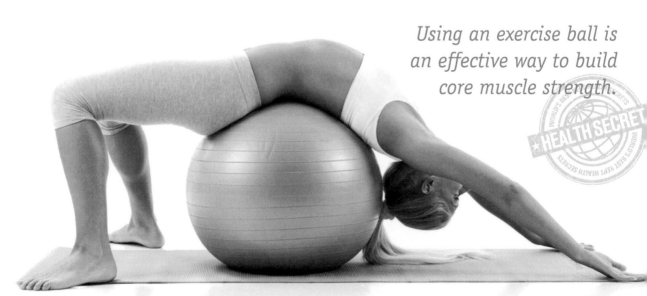

Using an exercise ball is an effective way to build core muscle strength.

HEALTH SECRET

of these medicines can cause you to excrete excess potassium, which can lead to cramps and muscle weakness. Ask your doctor if any drugs you have been prescribed are having this effect and whether a change of medication might be advisable.

● **Eat some beans** Eating beans and lentils, dairy foods, almonds, Brazil nuts, and leafy green vegetables, can ensure an adequate intake of calcium. This mineral, which is a major contributor to the health of your bones, also promotes effective muscle contraction.

● **Get pedaling** For an instant workout at home, try a pedal exerciser. Compact, lightweight, and portable, these convenient devices can be used to work leg muscles when placed on the floor or to exercise the muscles of the upper body when on a table or worktop. By using one of these devices, you can strengthen muscles and shed calories while watching TV or reading, or anything else you can do while sitting still.

● **Drink water to combat cramps**
If you get cramps during exercise, drink at least two cups (500ml) of water 2 hours before a workout. Take a water bottle with you and drink one cup (250ml) every 10–20 minutes while exercising. If you sweat a lot, try drinking a sports drink, which replaces lost minerals, instead of plain water.

● **Take a tonic** If you suffer from night cramps, drink a glass of tonic water before going to bed. Tonic water contains quinine and is a popular remedy that has now been backed up by research. However, steer clear of quinine tablets, which can have unpleasant side effects.

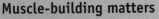

SECRETS OF SUCCESS

Muscle-building matters
Look after your muscles and they will look after you. Keeping them strong through exercise will provide the following benefits:

● **Help you stay slim** The amount of lean muscle in your body controls your resting metabolic rate, which in turn significantly affects the number of calories you burn. The more muscle you have, the easier it is to keep your weight under control.

● **Build up your bones** Over time, strength training has been found to increase bone density and therefore help reduce your risk of osteoporosis and fractures resulting from minor accidents and falls.

● **Make life easier** Strengthen your muscles and you'll need to exert less effort when you lift and carry.

● **Cut your chance of injury** The better your muscle fitness, the easier it is for you to carry out everyday tasks and physical activities without injuring yourself.

● **Enhance your sporting prowess** Muscle strength training has been shown to improve athleticism.

● **Help you stay independent longer** The stronger your muscles, the less likely you are to fall as you age. Falls in the elderly are a major cause of injury and hospitalization.

● **Reduce back pain** Keeping your core abdominal and lower back muscles strong will improve your posture and cut the risk of strain.

● **Boost your mood** Strength training has been shown to have a positive impact on levels of anxiety, depression, and self-esteem.

● **Watch where you're pointing** Try not to sleep with your feet bent so that your toes point toward the bottom of the bed, which can lead to cramps, and keep the bedsheets loose: If they are tightly tucked in, they may bend the toes downward.

The position of your feet in bed could be the cause of your cramps.

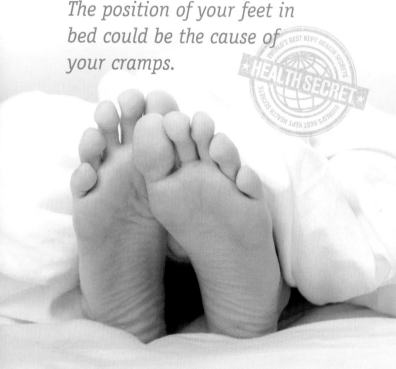

● **Solve it with soap** Many people swear that sleeping with a bar of soap in the bed prevents night cramps. Nobody has found a reason why this old wives' tale should work, but whenever a famous American advice columnist advocated this cure, she received huge numbers of thank-you letters. It can do no harm to give this simple and cheap remedy a try, and it may work for you.

● **Exercise for night cramps** Try the following simple fixes if you suffer from night cramps:

★ **Preventive stretching** Stretch against a wall three times a day, including just before bed. Stand about 2½ft (75cm) from the wall and place your palms on it, near eye level. Keeping your heels on the floor, gradually move your hands up the wall until you are stretching as high as you can. Hold, then return to the first position.

★ **For cramps of all kinds** When cramps strike, press the central point of the area affected with your thumb, the heel of your hand, or a loosely clenched fist. Apply the pressure for 10 seconds, ease off for 10 seconds, then press again. Repeat until the pain eases.

★ **For calf cramp** Stand with your legs apart, one (with cramp) behind the other, feet facing forward. Shift your weight to the front leg, bending it slightly, but keeping the back leg straight. Hold until the cramp eases.

★ **For front thigh cramp** Bend the cramped leg back while holding onto a chair. Grab the foot, bringing the heel as close to your butt as you can. Keep the knee pointing down. Hold the position until the cramp eases.

★ **For hamstring cramp** Place the heel of the leg with the cramp on a low stool or step. Slowly lean forward from the waist until you feel a stretch at the back of your leg and the cramp eases.

Looking after
YOUR JOINTS

To stay mobile and flexible for years to come, you need to keep your knees, hips, shoulders, and numerous other joints healthy and strong. Using them regularly—but not overusing them—and eating nutritious foods that enable the specialized tissues to repair themselves are among the joint-protecting measures we can take.

● **Eat plenty of green vegetables**
When researchers looked at the diets of nearly 700 people with an average age of 65, they found that the more vitamin K they consumed, the less likely they were to have osteoarthritis of the hand or knee. Among the best sources are vegetables from the cabbage family including kale, broccoli, and Brussels sprouts. Spinach and watercress are also excellent sources of this vitamin.

● **Go for what really works** If you've had joint aches and pains of any sort, the chances are that you've tried some form of complementary or alternative medicine. But do you know which treatments have been scientifically proven to work? A report on complementary treatments for arthritis, carried out by Arthritis Research UK, came up with some intriguing findings:

★ **Get chile** If you have osteoarthritis, try capsaicin gel or cream, which is made from chile peppers. It was the only product to score the full five points for effectiveness in osteoarthritis. In its review of research trials, Arthritis Research UK found that capsaicin was four times more effective at improving pain and joint tenderness than a placebo gel. It is available on prescription and works mainly by depleting Substance P, a pain transmitter in human nerves.

★ **Go for herbs** Phytodolor, a German herbal preparation available as a tincture

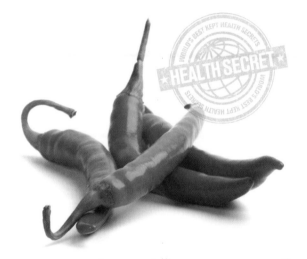

Capsaicin from chile peppers really does help arthritis.

from some pharmacies, scored well for effectiveness in treating osteoarthritis. In trials it helped to improve joint mobility and reduced pain.

★ **Try the SAMe remedy** The food supplement S-adenosylmethionine, known as SAMe, which stimulates the body to make joint cartilage, can relieve osteoarthritis pain as effectively as medications such as ibuprofen. But do not stop prescribed medication without your doctor's advice.

★ **Opt for omega-3** Supplements made from fish oil were the top-scoring product for rheumatoid arthritis (RA). Fish oils rich in omega-3 fatty acids block the release of elements in white blood cells that can encourage inflammation. They also form the building blocks for the production of anti-inflammatory substances in the blood called prostaglandins. Research suggests that fish oil supplements can significantly reduce joint pain, morning stiffness, and fatigue. And they can reduce the need for painkillers in those with RA. You can also get the benefits of omega-3s by eating plenty of oily fish such as salmon, mackerel, and sardines.

● **Try something different?** There is no scientific basis for the use of many supplements and traditional arthritis remedies, such as antler velvet (a dietary supplement made from deer or elk antlers), black currant seed oil, feverfew, flaxseed (linseed) oil, green-lipped mussels, selenium, and the antioxidant vitamins A, C, and E. But if you believe they may be helpful for you, ask your doctor's advice before you use them. And many people with arthritis swear

Swimming improves flexibility and reduces arthritis pain.

that they get pain relief from wearing magnets and copper bracelets. While good evidence for their benefits is lacking, they are safe and you may find they work for you. Acupuncture, in which fine needles are inserted into the skin, is another therapy that many arthritis sufferers find helpful.

● **Eat more garlic** Researchers have found that women whose diets are high in vegetables of the allium family such as garlic, onions, and leeks are less likely to develop osteoarthritis of the hip. The researchers analyzed the diet patterns of 1,000 female twins alongside X-ray images of their hips, knees, and spine. They found that those who ate a healthy diet with a high intake of vegetables of the allium family, had less evidence of early-onset osteoarthritis in the hip joint. One of the compounds in garlic appeared to block the action of cartilage-damaging enzymes. And if you're worried about bad "garlic" breath, chew some fresh parsley after your meal.

● **Don't give up on exercise** It may be tempting to rest when your joints ache, but the Arthritis Foundation (www.arthritis.org) recommends staying active. Benefits include easing stiffness, improving mobility, strengthening muscles and bones, and helping you lose weight, which will reduce strain on your joints. Here are some exercise tips for people with painful joints:
★ **Swimming** is an excellent exercise for people with arthritis because the buoyancy of the water makes it easier to move your

joints. Research shows it improves flexibility and reduces pain. Or you could find out whether your local pool runs aquarobic classes, which involve exercising in water without swimming.

★ **Walking** strengthens muscles, bones, and joints. Start gently and increase the distance gradually. Try some hills, too.

★ **Cycling** builds fitness and knee strength, but don't be overambitious, especially if you have knee pain. If your knees feel worse after cycling, try another form of exercise.

★ **Low-impact fitness gym training** is best for arthritis sufferers. Choose low-impact classes such as general fitness and yoga rather than high-impact aerobics. On the weights, start low and do lots of slow repetitions. Avoid jogging. It may jar your joints and make the pain worse.

● **Don't crack your knuckles** Repeated knuckle cracking does not lead to arthritis, but it can reduce the strength of your grip and cause joint swelling, so is best avoided. The crack comes about when you stretch the joint. The stretching at first causes nitrogen bubbles to appear in the fluid surrounding the joint, as the pressure inside the joint is lowered by the stretching—just as bubbles appear in a bottle of soda when the pressure inside is reduced by unscrewing the cap. As the stretching continues, the pressure drops so low that the bubbles burst into existence —and this produces the crack.

● **Get a new view of gout** If you and your doctor think you may have gout but the usual tests, which examine fluid drawn from joints using a needle, come back negative—consider asking for a CT scan. Gout occurs when the body cannot flush out excess uric acid produced by its own cells and by the breakdown of food, and crystals of uric acid accumulate painfully in

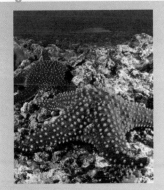
the joints. A US study has found that CT scans can help confirm the diagnosis, especially in those with the acute form of the disease. This new diagnostic technique is also helpful when joint fluid cannot be taken for any reason.

● **Take care of your heart** If you have rheumatoid arthritis (RA), it is important that you follow a heart-healthy lifestyle. This is because the inflammatory nature of RA means that the condition affects blood vessels as well as the joints and can put you at greater risk of a heart attack, and chances that any heart attack will be of the "silent" type are also higher. New drugs for RA can reduce the risk of heart problems, but if you have RA and have chest pains or pain radiating down your left arm, get medical help promptly.

For further tips on heart care see Chapter 1, *Protecting Your Heart*

Secrets of spa
TREATMENTS

The soothing power of water has long been used to treat ailments, especially in joints and muscles. Today, spas around the world offer many water-based therapies. While their value is debated, new studies show that contact with water often gives symptomatic relief.

From eastern Europe to North America and Japan, thousands of thermal spas around the world promise relief from osteoarthritis and rheumatoid arthritis, back pain, fibromyalgia, and trauma damage. Their claims are based on the healing properties of water, particularly mineral water from thermal springs and also seawater, such as around the Dead Sea. Together with water therapies, known as balneotherapy, spas may offer massage, mud baths, seaweed, and algae wraps, and exposure to natural gases.

How well do spa treatments work?

The effectiveness of spa treatments is difficult to quantify. There are few flawless trials and the therapies are known to produce a positive placebo effect. But a 2009 French study confirmed "a persistent improvement" in patients with various painful musculoskeletal conditions following spa treatments. And 2011 research from the University of Padua reported "clear, long-term benefits" to patients with ankylosing spondylitis who received a combination of spa treatments and rehabilitation exercises. Some of the most common therapies and their benefits are outlined here.

Spas are often located in mountain regions close to natural springs.

Massage has a proven range of health benefits, from lowering blood pressure and stress to easing migraines and musculoskeletal pain.

Lymphatic drainage massage may reduce swelling following lymph node removal. Macmillan Cancer Support endorses this form of therapy, emphasizing that the practitioner should be appropriately qualified.

Thalassotherapy Saltwater, algae, and seaweed therapies, like other spa treatments, involve touch—inducing a sense of well-being. A 2008 Brazilian study found that fibromyalgia sufferers got more benefit from exercise in saltwater than in standard pool water.

Warm-water pool Warmth relaxes muscles, eases joint pain, and aids circulation; buoyancy extends range of joint movement; resistance aids muscle strength. Warm water exercise is a key element of spa-based balneotherapy. But it is effective even without the mineral content of spa waters; warm water pools are now standard in UK hospital physiotherapy departments.

Wraps Mud, seaweed, and clay wraps are used for the relief of a variety of arthritic conditions. A 2007 study by Italian researchers confirmed the efficacy of mud treatments for fibromyalgia.

Preventing and
TREATING INJURIES

Strains, sprains, and in more serious cases, fractures are among the most common types of damage to the muscles, joints, and bones. While such injuries are almost always unexpected and accidental, there's plenty you can do to prevent them—and to hasten recovery.

● **Warm up ...** Preparatory moves can help prevent strains caused by strenuous physical activity by gradually "tuning up" your circulation, increasing blood flow to your muscles, and raising your body temperature. Stretches can improve flexibility. Here are some pointers:

★ **Pay attention** to the large muscle groups such as hamstrings and back, making sure to stretch the muscles you'll be using during your workout.

★ **Stretch muscles** gently and slowly to the point of tension, but not pain, and hold for 30 seconds. Keep as still as possible.

★ **Tailor exercises** to your specific sport or activity. For example, if you are doing a brisk walk, start by walking slowly for up to 10 minutes. For a run, walk briskly for the same amount of time. If you're working with weights, mimic the movements you'll do but without the weights. In the pool, begin with a few gentle laps before starting your main workout.

● **... then cool down** Did you know that cooling down after exercise is as important as warming up in terms of protecting your body from injury? Cooling down will help to gradually reduce the temperature of your muscles and regulate blood flow, especially if you've had an intense workout. This can help reduce

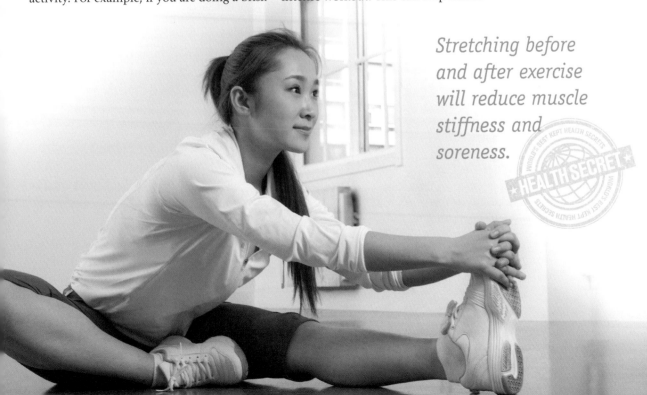

Stretching before and after exercise will reduce muscle stiffness and soreness.

muscle injury, stiffness, and soreness. Just slow your workout to a gentler pace—for example, by doing a few leisurely laps in the pool or a few minutes of slow revs on your exercise bike. Do some stretches to put your muscles and joints through their full range of movement.

● **Have a snack** After exercise replenish your stores of glycogen (the glucose stored in the liver that provides energy to the muscles) with some carbohydrate plus protein to help build and repair muscle tissue. Eating a fruit yogurt, energy bar, or a handful of dried fruit and nuts should provide the nutrients you need.

● **Get the right shoes** For all exercise activities make sure you wear shoes that are appropriate for the activity to help prevent

BELIEVE IT OR NOT!

Shock for soft-tissue injuries

The idea of passing electrical waves through your skin may sound "shocking"—but this treatment is now offered in the UK by some hospitals as an alternative to surgery for conditions such as frozen shoulder and tendonitis.

Extracorporeal shock wave therapy (ESWT) consists of a series of short sessions during which low-energy shockwaves are sent through the skin. This prompts an inflammatory response in the injured tissue and the body reacts by increasing blood circulation to the area, which hastens healing by dissolving calcium deposits and promoting cell regeneration.

It's not yet clear whether ESWT is better than other treatment options, but if you are interested, discuss the pros and cons with your doctor.

injury. In particular, take care to choose shoes that fit properly, are stable and supportive, and that have soles designed to absorb shock.

● **Avoid repetition** You may think of repetitive strain injury (RSI) as a work-related problem, but as we spend more time on game consoles, tablets, and mobile phones, our leisure activities also put us at risk. Children and teenagers are especially vulnerable, as are people who work at a computer all day. Take the following precautions if you can't avoid long periods of computer use:

★ **Be posture aware** At a computer, make sure your chair, screen, and desk are at the right height for you. Your eyes should be in line with the top of the screen.

★ **Watch your wrists, arms, and shoulders** Keep your wrists comfortable and your upper arms resting against your body rather than reaching forward. Keep your shoulders relaxed.

★ **Break it up** Avoid doing the same thing for too long by taking a break twice an hour —get up, move around, and do some stretches. Turn your head from side to side; loosen your wrists, make a fist then spread your fingers; bring your shoulder blades together to open your chest, and round your shoulders to stretch your upper back.

● **Soothe it with pineapple** If you've suffered a strain or sprain, try eating fresh pineapple. It's a favorite treatment among nutritional therapists looking after athletes with sports injuries. The fruit contains the enzyme bromelain, which is thought to speed up tissue repair.

● **Get support—for plantar fasciitis** An orthotic (an artificial support inserted into the shoe) is often prescribed for this painful inflammation of the connective tissue supporting the arch of your foot. A recent Canadian study looked at different areas of the foot and discovered that over-the-counter orthotics reduced strain on the affected tissues by an impressive 34 percent. If you suffer from this problem, try putting supportive inserts in your shoes.

● **Exercise your neck** Simple exercises might make a difference if you suffer from neck pain. Researchers have found that patients with neck pain who did gentle exercises at home up to eight times a day, following instruction from a coach, felt better than those on medication such as aspirin or ibuprofen. If you suffer from neck pain, ask your doctor for exercise advice or for a referral to a physiotherapist.

● **Don't be hard on yourself** If you have back pain and a firm mattress, think about changing it for something slightly softer. In the past, back pain sufferers were often told that it's best to sleep on a hard mattress, but research doesn't agree. A study of people with chronic low back pain showed that after 90 days those who slept on a medium-firm mattress had less pain in bed and on rising and less disability than those who slept on firm mattresses. So pamper yourself and go for something with a bit more "give" in it.

● **Say "yes" to yoga** A large UK study of the health benefits of yoga suggests it is more effective for chronic lower back pain than conventional approaches. The study found that people offered a specially designed 12-week yoga program had bigger gains in back function and more confidence in doing everyday tasks than those offered standard care by their doctor. After three months, members of the yoga group found

they were able to undertake 30 percent more activities on average than those in the standard care group.

If you have chronic lower back pain, and want to try a yoga class, first consult your doctor or physiotherapist, and ideally, look for a yoga teacher trained in back care.

The enzyme bromelain in pineapple can speed up tissue repair.

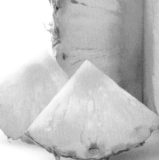

HEALTH SECRET

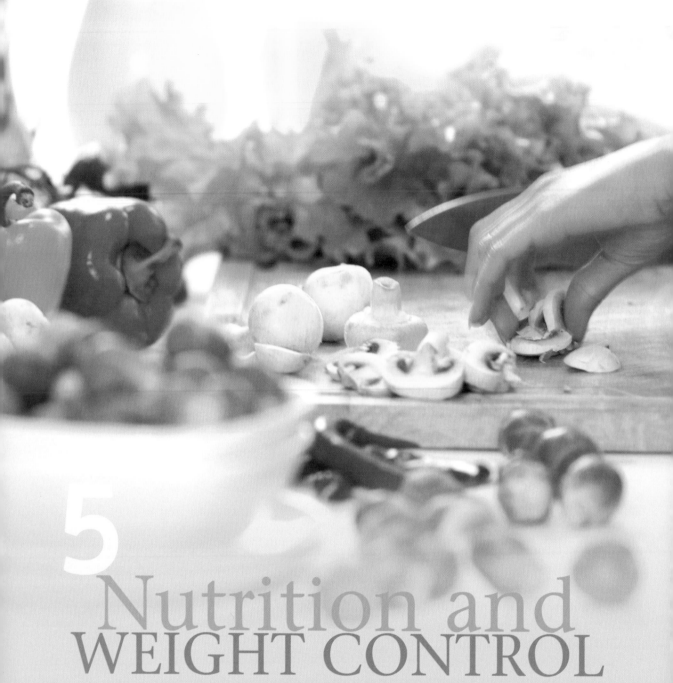

5
Nutrition and
WEIGHT CONTROL

The type of food we eat and the range of nutrients it supplies are among the most important factors determining our overall state of health—yet even people in highly developed societies can be lacking in key vitamins and minerals. Here are some ideas for ensuring that you and your family get all the nutrients you need without gaining excess weight.

Your
DAILY DIET

Many of us think we know the basics of healthy eating. But the science of nutrition is developing all the time, and we may underestimate the need for certain nutrients or overlook the value of some everyday foods. Here are some useful and sometimes unexpected tips for boosting your health through diet.

● **Eight is better than five** Experts suggest that eight portions of fruit and vegetables a day is even healthier than the standard recommendation to eat five a day.

★ **Get a multi-hit** by combining several different fruits in smoothies and adding a mix of vegetables to soups and stews.

★ **Vary your intake** because no single fruit or vegetable has all the nutrients you need.

● **Check your portion size** A portion of fruit and vegetables weighs about 3oz (80g), which equates to a small banana, a medium-size apple, or a small carrot. With this guideline in mind, it shouldn't be difficult to get the amount of fruit and vegetables you need to stay healthy.

● **Go for clean, bagged vegs** If you can't be bothered with scrubbing, peeling, and chopping vegetables, you'll be pleased to know that ready-prepared and bagged ones are just as healthy. Look for washed salad leaves as well as ready-to-cook green beans, asparagus, carrots, baby corn, peas, and lima beans. By using these products, you can cut the preparation time and still have a healthy diet—even if it is a bit more expensive.

● **Give carrots a roasting** Cooking carrots with a little oil increases the available levels of the antioxidant beta-carotene, because this vitamin is soluble in fat. A 2011 study found that our bodies can absorb just 11 percent of the beta-carotene from raw carrots but this figure rises to 75 percent when they are stir-fried. Add carrots to stews, soups, casseroles, and roasts.

● **Have a herbal cup** Herbal teas have proven health benefits. Scientific studies have found that:

★ **Chamomile** helps reduce inflammation and boosts the immune system.

★ **Peppermint** helps combat infections and harmful free radicals—by-products of reactions in the body's cells.

★ **Hibiscus** helps to lower blood pressure.

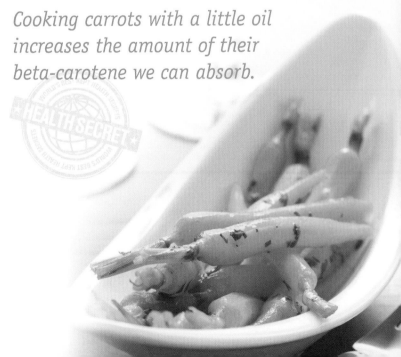

Cooking carrots with a little oil increases the amount of their beta-carotene we can absorb.

HEALTH SECRET

● Fight inflammation with nuts

Spanish scientists have discovered that a diet high in nuts, especially almonds, walnuts, and hazelnuts, can help reduce the risk of metabolic syndrome—a cluster of symptoms that increases your risk of type 2 diabetes and heart disease. This is the first study to show that a diet rich in nuts cuts the levels of substances associated with inflammation and other risk factors for these conditions. Try snacking on nuts between meals, and find ways to include them in your recipes.

● Swap roast beef for a nut roast

Replacing your Sunday roast with a healthier nut or lentil loaf could lengthen your life. Researchers have found that every extra daily portion (about the size of a deck of cards) of lamb, beef, or pork pushes up the risk of early death by 13 percent. Swapping red meat for fish, poultry, and plant-based proteins such as nuts and beans, however, contributes to a longer life. Aim to cut red meat consumption to about 1½oz (40g) a day—save the steak for the occasional treat and eat more healthy plant-based proteins.

● Be cautious with "lite" foods

Take care if opting for "lite," "low-fat" or "healthy eating" meals on the grounds that they are healthier. "Lite" meals can be very high in calories, and "low-fat" meals are often packed with unhealthy levels of salt (sodium). US researchers found that snacks labelled as low-fat encourage people to eat up

→
SURPRISINGLY EASY
→

Make canola oil a staple

Canola (rapeseed) oil has the lowest level of saturated fatty acids of any vegetable oil. It's rich in healthy monounsaturated and polyunsaturated fatty acids and consists of 11 percent heart-friendly omega-3 fatty acids. It also contains the antioxidant vitamins E and K, making it one of the most nutritious oils around. What's more, it's one of the cheapest oils on the shelves. Look for it in supermarkets—it's often labelled simply as vegetable oil.

Canola oil has the lowest level of unhealthy saturated fats of any vegetable oil.

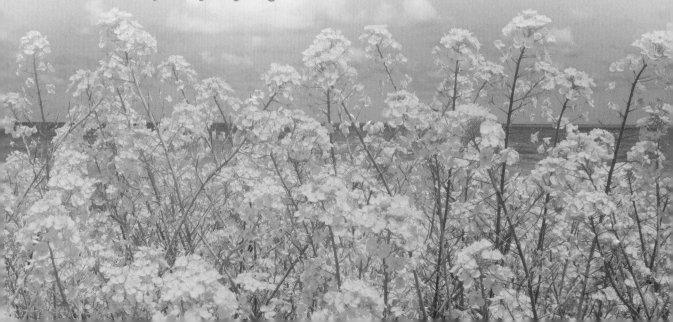

to half as much again as snacks that carry no low-fat claim. Unless your doctor has advised a low-fat diet, it's often better to opt for regular or full-fat foods but eat less of them. Some common claims on food labels are:

★ **Reduced fat/sugar/salt** At least 25 percent less than the standard version, these foods may still be high in fat.

★ **Low fat** No more than 3g fat per 100g for solids; 1.5g fat per ⅓ cup (100ml) for liquids (low-fat milk: 1.8g fat per 100ml).

★ **No added sugar** May still be high in naturally occurring sugars; products with added milk will contain milk sugar and fruit juices will contain fruit sugars.

★ **Lite/light** 30 percent lower in at least one typical value, such as calories or fat, than standard products of the same brand. But a "lite" version of one brand may contain the same amount of fat or calories as the standard version of another. Compare products by checking calories per 100g.

● **Read the label** People who make a habit of reading the nutritional information on food packaging eat around 5 percent less fat than those who don't bother, according to US researchers.

● **Fortify yourself with juice** A glass of orange juice taken after dinner is better for you than tea or coffee. Plant compounds in tea and coffee can tie up iron in the gut, making it unavailable for your body to use; vitamin C, by contrast, enhances iron uptake, helping to prevent anemia. Resist the caffeine craving and boost both your vitamin C and iron levels.

● **Choose brown over white** When it comes to rice, color counts, say American researchers. They found that the risk of type 2 diabetes rises by 10 percent for each daily portion of white rice eaten. The reason is unknown, but much white rice has a higher glycemic index (GI) than brown, pushing up blood glucose levels more steeply. White rice also has fewer B vitamins and less insoluble fiber and magnesium—components that reduce the risk of diabetes. Choose brown rice whenever you can.

● **Start with asparagus** This delicious vegetable is a rich source of oligofructose, a natural soluble fiber that can curb appetite and trigger the sensation of being full. Dutch scientists found that oligofructose triggers the release of gut hormones that govern appetite and that people who took it as a supplement ate 11 percent fewer calories after just 13 days. Oligofructose is also found in bananas, onions, chicory, barley, wheat, and tomatoes. See if eating these foods reduces your appetite.

● **Steer clear of sugar** Sugar rots your teeth and provides only calories with no additional nutrients. What's more, too much sugar raises the levels of damaging triglyceride fats in the blood. These fats are associated with lower levels of high-density lipoproteins (HDL), or "good" cholesterol— the form of cholesterol that protects against heart disease. Here are some ideas to help you cut down your sugar intake:

★ **Avoid** soft drinks, sweets, high-sugar breakfast cereals, and other foods that contain added sugars such as dextrose, fructose, invert sugar, maltose, and syrups.

★ **Check** the sugar levels in any processed product, such as frozen dinners, pasta sauces, desserts, and bread.

★ **Eat** only natural sugars that are found in fruit and vegetables.

★ **Choose** breakfast cereals that have no more than about 8g of sugar in a serving.

★ **Use** spices—such as vanilla, cinnamon, and ginger—in place of sugar.

Secrets of
PHYTONUTRIENTS

For decades scientists have thought that vitamins and minerals, together with fiber, were the most important health-giving components of fresh fruit, vegetables, whole grains, nuts, and seeds. But new studies are revealing that a variety of other plant compounds have equally important healing powers.

One of the first scientists to discover the properties of plant compounds known as phytonutrients was Dr. James Joseph, of the Human Nutrition Research Center on Aging at Tufts University. In 1999, he and his team first reported that eating blueberries may improve motor skills and reverse short-term memory loss, and in 2003 they announced that the same fruits could help people overcome a genetic predisposition to Alzheimer's. These findings were part of an ongoing process of identifying more than 5,000 chemicals (so far) that protect plants against attack by insects, animals, and disease, and of analyzing their effect on human health. Scientists now believe that phytonutrients are responsible for many of the benefits of fruit and vegetables.

Changing nature

Certain phytonutrients taste bitter, causing some people, especially children, to dislike the flavor of foods such as broccoli, Brussels sprouts, cabbage, cauliflower, and kale that contain them. This led the food industry to spend decades producing less bitter hybrids and to develop "debittering" processes for their vegetables to encourage us to eat more of them; you may have noticed a change. Today, as a result, such vegetables contain much smaller amounts of these healthy chemicals. Now food scientists and plant breeders have begun working together to identify old, nutrient-rich vegetable varieties and cross-pollinate them with commercial ones to produce hybrids that not only contain more of these life-giving chemicals but also taste good. A broccoli hybrid launched in the UK in 2011 contains two to three times the normal level of the beneficial phytonutrient glucoraphanin.

Phytonutrient families

Studies have identified several main groups of phytochemicals, including:
● **Anthocyanins**, found in blue or purple foods. These have a wide variety of actions, such as helping combat the inflammation thought to lie behind many diseases, from Alzheimer's to diabetes and heart disease.

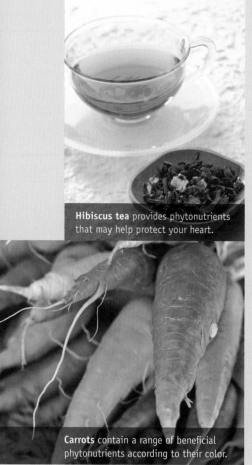

Hibiscus tea provides phytonutrients that may help protect your heart.

Carrots contain a range of beneficial phytonutrients according to their color.

- **Carotenoids,** which are linked to a lower risk of heart disease and some cancers and occur mainly in orange fruit and vegetables. Carotenoids in foods of other colors include lycopene (linked to a lower risk of some cancers, especially prostate cancer) in red fruits; and lutein (present in the lens of the eye, which may help to prevent cataracts and age-related macular degeneration) in green, orange, and yellow fruit and vegetables.
- **Glucosinolates,** which occur in vegetables of the cabbage family. These have been shown to protect against breast and prostate cancer.
- **Polyphenols,** which have anti-inflammatory properties and protect nerve cells. Some may also help prevent cancer and Alzheimer's. They are present in tea, wine, coffee, and blue and purple fruit and vegetables.
- **Resveratrol**, found in red wine and grape products, which may protect against some cancers, heart disease, metabolic syndrome, and degeneration of nerve cells.

Figs are rich in anthocyanins, which may counter age-related diseases.

Green leafy vegetables are among the best sources of lutein, a phytonutrient that benefits the eyes.

Eat a cocktail of phytonutrients

So far there is little scientific consensus about the exact benefits of various phytonutrients. But every year numerous studies find that certain fruits or vegetables, or groups of these foods (such as color groups), appear to offer some protection against particular diseases that tend to develop with age. To obtain a healthy mix of phytonutrients, eat a variety of differently colored fruit and vegetables every day—a plant's color reflects its mix of phytonutrients. Target foods in these color groups:

Red and pink Red and pink fruit and vegetables, such as tomatoes, watermelons, papaya, pink guavas, and pink grapefruit, are rich in lycopene. Cooked tomatoes, including tomato purée, are the best source.

Orange Carrots, sweet potatoes, squash, pumpkin, papaya, mango, and cantaloupe are all rich in carotenoids. Carotenoids are best absorbed with a little fat, so cook them in a little unsaturated oil if possible.

Yellow The yellow spice turmeric—so delicious in curries—contains curcumin, one of the polyphenol family of phytonutrients.

Blue and purple Eggplant, blueberries, blackberries, grapes, plums, raisins, tart cherries, figs, purple potatoes, sweet corn, red wine, grape juice, and purple teas such as hibiscus are all rich in anthocyanins, which form a complex phytonutrient cocktail. Red wine, purple grape juice, dark grapes, and some berries also contain resveratrol, a polyphenol.

Green Many green vegetables and fruit, such as kale, spinach, chard, watercress, garden peas, and avocado, are rich in lutein.

Vegetables of the cabbage family, such as broccoli, Brussels sprouts, and cauliflower, are a good source of glucosinolates.

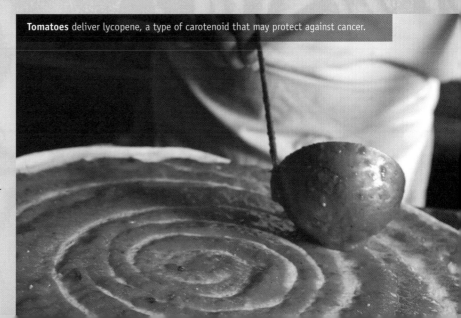

Tomatoes deliver lycopene, a type of carotenoid that may protect against cancer.

Nutrition
THROUGH LIFE

Our dietary needs and eating habits change throughout life, from infancy to old age. One of the keys to good health is to adapt your diet and pattern of meals to maximize your intake of the nutrients you need at each stage of life. You'll find out more here.

● **Breast is best** to protect your baby's gut. Here is yet another benefit breastfeeding brings—it helps to increase your baby's healthy gut bacteria. These bacteria play a vital role in digestion, building up the baby's immunity and determining whether extra calories are stored as fat. Breast milk contains special starches that feed "good" gut bacteria and reduce the number of "bad" bacteria that can cause bacterial pneumonia, middle ear

infections and meningitis. Breast milk also contains enzymes, hormones, and infection-fighting antibodies that formula milks do not.

● **Give your baby fewer calories**
Breast milk is 15 to 20 percent lower in calories than formula, which can help to prevent your baby gaining excess weight. And overweight babies are more likely to have health problems in later years.

● **Wean earlier?** Exclusive breastfeeding beyond four months may not reduce the risk of allergies as was once thought; indeed, it may even increase the risk, according to a review in the *British Medical Journal*. The review also suggests that babies exclusively breastfed for six months or longer may not get enough iron, which is vital for mental, physical, and social development. Discuss the right time to introduce your baby to solids with your doctor.

Babies who feed themselves are more likely to enjoy healthy foods.

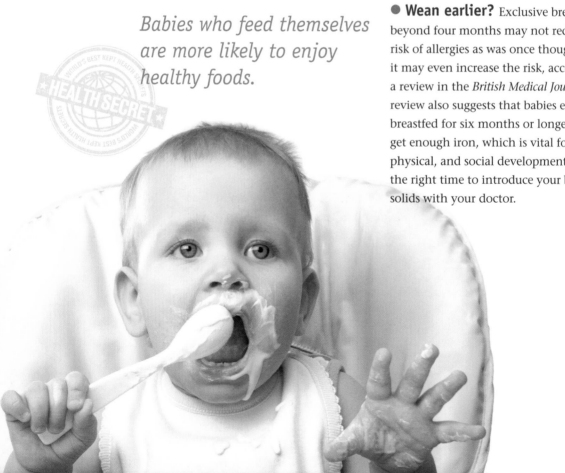

● **Help yourself** Encouraging your baby to eat finger feed could prevent future weight gain and foster a natural liking for healthy foods, say UK psychologists. They found that babies who were encouraged to feed themselves from a range of solid finger foods when weaning were more likely to have a healthy diet. By contrast, spoon-fed babies had a sweeter tooth and were more likely to be overweight.

● **Practice the rule of six** If your preschooler doesn't like greens, serve them at least six times. So says a US study in which children were encouraged to take small repeated tastes of two vegetables that they initially disliked, one with a tasty dip and one without. In both cases the children liked the vegetables by the sixth tasting. Most young children don't eat enough vegetables, and this study suggests that this is because it takes time to develop a taste for them. Give gentle encouragement, and a dip if you want, and see them down the treat.

● **Eat rainbow foods for a healthy glow** A Scottish study has revealed that people who eat red, green, yellow, and orange fruit and vegetables achieve a healthy glow that attracts members of the opposite sex. The glow comes from the yellow-red pigments (carotenoids) that give orange and red fruit and vegetables their hue and which are also found in many dark green vegetables. These build up in the skin in just a few weeks and alter its color—eating just three portions a day makes people look healthier and boosts attractiveness. Tell that to any fruit and vegetable-hating teens you have.

● **Don't clam up on clams** Clams are among the shellfish that may be beneficial if you're trying to have a baby. They are good

SECRETS OF SUCCESS

Preventing fuss

Breastfed babies often have more adventurous palates than formula-fed babies as they get older. This is because breastmilk provides a kaleidoscope of taste sensations that changes according to what the mother eats. Researchers from the University of Copenhagen in Denmark found that breastfed babies prefer stronger flavors than those fed on formula.

It's not quite as simple as babies picking up a taste for whatever their mother eats. What seems to happen is that the constant small flavor changes in breastmilk make breastfed babies more receptive to new flavors and therefore more willing to try a wider variety of foods once they start solids.

If you are bottle-feeding, experiment with different types of formula milks as flavors do differ between brands. That way your baby will also become used to a variety of different tastes.

sources of iodine, which is vital for the health of the thyroid gland in both mother and baby and for the development of the baby's brain and nervous system. A deficiency can lead to a lack of hormones produced by the baby's thyroid (hypothyroidism), which in turn can lead to mental problems—one reason why babies are tested for thyroid function at birth. Hypothyroidism in the mother after giving birth produces symptoms that are virtually indistinguishable from postnatal depression. For your health and that of your baby:

★ **Eat fish and shellfish** Ocean fish (especially oily ones) are excellent sources. Shellfish must be well cooked until they

For further tips on looking after your thyroid gland, see Chapter 8, *Healthy Hormones*

DIET AND PREGNANCY

Some foods are best avoided during pregnancy because they could harm your unborn baby. All cereals, fresh fruit, and vegetables that you would normally eat are safe. The following guidelines apply mainly to meat, fish, shellfish, and dairy products.

Foods that are safe:
- Hard cheeses
- Soft cheeses (pasteurized only)
- White fish, if not from polluted waters

- Oily fish (up to 2 portions a week)
- Eggs (cooked until solid)
- Cooked shellfish (only if shells have opened during cooking)
- Sushi, if the fish has been frozen first.

Foods to avoid:
- Soft cheeses (unpasteurized, mold-ripened, or blue-veined)
- Raw or undercooked eggs and foods that contain them, such as homemade mayonnaise

- Raw (unpasteurized) cow, goat, or sheep's milk (unless boiled)
- Unpasteurized juice
- All pâtés, including vegetable pâtés
- Raw or undercooked meat
- Liver or liver products
- Shark, marlin, and swordfish
- Raw shellfish.

If in doubt, consult your doctor or midwife.

---

open—discard any that remain closed. Other sources of iodine include milk and milk products, cereals, fruit, and vegetables.

★ **Avoid kelp and iodine supplements**, which may contain dangerously high levels of iodine.

● **Try some crispy tofu** Soy products such as tofu may help to relieve menopausal symptoms such as hot flashes, according to some, though not all studies. Try a tasty snack of tofu chunks, rolled in sesame seeds and fried in a little canola oil.

● **Eat more ricotta** An adequate protein intake helps to keep muscle tissue strong and guards against age-related muscle loss. Research suggests that consuming whey, a naturally occurring milk protein, is one of the best ways to encourage the body to build muscle. Italian ricotta cheese is one of the best sources. Mix it with tomato sauce for a creamy pasta topping or use in desserts. But all milk products contain whey.

● **Go for convenience** Frozen vegetables can help you meet your nutritional needs when you have less energy for shopping and cooking. Frozen, precut vegetables that can be resealed, and single portions of canned fruit, are easy to prepare and have a long shelf life. So make life easy on yourself and don't turn your nose up at frozen vegetables.

● **Supplement if necessary** As you grow older, you may need more of certain vitamins and minerals. But it can sometimes be difficult to get enough from food alone. Look for a supplement designed for older adults—it will include calcium and vitamins D and B12.

● **Have a dental checkup** Dental problems or poorly fitting dentures can make it hard to chew fruit, vegetables, and whole-grain bread, which may mean you avoid these healthy foods. Get dental treatment, but meanwhile eat soft fruits and vegetable soups and purées.

Losing EXCESS WEIGHT

Being overweight is now thought to be one of the most serious threats to health in the West. Plentiful cheap food has sparked an epidemic among rich and poor alike, fueling the incidence of heart disease, stroke, diabetes, and other major disorders. It's harder than ever to maintain a healthy weight but vital for your well-being. Here are some guidelines.

● **Eat whenever you like** Eating late at night won't make you fat. It's what you eat, not when you eat, that matters, say the experts. If calories-in exceed calories-out, then the excess is stored as fat whatever the time of day. The message is simple: Whenever you feel like a snack, have soups, salads, or fruit rather than chips or cake.

● **Start with soup** Soup can be your secret weapon when it comes to dropping a few pounds. A US study suggests that eating soup before your main course curbs your appetite so that you reduce your total calorie intake at that meal by more than 20 percent. This may be because soup takes a relatively long time to leave the stomach and is thought to help quieten appetite-stimulating hormones. So make this your starter of choice, but avoid creamy soups as they are likely to be high in calories.

● **Choose boiled potatoes not fries**
Swapping high energy-dense foods for low energy-dense foods is one of the best ways to get and stay slim. It's the difference between eating 3½oz (100g) of fries and 3½oz (100g) of boiled potatoes—they weigh the same but the fries have more fat and calories. Eating more low energy-dense foods will help you feel full and stay feeling full longer—the pounds should roll off. Good options are fruit, vegetables, soups, casseroles, and foods such as brown rice and pasta that soak up lots of water during cooking. Steer clear of foods high in fat or sugar.

● **Go coco loco** A daily dose of coconut oil may help you shed hard-to-lose pounds. Coconut oil is rich in medium chain fatty acids (MCFAs), a type of fat that can speed up metabolism. A Brazilian study showed that women who followed a healthy lifestyle and consumed 1oz (30ml) of coconut oil a day had more slender waists, higher levels of "good" HDL cholesterol, and lower levels of "bad" LDL cholesterol after just 12 weeks. Eat a teaspoon or two of coconut oil a day

A daily dose of coconut oil may help to lose the pounds.

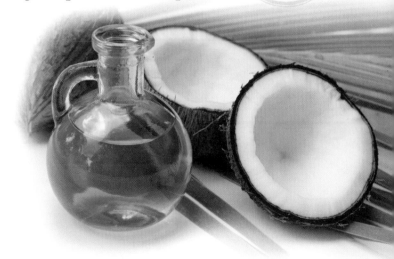

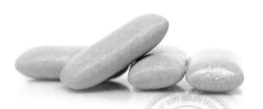

Chewing gum helps put a stop to sweet cravings.

and use it in your cooking—as with any fat, it should be used sparingly. If you have high cholesterol, ask your doctor's advice first.

● **Take it slowly** US researchers report that how quickly we eat affects how much we eat. In one study, fast eaters consumed about 3oz (90g) of food per minute, medium-speed eaters 2½oz (70g), and slow eaters just 2oz (60g). It takes at least 20 minutes for the stomach to alert the brain that you are full, and faster eaters are more likely to overeat before this happens. Pause between mouthfuls and chew well; you may find that you lose a few pounds.

● **Forget diet pills** The magic pill that will help you lose weight and keep it off does not exist, according to a study reported

SURPRISINGLY EASY

Pep it up
Spicing up your diet with a sprinkling of chopped-up chile peppers can help curb appetite, according to researchers from Indiana. It seems the sensory experience of eating chiles aids digestion and cuts down cravings for fatty, salty, or sweet foods, especially in people who don't often eat spicy food.

in the *International Journal of Sport Nutrition and Exercise Metabolism*. The researchers found no proof that any single product results in significant weight loss without diet changes and regular exercise. So stop hoping for a quick fix and eat more whole grains, fruits, vegetables, and lean meats, cut back on high-fat foods, and make sure you exercise every day.

● **Be a gum chewer** Chewing gum may help quell sweet cravings suggests a US study. People who chewed sugar-free gum for 15 minutes an hour for 3 hours and then indulged in a variety of snacks reported feeling significantly less hungry and had fewer cravings for sweet foods than those who did not chew gum before snacking.

● **Drink up to drop pounds** If you're trying to eat fewer calories, drinking just two glasses of water before each meal will help you, say US researchers. Water is effective because it fills up the stomach with a calorie-free liquid, giving a calorie-free sensation of fullness. So drink up before every meal—water could be the magic potion you've been looking for in the battle of the bulge.

● **Go for good carbs** Low-carbohydrate diets such as Atkins and The Zone have spread the idea that carbohydrates should be avoided if you want to lose weight. But carbohydrates with a low GI (short for glycemic index—a measure of how fast food raises blood glucose levels), such as oatmeal, beans, nuts, seeds, whole-wheat pasta, and bulgur are an exception. They keep you feeling satisfied for longer by releasing their energy slowly, resulting in eating less. So have oatmeal for breakfast, bulgur salad for lunch, and whole-wheat pasta for dinner.

Curb appetite—indulgently

Thinking that what you eat is high in calories could help to control your appetite. In a US study, 45 healthy volunteers were given the same 380 calorie milkshake, but were either told it was a low-cal choice or an indulgent high-cal treat. Levels of the hunger-hormone ghrelin were measured before and after drinking the shake.

The researchers found that ghrelin levels dropped most in the group who assumed that they had indulged. These results suggest that merely thinking you have eaten something "naughty" or high in calories can quell hunger pangs.

● **Keep a food diary** Recording what you eat is one of the most effective ways to help you lose weight according to US research—it seems that it can enable you to double your weight loss. The simple act of writing down what you eat, when you eat, and whom you eat with encourages you to consume fewer calories. Keep a food diary for a few weeks and see if it helps you.

● **Pack some protein** Eating some protein at every meal can help to keep your weight steady on the scales—it is one of the best types of food for triggering that "I've had enough now" feeling that controls appetite. Protein also stimulates fat burning and helps to build or maintain lean tissue. Besides meat and fish, you can get this vital component of a healthy diet from beans, lentils, nuts, seeds, eggs, and soy products.

● **Feel calm to stay slim** Feeling stressed about everyday anxieties may exhaust you, but it won't make you thin.

When you produce high levels of the stress hormone cortisol, your body reacts by storing fat—an ancient survival mechanism in emergencies. If you feel under constant pressure, a persistently raised level of cortisol continuously encourages fat to accumulate in your abdomen—the most risky kind of fat. Soothe your anxieties with stress-busting methods, and you'll give yourself the best opportunity to lose weight.

Recording what you eat could boost the amount of weight you lose.

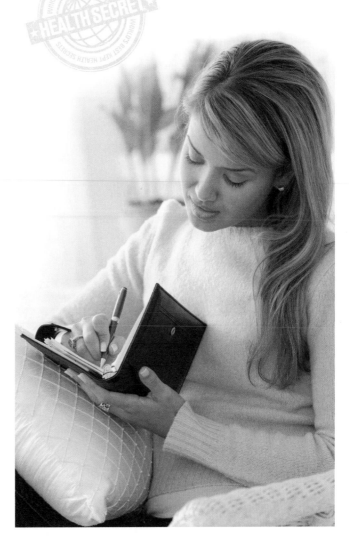

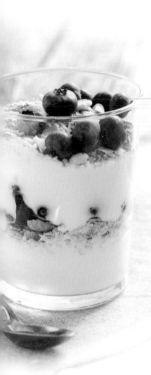

● Eat and drink dairy Dairy foods may help prevent women from gaining weight and allow them to reduce their overall body fat. US researchers found that young women of normal weight who had 1,000mg of calcium every day from dairy sources—the amount of calcium found in 1.8 pints (about a liter) of low-fat milk—lost 6 lb (about 3kg) over two years.

Low-fat yogurt can help you lose weight.

Aim for three servings of dairy food a day, such as a glass of milk, a small container of low-fat yogurt, and a matchbox-sized piece of cheese. But for this strategy to work, be sure to also follow a calorie-controlled diet.

● Change your habits in six stages

Knowing how to lose weight is one thing, but actually doing it is another. To lose weight, you need to break the habits that made you put it on in the first place. James Prochaska, Professor of Psychology at the University of Rhode Island, has identified the following six stages of successful habit-changing:

KNOW YOUR BMI

To bolster your resolve to tackle excess weight, it's useful to have an objective indicator of the seriousness of your weight problem. Plot your height and weight on this chart to find out whether your BMI is putting your health at risk. Note: This chart

may not reflect the health risk for those who are lean but heavily muscled. To calculate your precise BMI, use the formulas at the Centers for Disease Control's website at www.cdc.gov/healthyweight/assessing/bmi/adult_bmi/index.html.

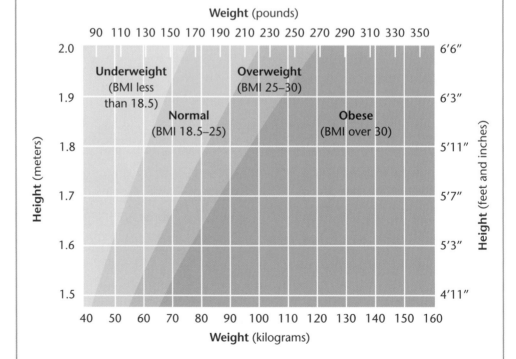

★ **Be candid** Take an honest look at yourself then make up your mind to get started on a program of weight loss.

★ **Ponder the positives** Visualize the improvements to your health, energy levels, and looks that you will experience when you have lost weight.

★ **Get ready** Make a detailed plan that includes a start date and realistic goals for each day, each week, the first month, and three months from now. These goals can be small and specific, such as buying a kitchen scale or swapping an unhealthy snack for an extra piece of fruit. Add goals for six months and one year. Tell your friends, family, and colleagues about your intentions and enlist their support.

★ **Take action** Create weekly menus, write shopping lists, and stick to them. Exercise—ideally with a partner to boost your motivation. Make sure you include small treats, such as a an occasional piece of chocolate, to reward yourself for sticking to your plans. Be patient—new habits take time to feel natural.

★ **Maintain your resolve** To cement your new habits, start thinking of yourself as a healthy eater and and regular exerciser.

★ **Congratulations!** Now that you are a fitter, healthier person, an occasional lapse won't derail your new outlook.

Sticking rigidly to shopping lists and meal plans are sure-fire ways to lose weight.

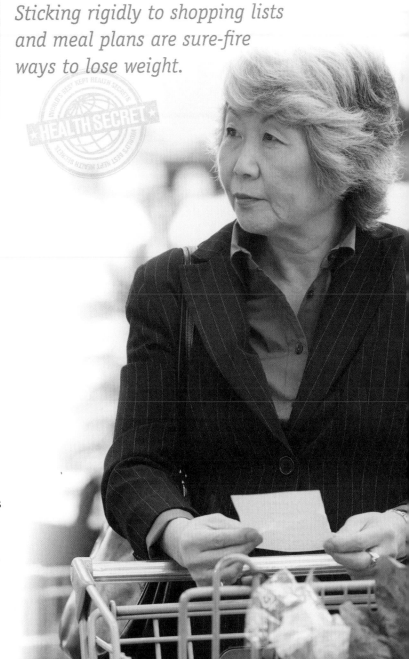

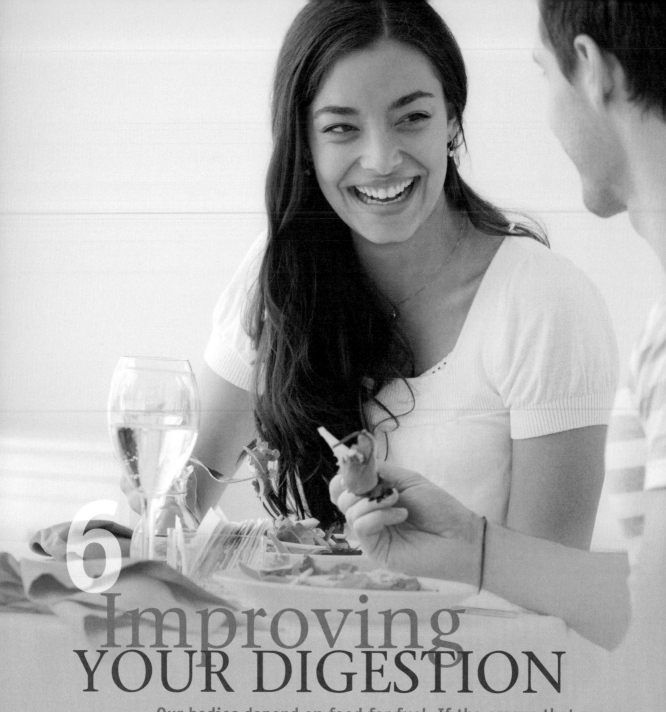

6
Improving
YOUR DIGESTION

Our bodies depend on food for fuel. If the organs that process what we eat don't function properly, our well-being is at risk and we may also suffer discomfort and pain. But modern scientific know-how and tried-and-tested methods can provide solutions to most digestive disorders.

Stomach CARE

Acids produced in the stomach break down the food we eat to release essential nutrients. Although natural and necessary, stomach acid can cause problems, especially when combined with the action of bacteria on the stomach wall, which can lead to peptic ulcers. The following tips can help to prevent or relieve a variety of stomach disorders.

● Heal your stomach with sleep

Every night while you sleep, your body repairs damage to the stomach lining. It does this by increasing production of human trefoil protein (TFF2), which aids the repair of damaged areas of the linings of the stomach and intestines, and is fully effective only while you're asleep. For optimum stomach health, make sure you sleep for 7–8 hours each night.

● Sip a strawberry stomach soother

Everyone's favorite summer fruit also soothes a troubled stomach, new research suggests. Strawberries are thought to help prevent stomach ulcers by reducing damage done to the stomach's mucous membrane. The findings are still unconfirmed, but you'll do yourself no harm by enjoying this delicious preventive remedy whenever strawberries are available.

● Eat to boost ulcer treatment

Choosing the right foods can make the treatment your doctor prescribes for your peptic ulcer more effective. A seven-day course of "triple therapy"—two kinds of antibiotics plus a drug known as a proton pump inhibitor—is a common regimen. While the treatment does its work, cranberry juice, probiotic yogurt, and turmeric may all help it heal the stomach lining, as will oily fish and plenty of dark green vegetables.

BELIEVE IT OR NOT!

Worry doesn't cause ulcers

Myths abound about the cause of peptic ulcers, which typically occur in the stomach or small intestine. One common belief is that chronic anxiety or anger leads to the painful disorder. It is possible that strong emotion may constrict the blood supply to tissue, eventually leading to ulceration—but this is rare.

It's certainly true that aspirin, ibuprofen, and some prescription drugs cause ulcers. But the trigger for most peptic ulcers is *Helicobacter pylori*, a type of bacterium that infects nine out of ten people who develop an ulcer. Getting rid of the bacteria with an antibiotic, while suppressing the production of acid in the stomach, is a simple and speedy way to cure the problem.

● Breathe away the burn
Try deep breathing to relieve heartburn. It reduces the amount of stomach acid that leaks into the esophagus, scientists claim. If you have chronic heartburn, engage in conscious deep breathing for 30 minutes a day to improve your quality of life and reduce your need for drugs. As a bonus, you'll experience a soothing state of relaxation.

● Rest your fork
If it were a drug, this technique would make millions: Simply put down your fork between each mouthful, take time to chew, and don't be in a hurry to pick the fork up again—perhaps chat, read a

● **Chew away heartburn** If you have heartburn, try chewing gum. The chewing action creates saliva, which coats the esophagus with a protective gel, preventing heartburn. Don't overdo it, though. Too much chewing creates excess stomach acid, increasing the risk of a stomach ulcer.

● **Go Japanese** Nori, wakame, and kelp—seaweeds used in Japanese cooking—have been found to form gels in the stomach that help to prevent heartburn.

● **Add some acid** Drink a teaspoon of cider vinegar in half a glass of water before or after a large meal to aid digestion. The vinegar boosts acid levels in the stomach, which may help to break down food. This could help people who don't produce enough stomach acid, which causes belching after meals, feeling too full, and abdominal pain. Don't try this if you have a disorder related to excess stomach acid, such as gastroesophageal reflux (GERD).

book, or listen to the radio. The pause gives your digestive juices more time to work, and gives your stomach the chance to signal to the brain that you're full before you've eaten too much. Aim to take more than 20 minutes for a meal. Chew well and eat slowly to reduce heartburn, avoid overeating, and enjoy mealtime even more.

● **Have a glass of wine—if you like**
A glass of wine with a rich meal does not increase your risk of gas or heartburn, say Swiss scientists. They assessed the speed and quality of digestion in healthy people who ate a meal of cheese fondue and drank either black tea or wine and a glass of brandy. Those who drank alcohol digested food more slowly—alcohol slows stomach emptying. But neither group was more likely to have gas or heartburn.

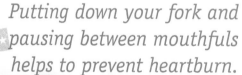

Putting down your fork and pausing between mouthfuls helps to prevent heartburn.

● **Calm it with caraway** This aromatic seed has powerful antispasmodic and antibacterial properties. A key ingredient in old-fashioned gripe water for colicky babies, caraway seed is an ideal home remedy to relieve the symptoms of indigestion. Use it in bread, cookies, cakes, curries, and stews.

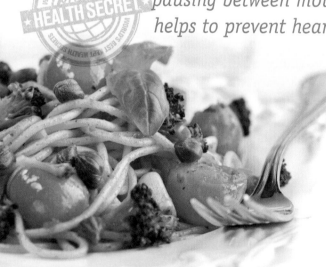

Keeping the juices FLOWING

As food passes through the digestive tract, it undergoes many processes to enable its nutrients to be absorbed. The action of bile, a digestive juice made in the liver, is vital for fat digestion. The gallbladder, which stores bile, can become inflamed or its ducts can be blocked by stones. The tips that follow will help you reduce your risk of trouble.

● **Don't go fat-free** If you have gallstones, the conventional advice to follow a virtually fat-free diet is probably a step too far, experts now say; following healthy guidelines for including some fat in your diet is unlikely to cause harm. That means choosing olive oil over animal fats, avoiding high-fat fast food, and limiting store-bought prepared meals. It's very important that you eat at least five portions of fresh fruit and vegetables a day and avoid high-fat and high-sugar foods.

● **Hit the caffeine** Many doctors warn people with gallbladder problems to avoid coffee, which has a reputation as a trigger for pain. A new study found that people who drank at least four cups a day were least likely to develop gallbladder disease because caffeine in coffee boosts the flow of bile. However, coffee isn't good for everyone, so if you are at risk of gallbladder problems, talk to your doctor about the pros and cons of this approach.

● **Breathe away bloating** If you experience bloating and indigestion after a heavy meal, try deep breathing. Bloating occurs when the lymphatic system can't move food proteins and fat molecules through the system for detoxification. Deep breathing requires deep movements by the diaphragm, which massage the liver and stomach and stimulate the lymphatic system to clear unwanted substances from the body. Breathe in deeply and out again very slowly and repeat several times.

Coffee may protect against gallbladder disease.

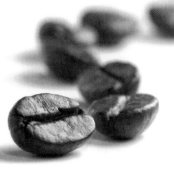

HEALTH SECRET
WORLD'S BEST KEPT HEALTH SECRETS

SURPRISINGLY EASY

Abdominal massage
To relieve indigestion, massage your lower abdomen in a clockwise direction—from right to left across the top of your abdomen and from left to right across the bottom—to promote blood flow to the area. The direction of movement matches the flow of the digestive system and helps to push trapped air and food residues through the large intestine. For extra benefit, use massage oil to which you've added a few drops of peppermint essential oil.

Milk thistle may help flush away gallstones—naturally.

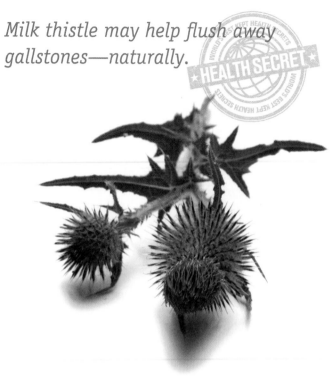

● **Make more of mint** This common herb can provide valuable protection for your gallbladder. Peppermint oil stimulates the secretion of bile from the liver, which reduces the risk of developing gallstones. To get the benefits safely, take medicinal peppermint oil in the form of delayed release capsules, such as *Colpermin*, with a special coating that protects the stomach from the irritating effect of the oil.

● **Go easy on sugar** Cut down on sugar and refined carbohydrates. A diet high in these foods increases the risk of most digestive disorders and is one of the major risk factors in inflammation of the gallbladder (cholecystitis), an unpleasant condition. Protect your gallbladder by swapping sugar and white flour for high-fiber, unrefined carbohydrates.

● **Eat more oranges** or plenty of any foods rich in vitamin C to help prevent gallstones and protect the digestive system

as a whole. Vitamin C converts cholesterol into bile acids, and research shows that people who don't get enough have an increased risk of gallstones. Stock your fruit bowl with vitamin C-rich citrus fruit and kiwifruit and fill your vegetable bin with peppers and broccoli.

● **Try herbal help for gallstones** If you have painful gallstones, you may need surgery to remove the gallbladder. First, try these natural ways of preventing the pebble-like formations, which work by stimulating the gallbladder to expel bile:
★ **Dandelion or milk thistle** Try tincture or capsules to help flush out gallstones.
★ **Conjugated linoleic acid** Derived from safflower, this stimulates bile production.
★ **Lecithin** This naturally occurring fatty compound found in liver, egg yolks, and soybeans is a major component of bile. Taken as supplement, it helps to break down fat in food and inhibits stone formation.

● **Have regular meals** If you have gallbladder problems, it may not be a surprise to learn that you'll need to pay special attention to what you eat. What you may not realize is that you could also benefit by adjusting *when* you eat. Regular meals throughout the day, starting with breakfast, stimulate the release of bile into the small intestine—ensuring that the bile does not stagnate in the gallbladder, a risk factor for gallstone formation.

● **Go veg for digestive health** Vegetarians have fewer digestive problems than meat eaters, largely because vegetables are high in fiber, so food residues pass through the gut quickly. Vegetarians rarely have constipation and are 60 percent less likely than meat eaters to have gallstones. There are good nutritional reasons to include some meat in your diet, but there's plenty of evidence that people in Western countries eat too much meat—especially red meat—and would have a healthier digestion if they ate less meat and more vegetables.

● **Know and act on your risk** Be aware of your risk of gallbladder disease so that you can take preventive measures if you're susceptible. The maxim that people with gallstones are often "fat, fertile, fair, and forty" is partly true. Fair skin or hair are not risk factors—but the other characteristics are, so here are some helpful action tips:

★ **Reduce your cholesterol** Gallstones can develop if too much cholesterol builds up in the bile, which is more likely in women, due to the effects of estrogen. Your diet should be low in saturated fat and refined carbohydrates such as sugar.

★ **Tackle excess weight** Being overweight leads to the liver over-producing cholesterol. Try to lose any excess weight by having a healthy diet and getting plenty of regular exercise. Gallstones are more of a problem for people between the ages of 55 and 65. If you're in this age group, pay extra attention to your diet and lifestyle.

● **Don't crash** While it's healthy to lose excess weight, it's important not to do so too quickly. Crash diets involve losing at least 3 lb (1.5kg) a week and are a leading cause of gallstones and also turn "silent" gallstones into painful ones. Up to one in four people who go on very low-calorie diets develop gallstones, and one in three of those require gallbladder surgery. Overly aggressive weight-loss causes the liver to secrete extra cholesterol into bile, leading to gallstones formed from cholesterol. If you have excess weight, follow a healthy, balanced diet and exercise program to help you lose it without increasing your risk of gallstones.

● **Consider a gallbladder flush** if you think you may be developing a gallstone. Drinking ¼–½ cup (50–125ml) of olive oil may stimulate the gallbladder to release more bile than usual, which may flush out any small stones that have formed. Ask your doctor about this treatment before using it.

SECRETS OF SUCCESS

Fish oil may prevent gallstones

We all know of the health benefits of the Mediterranean diet, but what of the benefits to the gallbladder of an Arctic diet? Indigenous peoples in Canada and Alaska, for example, have a diet that is very high in fatty fish, and the fish oil content is thought to be behind the very low incidence of gallstones in people who follow this traditional diet. Specifically, it is the omega-3 fatty acids in oily fish that scientists think prevent cholesterol from solidifying into hard stones in the gallbladder.

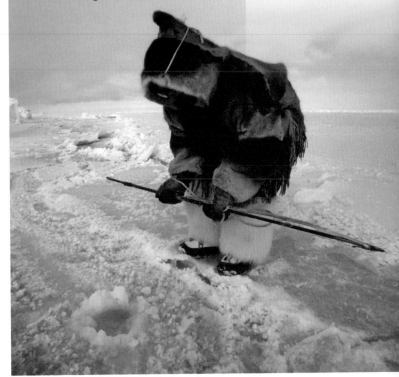

Secrets of
AYURVEDIC MEDICINE

The virtues of holistic medicine—treating the body, mind, and spirit—
have become increasingly accepted in the West. Discover here how one
of the most respected ancient healing systems, Ayurvedic medicine,
uses an integral approach to promoting well-being and the special
benefits this can bring to digestive health.

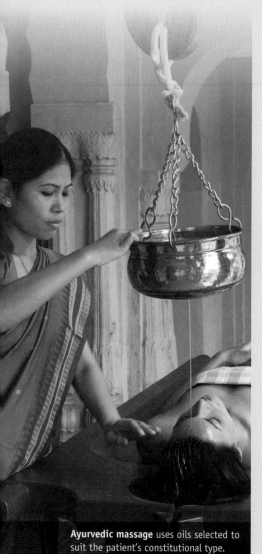

Ayurvedic massage uses oils selected to
suit the patient's constitutional type.

Around 5,000 years ago, Ayurveda emerged from the healing
tradition of India's great seers who, it is said, once departed for the
Himalayas to meditate on the secrets of health and longevity. Named from
the Sanskrit *ayur* meaning "life" and *veda* for "knowledge," Ayurveda
emphasizes the unity of mind, body, and soul, and gives equal weight to
the prevention of illness and its cure.

To determine an individual's *prakriti* or constitution and therefore
the most suitable treatment for any ailment or disorder, an Ayurvedic
practitioner will take a careful note of medical history, diet, and lifestyle.
He or she (as women are now entering this traditionally male discipline)
will also conduct a physical examination, observe a patient's eyes, voice,
skin, teeth, and tongue, and check urine and bowel movements.

Holistic treatment for digestive disorders

Ayurvedic medicine seeks to treat illness by discovering the nature
of an individual's *vikruti* (imbalance), then prescribing appropriate
measures, such as herbal remedies, as well as lifestyle and dietary
changes. Practitioners believe that a holistic approach is particularly
relevant for digestive problems and that many disorders identified in
Western medicine are the result of poor eating habits and inappropriate
food choices.

Herbs, plant oils, and spices play a major role. A number of those
prescribed for digestive disorders, including triphala (a combination of
three Indian herbs) and the spice turmeric have now been shown to be
effective in clinical studies.

Some of the lifestyle and dietary precepts echo Western advice. The
California College of Ayurveda suggests that "the largest meal of the
day should be taken near the noon hour when the sun is high and the
agni (digestive fire) strongest." It advocates quiet and calm when eating,
with no distractions such as television or "excessive conversation."
Food should be "chewed well," "one should never overeat" and rest is
recommended after a meal to allow food to digest.

Ayurveda in the kitchen

To find a reputable Ayurvedic practitioner, contact an organization such as the National Ayurvedic Medical Association (www.ayurvedanama.org), which represents the Ayurvedic profession in the United States. It is advisable to consult your own doctor before undergoing any Ayurvedic treatment. But many of the top Ayurvedic herbs and spices can be freely used in everyday cooking, since they taste delicious and can only do you good. Those readily available in supermarkets include:

Cardamom Used in sweet as well as savory dishes, this flavoring is good for treating sore throats, and for heart health and digestion.

Chile This key curry ingredient is a circulation booster that increases metabolism and enhances appetite.

Cinnamon A fragrant and warming stimulant that wards off fatigue and digestive ills. Add to desserts, cookies, and cakes.

Coriander seed improves the absorption of food; it helps treat diarrhea and has antibacterial properties. Use in curries of all kinds.

Cumin An important ingredient in curries as well as in many Greek and Latin American dishes, cumin aids digestion and combats nausea. It is also effective for pain relief and promotes tissue healing.

Fennel seed combines perfectly with fish of any kind, but is also good with meat. Chewed after meals, seeds cool and calm the stomach, soothing digestion.

Fenugreek is recommended for anyone with arthritis. May help lose weight or control type 2 diabetes by raising metabolism and helps lower blood sugar. Good with meat, fish, and in cakes.

Ginger A versatile ingredient for savory and sweet dishes of all kinds, ginger aids digestion and relieves the symptoms of colds, flu, headaches, and arthritis.

Mustard seed Add these to stir-fries and curries and to any vegetable dishes including brassicas and beets. They boost the appetite, relieve muscular pain, and promote better sleep.

Tamarind Widely used in curries, chutneys, and samosas, this sour spice is valuable as a laxative and is used to promote tissue healing.

Turmeric This curry spice is renowned for its medicinal properties, from wound healing to the treatment of respiratory problems; it also stimulates the immune system.

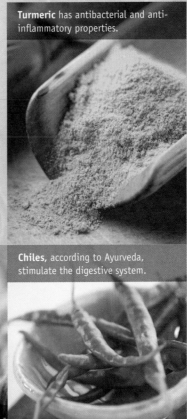

Turmeric has antibacterial and anti-inflammatory properties.

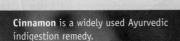

Cinnamon is a widely used Ayurvedic indigestion remedy.

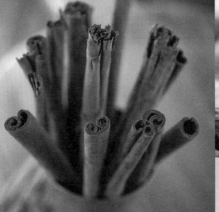

Cardamom is a standard Ayurvedic remedy for flatulence.

Chiles, according to Ayurveda, stimulate the digestive system.

It's a question OF RHYTHM

Food residues are normally propelled through the intestines by regular contractions that are hardly noticeable. But when that rhythm is disrupted for any reason, pain, constipation, or diarrhea can result. You'll find plenty of tips here for restoring healthy bowel action.

● **Get toned** A toned tummy isn't just about looks. As well as aiding posture and a robust pelvic floor, strong abdominal muscles help healthy digestion, squeezing the intestines as they contract and relax, helping to move along the contents of the large intestine. Find some exercises to firm up your tummy and reap the benefits for your digestion.

● **Fill your plate with fiber** Eating plenty of fiber is essential for healthy digestive systems to reduce the risk of problems ranging from constipation to bowel cancer. The USFDA recommends an AI (adequate intake) of fiber per day of 25g for women and 38g for men, but the average intake of most Americans is only 15g. Here are a few tips to help add fiber to your diet.

★ **Choose** whole-wheat bread over white, and brown rice over white rice.
★ **Add** seeds, especially flaxseed (linseed) to breakfast cereals.
★ **Include** beans and legumes in soups, chili, and casseroles.
★ **Snack** on fruit.

Don't forget to increase the intake of fluids when you increase the amount of fiber in your diet.

● **Choose the right fiber** Not all fiber aids digestion, and for some people, a diet that contains too much of one type of fiber can be harmful. Research published in the *British Medical Journal* showed that eating insoluble fiber (in whole grains such as brown rice and whole-wheat bread) can cause severe discomfort in many people

For some of us, white bread is actually better than brown.

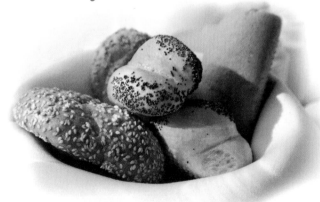

SECRETS OF SUCCESS

Stimulating beverages
Most people know that a cup of coffee moves the bowels, but fewer realize that this effect occurs because caffeine stimulates the colon. Be careful not to drink too much of it—it's a diuretic and will eliminate fluid from your body. Instead, try herbal or decaffeinated tea with hot water and the juice of a lemon as a gentle prompt for your bowels.

who suffer irritable bowel syndrome. If you suffer a painful reaction after eating such foods, stick to sources of soluble fiber such as lentils, apples, strawberries, and oats.

And a word of warning, young children, especially those under two, and those with poor appetites should not be encouraged to fill up with fiber—it won't provide the kind of balanced diet needed for optimum health and energy.

● **Try a low FODMAP diet** Researchers have pinpointed a range of foods that are thought to be responsible for up to 75 percent of gut disorders. These include pears, onions, garlic, baked beans, pork, breaded fish, alcohol, barley, and wheat. They all contain "short-chain" carbohydrates, or FODMAPs (fermentable, oligo-, di- and monosaccharides and polyols). Such foods are likely to ferment in the gut, producing hydrogen and methane in susceptible individuals and leading to pain, bloating, and diarrhea. There's no need to eliminate FODMAPs entirely, it seems. The problems occur only when the gut is overloaded with such foods. If you have symptoms, ask your doctor if a FODMAP diet might be advisable.

● **Don't blame your age** if you are often constipated. Although four out of ten older people have chronic constipation, the usual reasons are that they are less active, have unhealthier diets, and take more medication than those whose digestion is in better shape. Ask your doctor about changing any drugs you take regularly—and think of ways

Working on your abs could improve your digestion.

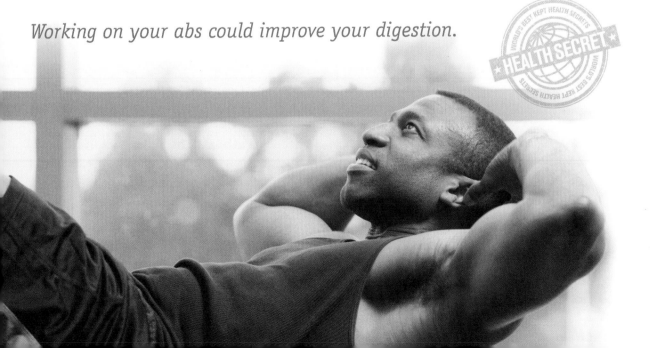

HEALTH SECRET

Inflamed response

People who have the inflammatory bowel disorder Crohn's disease are increasingly likely to be prescribed a medication that is also used to treat rheumatoid arthritis (RA). The relatively new drugs, which are known as TNF (tumour necrosis factors) blockers, have been shown to be successful in treating Crohn's. In earlier research they slowed down and even halted the disease process in RA. The connection between RA and Crohn's disease is inflammation—of the joints in the case of RA, and of the digestive tract in Crohn's disease. The new drug treatment means that people with Crohn's disease are less likely to undergo surgery.

to be more active and make better food choices, to encourage improved digestion as part of a balanced diet and lifestyle.

● **Brew a soothing beverage** If you have an intestinal problem such as irritable bowel syndrome or Crohn's disease, try peppermint tea, tincture of passionflower, or crushed fennel seeds in boiling water—all soothing drinks that can calm unpleasant symptoms. Many natural remedies also help cleanse the colon, including psyllium husks, flaxseed (linseed), aloe vera, slippery elm bark, and buckthorn bark.

● **Don't become dependent** Some drugs cause constipation as a side effect, putting you at risk of becoming dependent

on laxatives for normal bowel function—which is bad for your health. Ask your doctor or pharmacist about alternative drugs that will not have this side effect. In the meantime, try a gentle alternative to laxatives, such as a glycerol suppository available over the counter—but this too should not be a long-term solution.

● **Be wary of colonic irrigation** Colon cleansing is an ancient practice that became widespread in the nineties—but new evidence shows that it may be dangerous. The procedure involves pumping warm water into the intestines to flush out the contents and supposedly boost the immune system and encourage weight loss. A US review of research found that people who underwent colonic irrigation often had side effects, such as nausea, cramping, vomiting, and even kidney failure. Seek medical advice before trying the therapy.

● **Cut out alcohol** if you have the condition known as small intestinal bacterial overgrowth (SIBO). Even small amounts can provoke the severe and unpleasant symptoms of bloating, gas, abdominal pain, constipation, and diarrhea that are caused by excess bacteria in the small intestine. SIBO is usually treated with antibiotics and, sometimes, probiotics. Experts now say that those susceptible to SIBO may be able to eliminate their symptoms by simply cutting out all alcohol.

● **Cultivate the right bacteria** Probiotics are so-called "friendly" bacteria that occur naturally in the gut and have been linked to many digestive health benefits, including easing irritable bowel syndrome

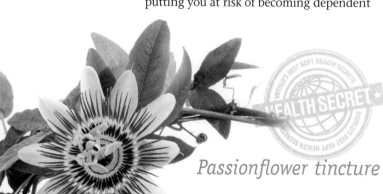

Passionflower tincture may calm an irritable bowel.

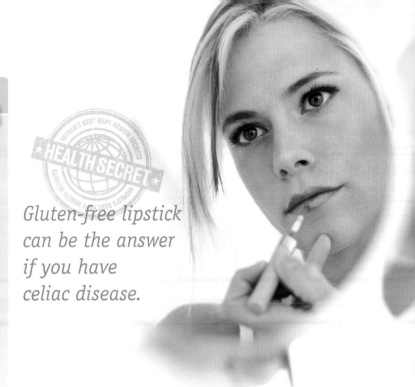

MIND POWER

The relationship between mood and digestive problems

If you have irritable bowel syndrome or chronic indigestion, resulting in symptoms such as stomach cramps, bloating, diarrhea, and constipation, your doctor may have advised you to consider ways to reduce stress in your life. Scientists have known for years that nervous tension can lead to gut disorders, and stress management is a common treatment option.

US researchers are now investigating whether the link also works the other way round, with gut problems leading to depression. Electrical stimulation of the vagus nerve—which extends from the abdomen to the brain—has been used to treat depression, and the researchers are hoping that this avenue may provide further treatments.

Gluten-free lipstick can be the answer if you have celiac disease.

and travelers' diarrhea. For bowel health, particularly after a course of antibiotics, try a probiotic supplement (available from health food stores) or live yogurt with probiotics—a good, natural source.

● **Get tested** You may not be able to tell the difference between celiac disease and irritable bowel syndrome (IBS) simply by checking out the symptoms: Both disorders cause much the same problems, including abdominal pain, bloating, diarrhea, and constipation. But celiac disease affects the small intestine and IBS is normally a disorder of the large intestine. Experts say that everyone with IBS should be tested for celiac disease—either with a blood test or by simply cutting out gluten to see if their symptoms improve. If you have IBS, ask your doctor to arrange for you to have a test.

● **Be careful with cosmetics** If you are suffering from the symptoms of celiac disease—digestive complications and rashes—despite rigidly following a gluten-free diet, your lipstick could be to blame. You may be so intolerant of gluten that you react to the minute amount used in some cosmetics. Even if you have scrupulously checked the ingredient list of your makeup and skincare products, you cannot be sure that gluten is not present. The only way to find out if a product contains the protein is stop using it and see if the symptoms disappear.

● **Retrain for regularity** Bowel retraining is a way of relieving chronic constipation that involves drinking plenty of water and eating as much fiber as your body can tolerate. This is combined with regular mealtimes and a regular time to visit the toilet each day—first thing in the morning or shortly after a meal—whatever feels right. It may help to eat a large fatty meal with a cup of coffee beforehand to stimulate bowel contractions. During the visit, keep your body at ease by practicing relaxation exercises or listening to music.

More gut
QUESTIONS

Scientists now know much more about the causes of bowel cancer— one of the most common cancers in the West—and by extension how to prevent it. Factors within our control, such as diet and lifestyle, are significant. Here are some further ways to protect your gut.

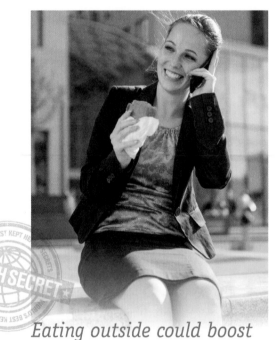

Eating outside could boost your digestive health.

● **Get up, stand up** It probably won't surprise you to hear that sitting down for hours at a time is associated with a higher risk of back pain, heart disease, deep vein thrombosis, diabetes, and obesity. But did you know that the inactivity associated with sitting for long periods without a break is now also linked with an increased risk of a number of cancers, and that colon cancer is at the top of the list? Sitting for prolonged periods leads to a build-up of inflammation in the body. Canadian research suggests that chronic inflammation is a predisposing factor for developing colon cancer and a number of other cancers. To reduce your risk, there are a number of easy self-help measures you can take:

★ **Take a break** If you work at a desk, make sure to stand up and take a short walk at least every hour—around the office, down the hallway, anywhere will do.

★ **Send fewer emails** If you can cross the room or walk upstairs to talk to a colleague instead of sending an email, take this opportunity whenever you can.

★ **Lunch outside** Don't sit at the desk to eat your lunch. Eat outside when the weather permits, and find a suitable indoors location when it doesn't.

★ **Walk and talk** If you spend a lot of time on the phone, stand up while you talk and, if possible, walk at the same time.

★ **Use pedal power** If it won't disturb others, you could invest in a compact pedal trainer to place under your desk. This will allow you to train and sit simultaneously.

● **Get out in the sun** The benefits of regular (but not excessive) exposure to sunshine extend to preventing colon cancer. It's essential, of course, to avoid sunburn, but your body needs plenty of vitamin D, produced when the skin is exposed to the sun, to stay healthy and prevent colon and other cancers. You need to expose limbs and face to sunshine on a regular basis, without the skin being covered in sunscreen. This exposure can be for up to 30 minutes, depending on your skin color, with darker skin able to be exposed for longest. Taking a vitamin D supplement as well as eating vitamin D-rich oily fish is also beneficial.

● **Consider double-dose aspirin** With growing evidence that aspirin can prevent cancer and possibly prevent it from spreading, some doctors advise that people at high risk of bowel cancer should take not just one dose per day—but two. People with a genetic link to bowel cancer have ten times the risk of developing it—and often do so at a young age. By taking two low-dose aspirin tablets a day, they can cut their risk by 60 percent. It's a controversial therapy that risks causing a peptic ulcer or anemia from chronic minor bleeding in the digestive tract. But in some cases, doctors believe the risk is worth taking. If bowel cancer runs in your family, talk to your doctor about this approach to prevention.

● **Beat bowel cancer with brown rice** The long-standing debate over whether high-fiber foods can help prevent bowel cancer appears finally to have been resolved conclusively. Following a major review involving nearly 2 million people, scientists have shown that eating plenty of whole grains and cereals—particularly rice and oats—does indeed protect against these cancers. If your digestion permits it, eat brown rice and oats as often as possible as an easy way to keep your bowels healthy.

● **Go for cancer-beating cabbage** A chemical produced when green vegetables such as cabbage are chopped, cooked, chewed, and digested has been shown to weaken cancer cells and prevent them from multiplying. The key chemical, known as singrin, is converted in the body to the anticancer substance allyl-isothiocyanate. But all you need to know is that eating your boiled greens really will help prevent cancer, including cancers of the digestive system.

● **Fill up on oily fish** to protect your digestive system. Omega-3 fatty acids are essential for good digestion, and the best sources are oily fish (such as sardines, mackerel, and salmon), flaxseed (linseed) oil, and fish oil. Studies show that taking fish oil reduces the number of episodes of Crohn's disease. What's more, people who eat oily fish every week cut their risk of cancers of the colon and rectum by up to 40 percent. The increased protection is dose-related: For every extra portion of fish consumed each week, the risk of developing cancer will be cut by a further 4 percent.

● **Time to quit** Smoking increases your risk of colorectal cancer—and this adverse effect appears to be more long-lasting in women. Researchers have shown that women who have quit for up to ten years still have a raised risk of colorectal cancer from smoking—while the impact has disappeared in male ex-smokers. Remember that it's important to mention your smoking history to your doctor when appropriate screening is being considered—and if you smoke, the sooner you give up the better.

Cabbage is a useful ally against digestive-tract cancer.

HEALTH SECRET

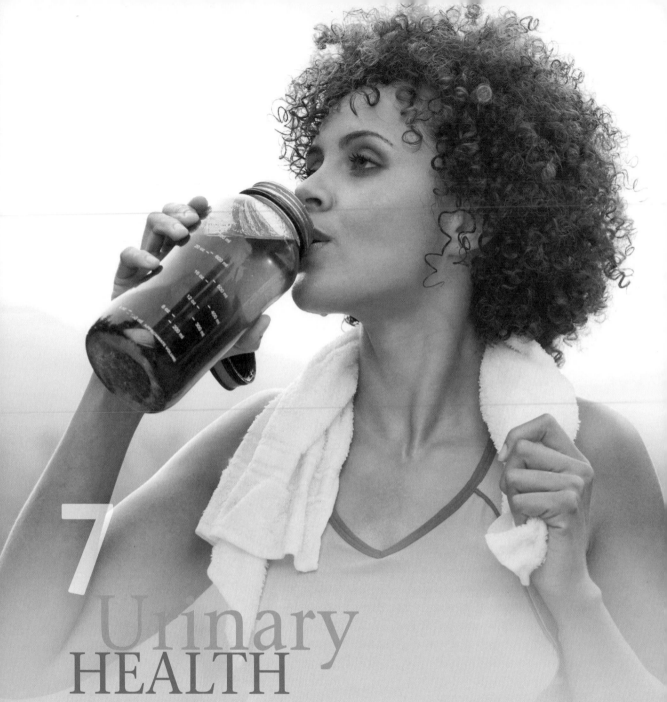

7
Urinary
HEALTH

The kidneys are among your body's most vital organs: They
filter the blood to keep its constituents in balance. Other parts
of the urinary system store then release the resultant waste
liquid—urine—from the body. There are many important ways
to keep this process functioning properly, which will benefit
your health and quality of life—at any age.

Kidney CARE

For reasons we don't understand, the incidence of kidney stones, an acutely painful condition, is increasing. It can be a recurrent problem, but whether or not you have been affected, try these tips for lowering your kidney stone risk and for keeping your bladder healthy.

● **Try an oriental wrap** According to ancient Japanese tradition, protecting your kidneys with a *haramaki*—an undergarment worn around the abdomen and lower back—aids digestion, eases menstrual cramps, brings restful sleep, and helps to prevent chills during outdoor activities. It may be worth trying and can certainly do no harm. Modern versions of this body-warming garment have become popular in the West as well as in Japan; they are sold on many Internet sites.

● **Avoid cola drinks** Drinking plenty of liquids, especially water, helps prevent all types of kidney stones. Tea, coffee, and alcohol were once thought to be stone makers, but the thinking has changed. And in moderation, beer and wine may actually be protective. But cola has been found to increase the risk of stone formation so is best avoided if you have a tendency to form kidney stones.

● **Move it, shake it** You may not feel like exercise when you have a kidney stone, but walking can help to dislodge it so that you pass it more quickly.

● **Don't cut out dairy foods** If you suffer from kidney stones composed of calcium phosphate or calcium oxalate, the advice used to be to avoid dairy products and other foods with a high calcium

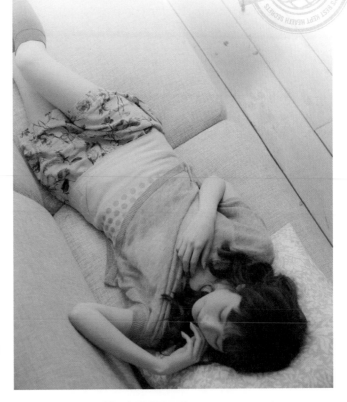

A Japanese haramaki, worn around the abdomen and lower back, can protect your kidneys and bring other benefits, too.

content. But recent studies show that dairy and high-calcium foods may actually prevent some types of stones. For calcium oxalate stones you should avoid high-oxalate foods such as rhubarb, spinach, nuts, and wheat bran.

● **Watch your salt intake** Although salt isn't a component of kidney stones, when sodium (the main component of salt) is excreted by the kidneys, it causes increased amounts of calcium to be expelled into the urine. High concentrations of calcium can combine with oxalate and phosphorus to form stones. So it makes sense for anyone susceptible to calcium-containing stones to cut down on salt intake—which will have the added bonus of helping to control blood pressure.

For further tips on keeping your salt intake low, see Chapter 2, *Blood and Circulation*

● **Need another reason to quit?** Recent research from Penn State College of Medicine suggests that smokers are twice as likely as nonsmokers to develop kidney cancer.

● **Or another?** Smoking is the cause of about half of all cases of bladder cancer in women—a far higher proportion than was previously thought. Studies now show that women face the same risk as men of developing bladder cancer if they smoke.

Citrus fruit may protect against calcium oxalate stones and uric acid stones.

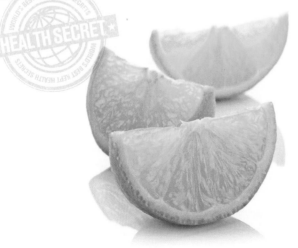

The new research suggests that current smokers are four times as likely—and former smokers are twice as likely—to develop bladder cancer as people who have never smoked. Visit the American Cancer Society at www.cancer.org for help to quit smoking.

● **Collect your kidney stones** This can help your doctor to identify the type of stone you make. If you are passing a kidney stone, urinate through a piece of gauze or a fine strainer to catch the stone, then take it to your doctor. Scientific analysis will determine what dietary advice you should follow.

● **Citrus dilemma** According to the US National Institutes of Health, citrus fruit or drinks may protect against calcium oxalate stones and uric acid stones. But they could be harmful for people who have a tendency to form calcium phosphate stones. The finding underscores the importance of knowing your stone type and getting appropriate advice.

● **Cut down on offal** A diet rich in animal proteins and purines—present in high levels in offal, fish, and shellfish—may make urine more acidic, which can increase the risk of uric acid stones. If this is your problem, keep your intake of these foods to a minimum.

● **Keep drinking** Drinking plenty of fluids may help protect against bladder cancer, according to a new study. The liquids may flush potential carcinogens (cancer-causing substances) out of the body before they have a chance to cause tissue damage that could lead to cancer. Researchers found that drinking more than 4½ pints (2.5 liters) of fluids a day was linked to a 24 percent lower risk of developing bladder cancer.

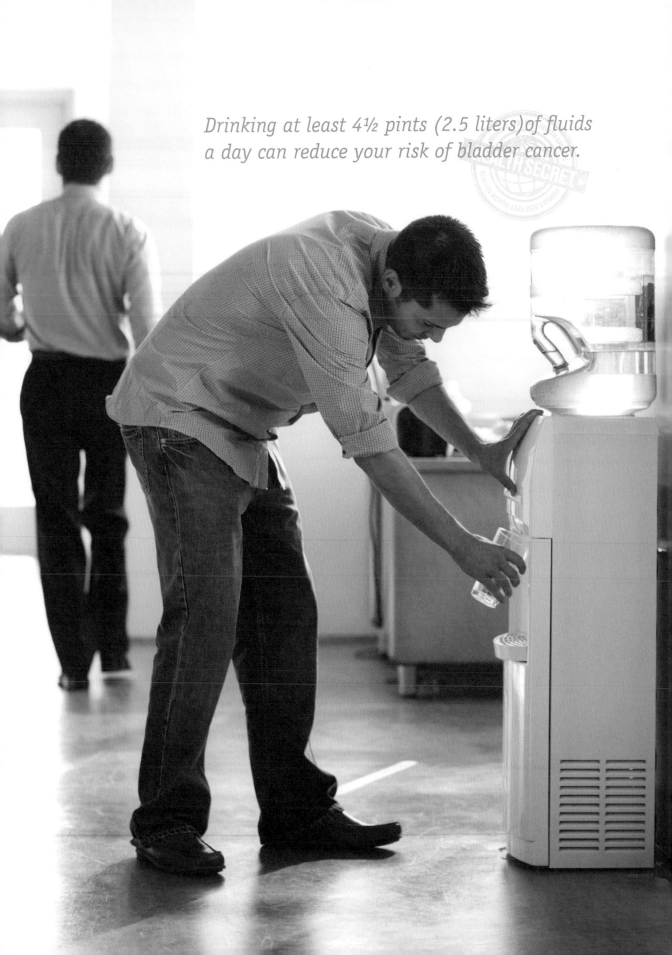

Drinking at least 4½ pints (2.5 liters) of fluids a day can reduce your risk of bladder cancer.

Combating
INFECTION

One woman in five suffers from a urinary tract infection—also known as a UTI or cystitis (when it affects the bladder)—at least once a year. Men get them less often because their "plumbing" is different. If you get a UTI, you may well be prescribed antibiotics by your doctor. Try these tips to shorten the infection and relieve the pain.

● **Reach for the bicarb** As soon as you sense that telltale sting when you urinate, reach for the bicarbonate of soda. First drink two glasses of plain water, then one-quarter teaspoon of bicarb dissolved in 4oz (125ml) of water. The bicarb makes the urine less acidic, so it's less painful when you urinate. Potassium citrate, available without prescription from pharmacies, works in the same way.

● **Pinpoint the pain triggers** Some food and drinks seem to irritate the bladder, so stay away from them during a bout of cystitis. These include tea, coffee, alcohol, fizzy drinks, citrus, and tomato juices, and spicy dishes. You may be able to figure out which foods make your symptoms worse, so you can avoid them during future bouts.

● **Go for live yogurt** A Finnish study found that women who often eat cheese and yogurt have fewer UTIs, perhaps because these foods contain friendly bacteria that keep the harmful bugs at bay. You may find that eating two or three containers of live yogurt a day is helpful for preventing attacks. And if you are taking antibiotics for a UTI, including live yogurt in your daily diet may help to restore the good bacteria that antibiotics destroy.

● **Get more garlic** Garlic is known as "nature's antibiotic" because it contains powerful antibacterial compounds. When you feel the symptoms of a UTI coming on, peel a couple of fresh garlic cloves, mash them and drop them in a cup of boiled water that has cooled a little. Let it steep for 5 minutes, then drink.

● **Try a herbal helper** Herbs have three roles to play in relieving UTIs: boosting the immune system, acting as a diuretic (a substance that makes you pass increased volumes of urine) to flush out bacteria, and soothing inflammation.
★ **Echinacea** is well known for boosting the immune system. Try echinacea tincture or have three cups of echinacea daily.
★ **Cleavers** This herb (also known as goosegrass) is a mild diuretic sold both as a tincture and in capsule form.

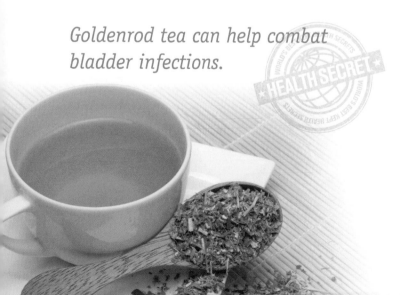

Goldenrod tea can help combat bladder infections.

★ **Lovage** is an anti-inflammatory and antibacterial herb with diuretic properties. Pour a cup of boiling water over two teaspoons of minced, dried root, steep for 10 minutes, then strain and drink.

★ **Nettle** is a natural diuretic. Take it as a tea, made from a teaspoon of dried nettle to a cup of slightly cooled boiled water.

★ **Goldenrod** This ancient remedy is enjoying a revival of popularity among herbalists. It is a diuretic, urinary antiseptic, and an immune-system stimulant. Infuse 2g of the herb in a cup of boiling water. Drink three cups a day.

● **Wash away UTIs** The way you launder your undergarments may reduce your risk of falling prey to UTIs. Here are some tips to help you avoid problems:

★ **Choose** nonbiological washing powder. The residues of biological products on fabrics can irritate your genital area, making it more susceptible to infection.

★ **Use** a hot setting. To beat bacteria, wash underwear at 140°F (60°C) or higher. Natural fibers such as cotton and linen, which are better for urinary-tract health, can withstand a hot wash. Check for color fastness.

★ **Rinse** thoroughly—if in doubt, run your laundry through an extra rinse cycle on your washing machine.

● **Conquer with cranberries** Make cranberry juice part of your strategy to protect yourself against UTIs. An authoritative review of research into the effectiveness of cranberries in preventing UTIs showed that drinking cranberry juice can reduce the number of episodes over a 12-month period, particularly for women who suffer from recurrent bouts. Some doctors suggest that women who are taking antibiotics for cystitis should also drink cranberry juice to prevent repeat infections.

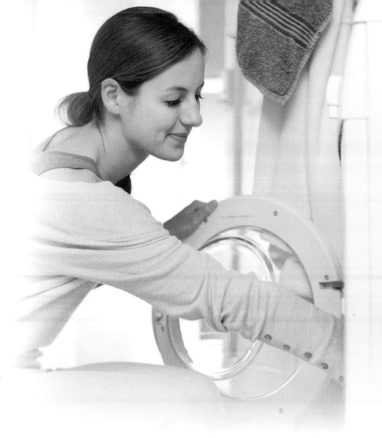

Using a hot wash for your underwear kills the germs that cause UTIs.

SECRETS OF SUCCESS

Cranberry juice

We've known for a while that cranberries contain a chemical that stops bacteria sticking to the wall of the urinary tract and may help prevent UTIs. But it has not been clear how the plant flavonoids thought to give cranberries their special powers should be taken. Should women drink copious quantities of juice, or simply pop a cranberry pill?

New US research suggests that you cannot isolate proanthocyanins (PACs) and put them in a capsule and expect it to do the same job as juice. A laboratory study has shown that cranberry juice is much more effective than PACs alone at preventing the formation of biofilm, which leads to UTIs.

Secrets of
PELVIC STRENGTH

For centuries, many otherwise healthy women suffered incontinence problems after giving birth. More than 60 years ago, one pioneering American gynecologist set out to discover why. He finally came up with a solution that has benefited thousands of mothers and is now helping men, too.

By 1948 Dr. Arnold Kegel, assistant professor of gynecology at the University of Southern California School of Medicine, had spent almost two decades pondering the incontinence that many of his patients experienced in the months after giving birth. The problem was usually treated with drugs or even surgery. But Kegel concluded that the weakness of a particular pelvic-floor muscle—the pubococcygeus, about which little was known—was the undoubted cause. This hammock-like muscle, which supports the pelvic organs, extends from the pubic bone at the front of the pelvis to the spine. In his revolutionary 1948 paper, Dr. Kegel outlined exercises that would treat incontinence by strengthening the pubococcygeus, which he described as "the most versatile muscle in the entire human body."

Various factors, besides childbirth, can weaken pelvic-floor muscles, including weight gain, aging and diabetes, and, in men, removal of the prostate gland. Dr. Kegel's brilliance was recognizing that these muscles could be exercised and strengthened like any others in the body. Doctors across the world now recommend his exercises.

The benefits of a strong pelvic floor

A number of medical trials, recorded in the prestigious Cochrane Database, have confirmed the efficacy of Kegel exercises for helping to prevent and reduce incontinence in pregnant women and new mothers. One small British study of men with an average age of 59 found that practicing the exercises regularly was as

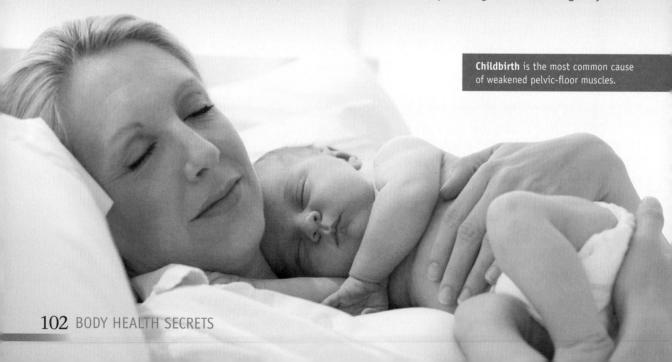

Childbirth is the most common cause of weakened pelvic-floor muscles.

effective for combating erectile dysfunction as taking Viagra.
To summarize, Kegel exercises can:
● Improve bowel and bladder control
● Prevent a prolapse
● Support and stabilize your spine
● Enhance your sex life by improving sensation in women and
combating erectile dysfunction in men
● Aid healing of the pelvic-floor muscles after childbirth by improving
circulation to the pelvic area.

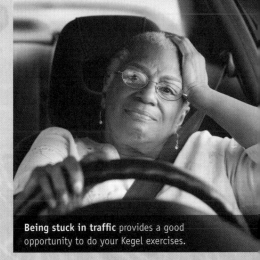

Being stuck in traffic provides a good opportunity to do your Kegel exercises.

Give your pelvic floor a workout

To keep your pelvic floor in good shape, give it a daily workout. First, you
need to locate your pelvic floor muscles; follow the steps below to make
sure you get this right.

Identify the muscles To find
the pelvic floor muscles, stop the
flow while passing urine. To avoid
exercising the wrong ones, do not:
● Hold your breath
● Squeeze your legs together
● Tighten your buttock, stomach,
or thigh muscles.

Then squeeze the muscles briefly,
and release. Repeat 10–15 times,
breathing freely. After some weeks,
hold each squeeze for 5 seconds,
building up to at least three sets
of exercises a day. When you find
this easy, move up to holding each
squeeze for 10 seconds.

When to work out Exercise
at the same time as a regular
activity—while working in
the kitchen, stuck in traffic, or
watching TV. If you exercise when
going to the toilet, wait until you
have fully emptied your bladder:
Don't stop and start the urine flow
as an exercise, since this can irritate
the bladder. If you suffer from
incontinence, aim to exercise six
to ten times a day.

Other strategies for women

Whether you have stress incontinence, in which activities such as
coughing or laughing may lead to leakage due to weakness in the pelvic
floor muscle, or urge incontinence, in which your bladder contracts
before you can reach the toilet, there are various options as well as
exercises. Talk to your doctor, who may refer you to a continence advisor.

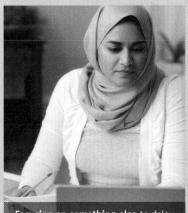

Focusing on something else to delay urination can retrain your bladder.

Put your mind to it If you
have urge incontinence, it's possible
to "re-educate" your bladder.
Bladder retraining programs involve
learning to distract yourself when
you feel the urge and only going to
the toilet at planned times. As you
regain control, you'll find you can
gradually increase the gap between
toilet visits until you go only when
your bladder is full. Ask your doctor
if a training program of this type is
available in your area.

Vaginal cones This equipment
comprises a cone with an adjustable
weight or separate cones of
different weights. You insert a
cone in your vagina and use your
pelvic floor muscles to grip it for
one minute. Start with the lightest
weight, work up to the next weight.
Once you can hold the heaviest
weight for 20 minutes, your pelvic
floor will be in good shape.

The PelvicToner This is a
spring-loaded device that you
insert into your vagina to increase
the effectiveness of a "pelvic
workout." It is available with a
prescription. Visit the website here:
www.pelvictoner.co.uk.

Avoiding
PROSTATE PROBLEMS

Most older men suffer from some kind of prostate gland problem. The gland naturally becomes larger and this can cause increased frequency of urination and problems with the flow. More seriously, this gland is also prone to cancerous changes. Luckily there's plenty you can do to keep your prostate in good health into your middle and later years.

● **Eat a few Brazil nuts each day**
These nuts are rich in selenium, a protective mineral. In a five-year American study, men who took 200mcg of selenium daily had 63 percent fewer prostate tumours. Brazil nuts are the best food source—just one nut can contain 75mcg.

● **Are your pills the cause?** Men who develop urination problems should ask their doctor to review the medicines they are taking for other conditions. A study has concluded that several common prescription medications—including antidepressants, antihistamines, bronchodilators, and diuretics—contribute to 10 percent of lower urinary tract symptoms in men. Before you accept treatment for difficulties with urination, be sure to ask your doctor if a change in your current medication might be a possible solution.

BELIEVE IT OR NOT!

Not just for wrinkles
For men with enlarged prostates who have urination problems, a shot of the antiwrinkle treatment Botox may be just what they need. A study has shown that it can reduce symptoms such as frequent urination and UTIs for up to a year without significant side effects.

● **Try the power of African pygeum**
An extract from the bark of this evergreen tree can help to shrink an enlarged prostate gland and, in France, has become one of the most widely used treatments for this condition. Pygeum is packed with anti-inflammatory phytosterols, which may be the reason for its effectiveness. Ask your doctor if this natural remedy could be of benefit to you.

● **Munch pumpkin seeds** These are a source of zinc, a mineral that scientists agree plays a significant role in boosting prostate health, protecting against enlargement and cancerous changes. Have a handful of unroasted seeds a day. Other foods that contain a plentiful supply of zinc include shellfish, meat, milk and dairy products, wheat germ, and whole-grain cereals.

● **Enjoy more mackerel** There are lots of good reasons to eat oily fish (a rich source of omega-3 fatty acids), such as mackerel or salmon, or take supplements of fish oil—and here's another. In a study, a low-fat diet with fish oil supplements eaten for four to six weeks before prostate removal was shown to slow the growth of prostate cancer. Those following the diet had fewer rapidly dividing cells in their prostate cancer tissue compared to those who were eating traditional, high-fat Western foods. Flaxseed oil is another excellent source of omega-3 fatty acids; add a tablespoon of the oil to your food every day for prostate health.

● **Eat more tomatoes** Men who had ten or more portions of tomatoes a week cut their risk of prostate cancer by more than 45 percent in one recent US study. Lycopene, which gives tomatoes their red color, interferes with the ability of cancer cells to multiply, spread, and invade body tissues. Canned and cooked tomatoes and tomato sauces seem to have the most potent anticancer effect.

● **Take a leisurely dip** Having a long bath is good for your prostate, reducing swelling and inflammation. So treat yourself to a relaxing soak in the tub for between 20 and 45 minutes a day.

● **Try croton oil** Researchers have discovered that that oil from the croton plant—a shrub native to Southeast Asia— kills prostate cancer cells and shrinks prostate tumors. Ask your doctor if this natural remedy could work for you.

SECRETS OF SUCCESS

Sling it—surgically

After prostate surgery, around 10 percent of men suffer stress incontinence—a loss of bladder control caused by triggers such as sneezing, coughing, or physical activity. A new surgical treatment involves inserting a sling across the urethra. The pressure of the sling closes the urethra, preventing embarrassing leaks. Early results for this technique look promising.

● **Chill out during surgery** If your doctor orders a transrectal prostate biopsy, get yourself some noise-cancelling headphones and play Bach. About 20 percent of men find the intrusive procedure highly stressful. In one US study, readings of diastolic blood pressure were taken from participants undergoing the biopsy; some had listened to Bach on headphones, others hadn't. The blood pressure readings of those who had no musical distraction were significantly higher.

A long, relaxing soak can reduce prostate inflammation.

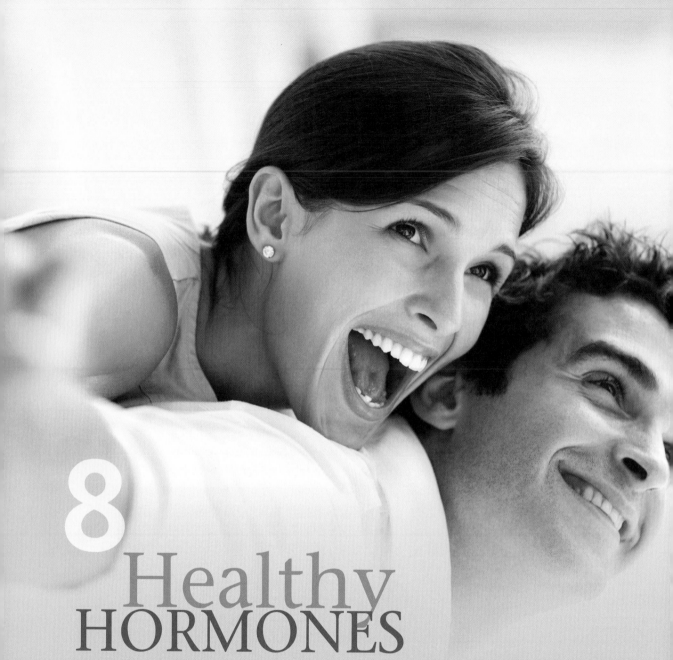

8
Healthy
HORMONES

We have dozens of hormones in our bodies. These chemical messengers, produced by our endocrine glands, travel in the blood and influence growth, metabolism, reproduction, and many other body processes. An imbalance or deficiency of a major hormone can cause serious health disorders. Here's how to spot symptoms and correct problems.

Get the better
OF DIABETES

This increasingly common condition occurs when the body produces too little of the hormone insulin to enable us to utilize the sugar (glucose) in the blood. There are two types: type 1 and type 2. Whichever type you have, careful attention to balancing diet and activity plays a key role in your long-term health.

● **Eat to beat it** The number of people diagnosed with type 2 diabetes—the kind that tends to develop later in life—is soaring: In the US, the figure has almost doubled since 2004 to 29 million. For the best chance of avoiding type 2 diabetes—and to help manage it if you already have the disease—try these four simple strategies:

★ **Eat breakfast** Starting the day on an empty stomach increases your risk of obesity and insulin resistance. What's more, breakfast eaters are better at saying "no" to fatty and high-calorie foods later in the day.

★ **Go for whole grains** Eating more fiber can improve your blood glucose control. As a bonus, it will also lower your risk of heart disease and help you lose weight by making you feel full. High-fiber foods include fruit, vegetables, whole grains, nuts, and seeds.

★ **Manage your carbs** Carbohydrate foods—bread, pasta, potatoes, noodles, rice, and cereals—also help you control blood glucose levels, so include some in each meal. Go for foods that are more slowly absorbed (have a lower glycemic index). Whole-grain varieties are best. Balance your carbohydrate

A nutrient-packed breakfast can help you say
"no" to unhealthy snacks later in the day.

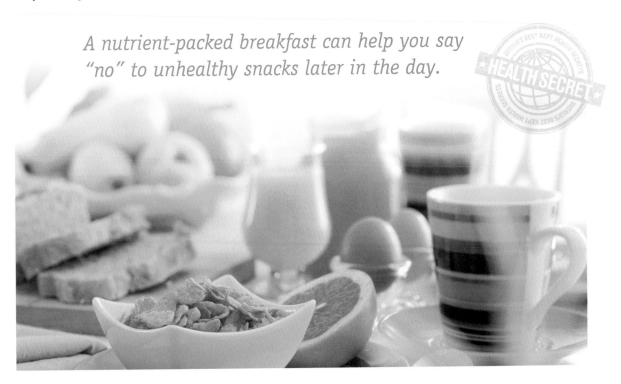

intake at each meal with foods of other types, such as dairy products, fruit, vegetables, and meat or fish.

★ **Trim the fat** Reduce the fat in your diet by choosing lean meat, eating less butter, cheese, and cream, and by grilling, broiling, and steaming instead of frying and roasting.

● **Keep moving** Some diabetics fear that exercise may upset their blood glucose control. In fact, physical activity combined with a healthy diet and medication will help you to manage your condition and prevent long-term complications, whether you have type 1 or type 2 diabetes. But be sure to get

TWEAK YOUR DIET

Try these simple food swaps to reduce your risk of developing type 2 diabetes. The "give up" foods have all been shown to impair good control of blood glucose, while the "pick up" alternatives have a positive benefit for those with diabetes or who are at risk of developing the disease.

Give up	Pick up	Why?
Corn oil	Olive oil	In a recent study, 17.9 percent of those on a low-fat diet developed diabetes, compared with 11 percent of those on a Mediterranean diet with ½oz (11g) of nuts a day and 10 percent of those on a Mediterranean diet that included up to 4 cups (1L) of olive oil a week (actual intake may have been less).
Sugary cereals	Oatmeal	Eating a 2oz (50g) serving of oatmeal five or six times a week can lower the risk of developing type 2 diabetes by 39 percent. What's more, oats are effective in reducing your blood levels of damaging LDL cholesterol.
Full-fat cheese	Low-fat cheese or avocado	Saturated fat impairs the action of insulin and makes blood glucose harder to control. Avocado is high in healthy monounsaturates.
Potato chips and other savory snacks	Unsalted nuts	You'll be swapping bad fats for good ones and keeping blood glucose levels steady. Nuts are high in calories, so a snack portion should be limited to about 1oz (25g)—roughly a handful.

advice before adopting a new exercise regime, especially if you:

★ **Are on medication**
★ **Are prone to attacks** of hypoglycemia
★ **Have any complications** of diabetes (such as foot or eye problems)
★ **Have another condition** that might affect your capacity for exercise, such as heart or lung disease.

Your family doctor or diabetes specialist will advise you on a sensible approach.

● **Drink water** Have around 2 cups (500ml) of water before you start exercising if you have diabetes. And take water bottle or a glucose drink with you.

● **Be safe alone** If you're undertaking strenuous activity on your own—jogging alone in open country, say—take a high-carbohydrate snack, your cell phone, and wear a medical tag or bracelet.

BELIEVE IT OR NOT!

Gastric bypass cures diabetes

Type 2 diabetes can be reversed by weight-loss surgery in a matter of days or even hours. Now scientists think they have discovered why. The operation—known as the Roux-en-Y gastric bypass, which makes the stomach smaller and bypasses part of the intestine—results in lower levels of nutrients called branched-chain amino acids in the bloodstream. This, in turn, reverses insulin resistance and restores blood glucose levels to normal. But gastric bypass surgery may not be suitable for everyone with type 2 diabetes. Ask your doctor for advice.

● **Continue testing** If you're on insulin, test yourself before, during, and after exercise to find out how activity affects your blood glucose and to make sure it stays

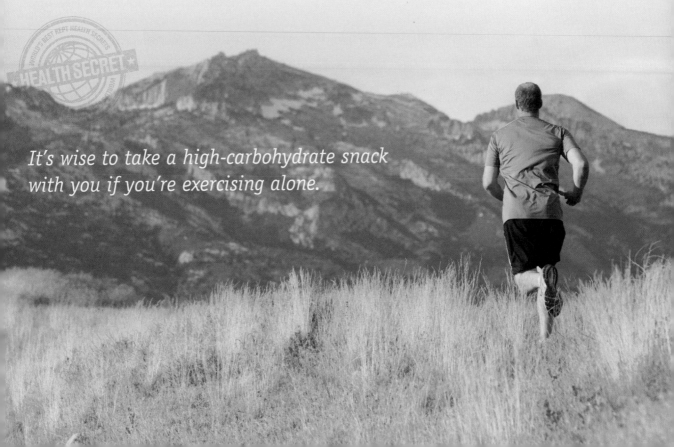

It's wise to take a high-carbohydrate snack with you if you're exercising alone.

within your target range. And check your blood glucose at intervals for several hours after exercise, especially if you have type 1 diabetes. Exercise requires an adjustment in the balance of insulin and carbohydrate intake (less insulin or more carbohydrate, or a combination of these adjustments), both on the day of exercise and for about a day afterward. You will need to monitor your blood glucose levels carefully in order to make adjustments that work for you.

● **Eat to protect your baby from diabetes** There are plenty of reasons for eating healthy while you're pregnant, but you may not know that a nutritious diet can reduce the risk of your child developing type 2 diabetes as an adult. Scientists think that a poor diet can cause the insulin-producing cells in the pancreas to develop abnormally. Poor nutrition may cause the cells to age prematurely, resulting in increased susceptibility to type 2 diabetes.

Smartphone apps can now help you to manage your diabetes.

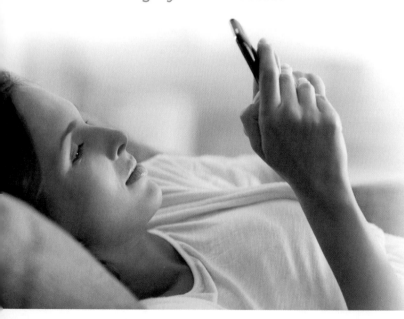

● **Are you at risk?** Did you know that there's a quick and reliable way of assessing your risk of developing type 2 diabetes without visiting your doctor? You can take the risk test of the American Diabetes Association at www.diabetes.org/diabetes-basics/prevention/diabetes-risk-test. Here are some of the key factors to take into account. You are most at risk if you:

★ **Have a close relative** (parent, brother, or sister) with diabetes

★ **Are over 35 years old**

★ **Are Asian, African, or Caribbean**

★ **Are overweight**, particularly if you have a large waist

★ **Had diabetes** during pregnancy

★ **Do little** physical activity

★ **Have high blood pressure** or have suffered a heart attack or stroke

★ **Have polycystic ovary syndrome**.

If the test results show you to be at risk, you can then assess how important it is to make lifestyle changes to reduce your chances of developing diabetes. You should also consult your doctor for further advice on reducing your risk of this disorder.

● **Enlist your smartphone** Modern technology is on your side. If you have diabetes, there are now a number of smartphone apps that can help you to manage your condition. A search of the internet will reveal a wide selection of apps for different smartphones which, among other features, will allow you to record blood glucose test results, weight, and calorie intake, to make notes of how you feel, and any other factors that affect your blood glucose levels. You can then refer to the stored data at your next medical consultation or even send the information directly to the health professionals in your diabetes care team.

● **Keep your feet happy** People with diabetes are more likely to get sores or ulcers on their feet. Here's how to cut this risk:

★ **Trim your toenails** straight across, to avoid ingrown nails.

★ **Wash your feet** daily in warm water with mild soap, and dry and examine them carefully for sores and broken skin.

★ **Moisturize after washing** to keep the skin supple, especially on the heels.

★ **Don't break blisters**, cut corns or calluses, or wear corn plasters.

★ **Keep the blood flowing** to your feet by rotating your ankles clockwise and counterclockwise and wriggling your toes. Repeat at intervals during the day.

★ **Wear well-fitting shoes,** preferably with socks or tights. If you run or practice a sport, wear appropriate footwear.

★ **Don't go barefoot**, especially if you have poor sensation in your feet. On vacation, remember that sand and pavement may be hot. Wear flip-flops or sandals on the beach and in the water.

★ **Ask a relative** or close friend to do the "Touch the toes test" with you to assess the sensitivity in your feet. You can find it at www.diabetes.org.uk.

★ **Have an annual checkup** with a chiropodist or podiatrist.

● **Beware of drug triggers** Some medications can occasionally interact and create unexpected problems. US scientists scanning patient databases have found that two common drugs—a selective serotonin re-uptake inhibitor (SSRI) antidepressant (paroxetine) and a statin cholesterol-lowering medication (pravastatin)—raise blood glucose levels when taken together, thus increasing the risk of developing diabetes. Neither drug has this effect when given alone. If you are taking both types of drug, ask your doctor whether your medications should to be reconsidered in the light of this information. Do not stop drug treatment you have been prescribed, except on medical advice.

● **Get vaccinated** You may be surprised to learn that a case of the flu can make your blood glucose more difficult to control. So if you have diabetes, do your best to avoid the illness by having a flu vaccination before the onset of winter.

● **Use your tape measure** You are at increased risk of developing diabetes, if your waist circumference is more than 37in (94cm) for men and more than 31½in (80cm) for women. The risk is higher still if your waist size is more than 40in (102cm) for men and more than 34½in (88cm) for women. Measure your waist this way:

★ **Find the bottom** of your ribs and the top of your hips and breathe out naturally.

★ **Put a tape measure** around your waist midway between these points, then read the measurement shown.

BELIEVE IT OR NOT!

Remote glucose checking
Pricking your finger each morning to get a blood glucose reading could become a thing of the past. Technology is currently being developed that will allow people with type 1 diabetes to check their blood glucose daily at home and then send the results wirelessly to a remote monitoring team, which will spot anything that looks amiss. In time, this technology may become more sophisticated. Eventually, you may simply wear an implanted device that can be read with a swipe of a smartphone, and the results transmitted to a base station for monitoring.

Thyroid and
ADRENAL CARE

Your metabolism—the speed at which your body works—is influenced by hormones released from the thyroid gland in your neck. The two walnut-sized adrenal glands on top of your kidneys release hormones that help your body to respond to stress. The tips below will help resolve problems associated with these hormones.

● **Screen yourself** If you think you may have the symptoms of an underactive thyroid, including tiredness, increased sensitivity to cold, and dry skin and hair, you can now check your levels at home with a simple blood-testing kit called ThyroScreen. Whatever the results of testing, if you suspect you have a thyroid problem, consult your doctor.

● **Time your medication** If you are being treated for an underactive thyroid gland (hypothyroidism), you can improve the effectiveness of your prescribed medicines by timing your consumption of certain foods. Wait 4 hours after taking your medication before eating high-fiber foods, foods that contain soy, iron and calcium supplements, and antacids containing aluminium or magnesium. This will ensure that they do not interfere with the absorption of your medication.

● **Ask about selenium** The protruding eyes characteristic of thyroid eye disease (TED) can be troublesome and disfiguring. A European study has recently shown that the trace element selenium can help. Six months of selenium supplements reduced symptoms of TED in the study's participants and improved their quality of life. The benefits were still seen at 12 months, and there were no side effects. If you have mild TED, ask your doctor about the supplements. TED occurs more commonly with an overactive than an underactive thyroid gland.

● **Don't take iodine** While lack of dietary iodine may sometimes trigger thyroid disorders, supplementation is a bad idea, as too much iodine can cause problems for people with an overactive or underactive thyroid. The same is true of kelp seaweed supplements, which are often promoted as being useful to "jump start" a sluggish thyroid. Because kelp extract has a high iodine content, such supplements may actually induce overactivity of the thyroid.

● **Pregnant? Get tested** A woman's thyroid hormone levels need to be just right during pregnancy. If the levels are too high

❊ MIND POWER

Thyroid hormones may make you SAD

Seasonal affective disorder—the "winter blues"—may be linked to the activity of thyroid-stimulating hormone, say Scottish researchers. The hormone seems to influence behavior and the secretion of other hormones. If proven, the finding could lead to new ways of treating seasonal depression.

Secrets of solving
IODINE DEFICIENCY

Lack of iodine—a compound that plays a key role in thyroid function—is a leading cause of mental disability worldwide. Yet it is easily preventable. In recent years, World Health Organization (WHO) programs to combat this problem have been successful in many countries, but some regions— including large areas of the developed world—are lagging behind.

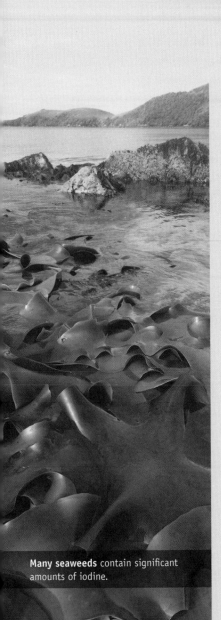

Many seaweeds contain significant amounts of iodine.

Europe, Australia, and the USA are surprisingly among the areas in which the incidence of iodine deficiency has been increasing. A 2011 UK study of about 740 girls aged 14–15 found that two-thirds had iodine levels below the acceptable minimum defined by the WHO, and a fifth had levels of less than half the minimum. Women with severe iodine deficiency are at higher risk of infertility, miscarriage, and of giving birth to a mentally disabled child. And, importantly, even mild iodine deficiency can affect the child's developing brain: According to the WHO, raising iodine levels in iodine-deficient communities boosts average IQ by 13 points. Deficiency may also lead to an underactive thyroid, causing tiredness, sensitivity to cold, and dry skin. It is more likely to occur in women than in men and is most common in pregnant women and adolescent girls.

Iodine sources

What you eat largely determines your iodine levels. Iodine is found naturally in seawater, rocks, and some types of soil. But even organic-rich soils, which are high in iodine, release the trace element only if the soil is acidic, so crops are not a reliable source.

To be sure you are getting enough iodine, take the following measures:
● Eat iodine-rich foods, such as dairy products—especially milk— seafood, oily fish, and eggs. But avoid supplements and over-consumption of seaweed (which may result in excessive iodine intake).
● Use only iodized table salt—no more than 6g (a teaspoon) a day.
● Avoid processed foods, which are often made with non-iodized salt.

Universal solution

Worldwide, the universal use of iodized salt would solve the problem of iodine deficiency, says the WHO. But this requires legislation to make sure that processed foods use only iodized salt and that all salt sold for culinary use comes in iodized form. The WHO recommendations are proving effective in the countries taking part, but implementing them worldwide is likely to take many years to complete.

or too low, there could be serious implications for the health of the baby, including mental impairment. Czech researchers say a blood test can pick up about a third of mothers-to-be who have no symptoms but will go on to develop thyroid disorders after the birth.

In the US, pregnant women do not routinely have a thyroid screening test.

Current UK recommendations are that women should have a thyroid function test before conception or at an postnatal appointment if they have:

★ **Type 1 diabetes**
★ **Previous history of thyroid disease**
★ **Current thyroid disease**
★ **Family history of thyroid disease**
★ **Goiter**
★ **Symptoms of an underactive thyroid (hypothyroidism).**

If you are in any of these categories, ask your doctor about getting tested.

● **Consider surgery** Removal of the lymph nodes in the neck during surgery on people with thyroid cancer may help prevent the disease from recurring, according to a new study at the University of California. Researchers found that only 1.5 percent of thyroid surgery patients who had had their central neck lymph nodes removed needed a second operation, compared with 6.1 percent of those who had undergone only thyroid removal. Ask your surgeon if this procedure might be appropriate for you.

● **Eat what you like** You may have read or heard that some foods, including soybeans, pears, peaches, and vegetables of the cabbage family, can reduce levels of thyroid hormone. The British Thyroid Foundation has dismissed such concerns, emphasizing that no foods contain sufficient amounts of substances known as goitrogens to have an adverse effect. So if you're

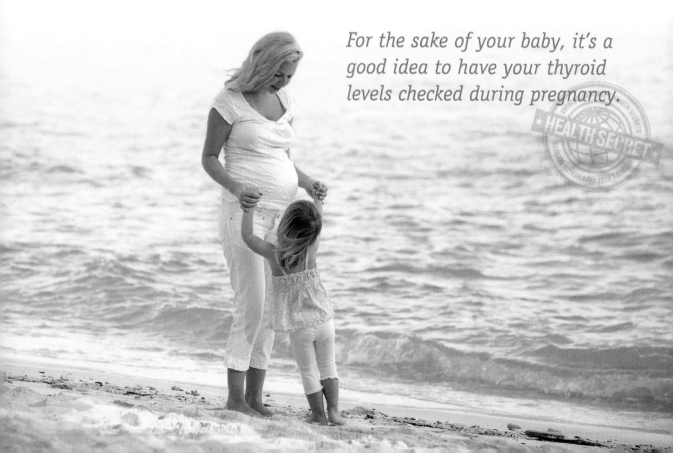

For the sake of your baby, it's a good idea to have your thyroid levels checked during pregnancy.

HEALTH SECRET

concerned about your thyroid gland, don't add to your worries by restricting your food choices unnecessarily.

● **Adrenal fatigue? Don't believe it**

If you visit a complementary practitioner and complain of exhaustion, stress, and insomnia, you may well be told that you have adrenal fatigue and be offered a supplement that is said to combat this problem. But according to the Society for Endocrinology, the professional body for hormone specialists throughout the world, there is no such condition. Adrenal glands cannot be "fatigued." Either they are fine and need no treatment or there is adrenal insufficiency due to adrenal or pituitary failure, which needs medical treatment. Many illnesses can cause the same symptoms as so-called adrenal fatigue; if you are worried, ask your doctor for a checkup.

● **Steer clear of germs** People with Addison's disease, a rare condition that affects the production of the hormones cortisol and aldosterone, are more likely to get infections, which may provoke a life-threatening adrenal crisis. Research indicates that people with this condition are 1.5 times more likely to contract an infection than the general population. If you have this condition, you will need to be especially careful to avoid colds and flu by keeping away from those who are infected and by keeping up to date with flu vaccinations.

● **Keep your kit handy** If you have been diagnosed with Addison's disease (see above), you should always carry an emergency kit containing a hydrocortisone injection. This can be given immediately if you suffer a sudden drop in your hormone levels—known as an adrenal crisis, which can occur as a result of injury, infection, or

MIND POWER

Soccer fever
We can all get emotional during a nail-biting sports match, but sometimes the problem is more serious.

A female soccer fan who suffered from anxiety, palpitations, panic, light-headedness, and a sense of impending doom toward the end of important matches, turned out to have Addison's disease. The woman's symptoms were particularly severe during crucial games when the outcome was in doubt until the very last minute. By contrast, symptoms were barely noticeable when the opposing team was at the bottom of the standings.

Doctors diagnosed a life-threatening manifestation of Addison's disease, in which the adrenal glands do not produce enough of the stress hormone cortisol. This can lead to very low blood pressure and even coma. The fan in question now takes medication halfway through important games and has not suffered further problems.

even emotional stress. Make sure your family, friends, and colleagues are aware of this and know what action to take. Always wear a MedicAlert tag in case you need emergency medical care while away from those who know about your condition.

A MedicAlert tag could save your life if you suffer from Addison's disease.

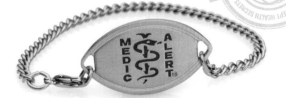

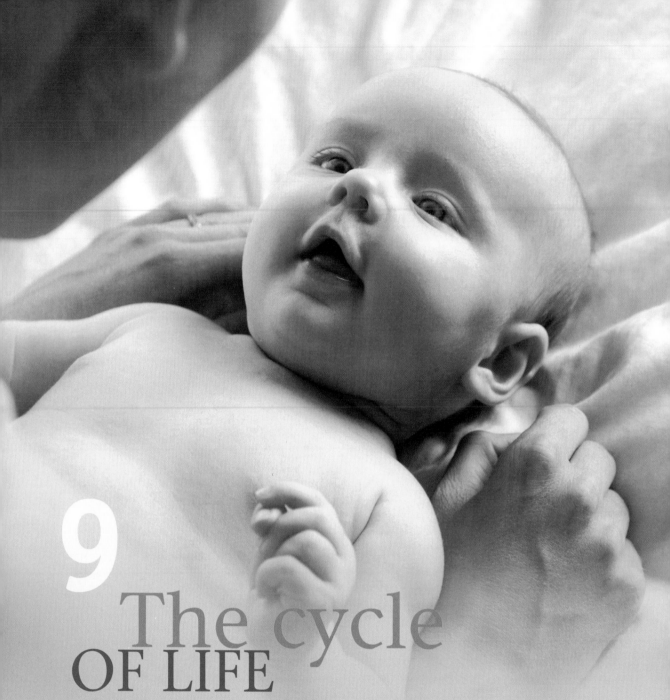

9
The cycle
OF LIFE

The drive to reproduce is among the strongest impulses in the animal kingdom—one that we humans share. From adolescence to old age, for both men and women, reproductive and sexual health is vital to both physical and mental fitness. Learn here about remedies—old and new—that can offer effective help for a range of problems that may arise.

Healthy REPRODUCTIVE SYSTEM

Lifestyle plays a significant role in the well-being of your reproductive system. A healthy diet and regular exercise are key and it's also important to be on the lookout for suspicious changes in the breasts and other reproductive organs that may signal problems. Although many of the tips are relevant only to women, men need to be aware of certain changes, too.

● **Be nipple aware** Formalized breast self-exams are no longer recommended, but "breast awareness" is judged to be the best way to ensure that you discover any worrying changes. The UK organization Breast Cancer Care encourages women of all ages to examine their breasts regularly and feel them gently (ideally in the bath or shower) so that you become familiar with how they normally look and feel. Women and men should report any unusual lumps or bumps, or changes in breast appearance to their doctor. In particular, look out for:
★ **Nipple changes**
★ **Discharge from the nipple**
★ **Puckering or dimpling of the skin.**

● **Eat less meat** You can lower your risk of breast cancer by eating more fruit and vegetables, which are rich in protective vitamin C, and less meat and other sources of animal (saturated) fats. One study suggested that women who consume the most saturated fat have twice the risk of breast cancer of those eating the least.

● **Protect with fiber** Increasing your intake of fiber will greatly reduce your chances of getting breast cancer, according to researchers at the University of Leeds in the UK. A study of those aged between 35 and 69 years revealed that women who ate 1oz (30g) of fiber a day (the amount in four servings of All-Bran) had half the risk of those who ate less than ¾oz (20g), with premenopausal women getting the most benefit. It is thought that fiber protects by regulating how the body produces and processes estrogen. To get 1oz (30g) of fiber you need to eat a high-fiber breakfast cereal, only whole-grain bread, and five portions a day of fruit and vegetables.

SECRETS OF SUCCESS

A beta way to beat breast cancer?

Beta blockers are widely used for lowering blood pressure and easing anxiety. Now research funded by Cancer Research UK has found that the drugs could also help to prevent breast cancer spreading around the body. Compared to people not taking beta blockers, those who took these drugs had half the risk of their cancer spreading and were 70 percent less likely to die from the disease over the next 10 years. The reason could be that the medication blocks adrenalin, which helps cancer cells to move around the body. If beta blockers are approved for the treatment of breast cancer, scientists say that six out of ten women with the disease could benefit.

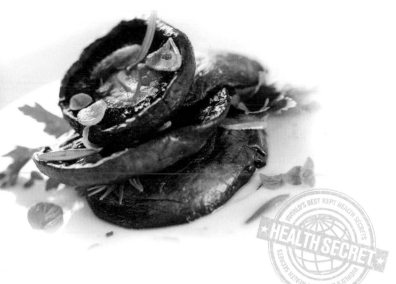

Eating a small portion of mushrooms daily could greatly reduce your risk of breast cancer.

● **Have more mushrooms** Eating a small portion of mushrooms each day could cut your risk of breast cancer by two-thirds. A Chinese study showed that women who ate at least 1/3 oz (10g) of fresh mushrooms a day were 64 percent less likely to develop this type of cancer than women who did not include mushrooms in their diet.

● **Weight control** Keeping your weight in check and doing regular exercise has been found to significantly lower your risk of developing breast cancer. When a woman is overweight (with a body mass index over 25), her body converts excess fat into estrogen, which can, in turn, be a trigger for breast cancer. Exercise helps lower estrogen, which is a good reason—on top of calorie burning—for exercising moderately for a minimum of 30 minutes five days a week.

● **Keep to the 3-glass limit** A 2011 study in the UK estimated that some 6 percent of breast cancers in women were directly linked to excessive alcohol intake. An intake of more than three units of alcohol (the equivalent of three small glasses of wine) a day can significantly increase the risk. The message is clear: Keep your drinking to a minimum and make sure you have at least two alcohol-free days a week.

● **Counter PMS naturally** There are a number of excellent herbal remedies for treating premenstrual syndrome (PMS), a collection of symptoms, including breast tenderness, headaches, bloating and nausea, that often precede a menstrual period. Always seek medical advice before using herbs, particularly if you are taking prescription drugs, or if symptoms persist.

★ **Evening primrose oil** Native American women have used this remedy for centuries. It's particularly effective for relieving breast pain. Evening primrose oil contains fatty acids that play an important role in the body's production of prostaglandins, which fine tune the action of estrogen and

❄ MIND POWER ❅

Meditation therapy

Following a diagnosis of breast cancer and treatment for it, many women feel depressed, stressed, and socially isolated. But a trial has found that transcendental meditation or TM can help improve mood and self-esteem and even offer pain relief in women affected by the disease. The technique, should be practiced for 15 to 20 minutes each day in a comfortable sitting position with the eyes closed. It produces deep relaxation and a state known as "restful alertness." As you relax, your thoughts quiet and your mind transcends or "takes over," producing a sensation of silence and calm.

progesterone, hormones that help to regulate the menstrual cycle. Take two 500mg capsules three times a day during the last ten days of your menstrual cycle.

★ **Chasteberry** Used since Greco-Roman times, chasteberry reduces the symptoms of PMS by its action on the pituitary gland, lowering estrogen levels and reducing bloating and breast pain. The usual daily dose is 175mg. Do not take chasteberry if you are taking birth control pills or are breast feeding.

● **Don't overdose on exercise** Vigorous exercise will undoubtedly keep you fit but women who overdo it—and also lose too much weight—can develop amenorrhoea (cessation of periods). Absence of menstruation is not a sign of fitness but a warning that the body is protecting itself from collapse. It's linked with lowered bone density and a risk of fractures and other injuries. If you're underweight (with a BMI of 19 or under) and your periods stop:

★ **Cut back** on exercise.

★ **Increase** your calorie intake by up to 15 percent (ideally with protein and unrefined carbohydrates).

★ **Take** calcium supplements.
If your periods have not returned within six months or you have other symptoms, it's vital to consult your doctor.

● **Conquer PCOS with (unrefined) carbs** Changing the kinds of carbohydrates you eat can form a key part of the treatment for women who suffer from polycystic ovary syndrome (PCOS)—a condition in which cysts grow on their ovaries, leading to weight gain, excessive hair growth, and problems with fertility. A switch from refined carbohydrates to those with a low GI (glycemic index), such as beans and whole-grain cereals, bread, and pasta, can help. PCOS makes the body resistant to insulin—the hormone that helps us to utilize sugar. When this happens, more insulin is then produced—along with excess testosterone, which encourages the cysts to grow. A low-GI diet slows the release of sugar into the bloodstream, which reduces levels of both insulin and testosterone, leading to the formation of fewer cysts.

Evening primrose is the source of a Native American remedy for PMS.

A gentle fix for fibroids

Fibroids—benign growths in the uterus—can be as small as a pea or a large as a watermelon. They are a problem for nearly half of all women of childbearing age, causing heavy bleeding, pain, and anemia. Hysterectomy—surgical removal of the uterus—was once the only permanent solution. But there's now a much less radical procedure available, known as uterine-artery embolization.

Under local anesthetic, fine particles are injected into the blood vessels supplying the uterus. These particles silt up the vessels, causing the fibroids to shrink away over a period of about 12 weeks. Women are usually able to return to normal activity after only two weeks.

● **Use feverfew to relieve menstrual pain** The plant, a traditional remedy, secretes substances called sesquiterpene lactones that have antispasmodic and anti-inflammatory properties. Feverfew is available in capsule form; the standard dose is 380mg of pure leaf extract, taken three times a day with food. You should consult your doctor before using feverfew, and do not take it with oral contraceptives.

● **Take it early** If you are prone to painful periods, here's a tip that may help. A review of 51 studies has found that starting NSAID pain-relief medication, such as ibuprofen, one to two days before the expected date of of the start of your period can successfully minimize pain. Continue the medication for the first two to three days of menstruation. NSAIDs work by reducing levels of prostaglandins, which trigger cramping.

● **Pop an aspirin** Just 75mg of aspirin a day may help keep ovarian cancer at bay. A UK study involving 250,000 women found that aspirin treatment cut their risk of the common cancer by at least a fifth.

Other research suggests that aspirin can also help prevent bowel cancer, but be sure to check with your doctor before taking it on a regular basis as there is a risk that it may cause internal bleeding.

● **Prevent it with the Pill** For premenopausal women, taking oral contraceptives for ten years or more has been shown to halve the risk of ovarian cancer. Of course, this reason alone isn't enough to warrant taking the medication, and your doctor will need to balance the pros and cons before prescribing this form of contraception for you.

● **Cut the risk by cutting out tobacco** A large body of evidence points to a strong link between smoking and cervical cancer, and the risk diminishes significantly after a woman stops smoking. It seems that smoking inhibits the body's immune system, allowing cancer cells to multiply. What's more, chemicals in tobacco smoke may make matters worse by turning off the genes that naturally suppress tumors.

● **Vaccinate for future health** There is more to the measles, mumps, and rubella vaccination (MMR) than simply avoiding the immediate effects of these diseases. It also safeguards the future fertility of boys and girls. In boys, mumps can permanently damage the testes; in girls, it can cause swelling of the ovaries and possible infertility. In addition, rubella (German measles) can have devastating effects on an unborn child if the mother catches it during the first 16 weeks of pregnancy, often causing blindness, deafness, and heart and brain damage. So be sure to take advantage of the protection that vaccinations can give. Seek your doctor's advice if you have any concerns about its safety.

Boosting
YOUR SEX LIFE

Everyday stresses and strains can often take their toll in the bedroom. But, there are many strategies for keeping your sex life active and healthy without resorting to medication. And if you are in good general health, there's no reason why you should not continue to enjoy sex well into your later years.

● **Fix your finances** Money worries come high on the list of stresses that can damage your sex life. A 2011 study of British couples found that anxiety over finance, added to increased working hours and the stress of juggling jobs and children were all cited as reasons for having less sex. Money worries were particularly significant in the reduction of men's libido. Balancing the books—and your priorities—can be a boost to your sex life.

● **Spice it up** Aphrodisiacs have been used for centuries to boost sexual appetite and enjoyment, with no scientific proof of their effectiveness. Now some are beginning to pass the scrutiny of 21st-century research:

★ **Coffee** A cup of coffee not only wakes you up but also increases your levels of dopamine, the neurotransmitter that is associated with the pleasure systems of the brain. It also increases sexual pleasure by increasing blood flow, an essential to achieving orgasm in both men and women.

★ **Ginseng** One of the most ancient aphrodisiacs, ginseng root has been reported to improve erectile function. Ask your doctor's advice before trying this remedy.

★ **Saffron** Reputedly used by Cleopatra in her bath, this is the most expensive spice in the world. Added to food, it is said to help erectile dysfunction and may boost estrogen levels in women.

> ### BELIEVE IT OR NOT!
>
> **"Love hormone" help for ED**
> US scientists are currently investigating the potential of the hormone oxytocin to combat erection problems in men. The "love hormone" as it is called, is released by both men and women during sex and by mothers during childbirth and breastfeeding, and it seems to play an important role in promoting feelings of attachment.

★ **Ginkgo biloba** The leaves of this ancient species of tree are used by herbal practitioners for a variety of effects, one

Favored by Cleopatra, saffron could enhance your libido.

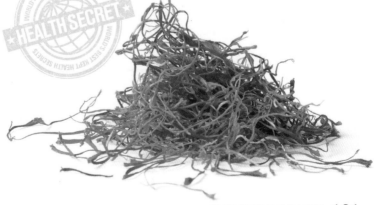

→ → SURPRISINGLY EASY →

Tone your pelvic floor for a better sex life

Strengthening your pelvic muscles with Kegel or pelvic floor exercises—originally developed to help bladder control—can greatly improve sexual satisfaction, helping women to reach orgasm more easily. For instructions on how to do these exercises, see *Secrets of Pelvic Strength*, page 102.

of which is improved blood circulation. This effect may improve blood flow to the penis, which could help to counter erectile dysfunction. But be aware of possible side effects such as diarrhea or irritability.

● **Change your medication?** Failure to achieve an erection (erectile dysfunction or ED) affects up to 25 percent of men over 65 according to the US National Institutes of Health. This common condition is often a side effect of prescription drugs that interfere with nerve signals to the penis. The top "culprits" are beta blockers, which are used to treat heart problems and high blood pressure, antihistamines, taken for allergies, and antidepressants. If you have been suffering from ED and suspect that a drug you are taking may be the cause, ask your doctor if an alternative medication that does not have this side effect might be suitable.

● **Don't worry about your heart** For most people, having an orgasm is no more likely to bring on a heart attack than a brisk climb up a couple of flights of stairs or a half-hour session in the gym. So try not to be overconcerned about having sex if you have a heart condition. What's most important is to keep fit and active so that you're able to cope easily with strenuous activities of all kinds—in and out of the bedroom. And there's also evidence that regular sex can benefit your heart health.

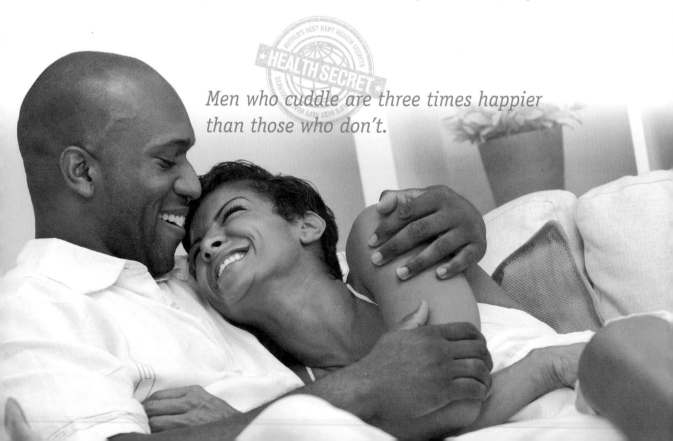

Men who cuddle are three times happier than those who don't.

● **Don't self-medicate** It's unwise to take drugs such as sildenafil (Viagra) to treat erectile dysfunction without advice from your doctor. He or she will explain how to use the drug safely to minimize the risks.

● **Get the right stuff** Be sure to choose a vaginal lubricant designed for the purpose. Oil-based products, such as baby oil or petroleum jelly, can quickly cause the latex in a condom used by your partner to fail or even dissolve, making it ineffective.

● **Have a hug—if you're a man**
When it comes to satisfaction in long-term relationships it turns out, contrary to expectation, that men need to cuddle more than women. In a US study of heterosexual couples carried out by the Kinsey Institute, men who reported frequent kissing and cuddling with their partners were, on average, three times happier with their relationships than those who did so infrequently. For women, what was more important was a long-term relationship accompanied by good sex.

● **Get sweaty four times a week**
Exercise not only helps you keep fit but can also significantly improve your sex life. A study has shown that among people who exercised four or five days a week, 88 percent of the women and 69 percent of the men reported their sexual performance as being above or much above average. Not only that, those who exercised more actually had more sex. For men, one of the main advantages of exercise is that it increases blood flow to the penis, helping to ward off erectile dysfunction.

● **Improve your sex life with yoga**
If you want to continue enjoying your sex life, consider taking up yoga. A small study

SECRETS OF SUCCESS

The allure of face paint
The most common forms of makeup tend to mimic the subtle changes in a woman's appearance that occur naturally during ovulation. At this time, when a woman is at her most fertile, her lips become a little larger and fuller. They are also redder (as during sexual arousal), an effect exaggerated by red lipstick. Another change that occurs at ovulation is that the skin around the eyes becomes a little darker, making them appear bigger, just as when eye make-up is applied. And blusher mimics the appearance of the cheeks during sex.

of 40 healthy women found that a 12-week program of yoga improved their sexual function in six areas (desire, arousal, lubrication, orgasm, pain, and overall satisfaction). And women aged over 45 seemed to experience the most benefit to their sex lives from this form of exercise.

● **Get a diagnosis by mail** If you're worried that you may have contracted genital herpes and feel reluctant to go to your doctor or specialist clinic, you can get a preliminary diagnosis by mail. Several online clinics will, on request, send you a tube in which you can return a urine sample for analysis then receive the results by email. Alternatively, you can request a lesion swab test. You take a sample from a sore using a swab, which is then sent back for laboratory analysis. It's important to refrain from sex if you have reason to suspect you may have contracted genital herpes—or any other sexually transmissible infection. Whatever the results, only a doctor can confirm the diagnosis and rule out other, potentially serious diseases.

Secrets of
BOOSTING FERTILITY

Societies throughout the world use folk remedies, including herbs and foods, to promote fertility and produce a longed-for baby. Some of the treatments from traditional Chinese medicine date back more than 2,000 years. Science is now finding evidence to support many of these natural solutions that can benefit both men and women.

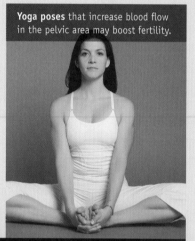

Yoga poses that increase blood flow in the pelvic area may boost fertility.

Symbols, ritual dances, and sacrifices to the gods are among the many ways that societies have sought to influence conception. Most have long disappeared, but certain age-old remedies are still recommended by today's herbalists (see opposite).

A combined approach

While modern medicine has developed a wide range of highly effective ways of tackling the myriad causes of infertility, these techniques can be costly and stressful. Many couples prefer to try a more gentle, natural strategy first and there is now evidence to support some of these remedies as a useful adjunct to conventional approaches.

In a 2010 Israeli study, for example, women undergoing intrauterine insemination (IUI) were also treated with acupuncture and Chinese herbs (including Szechuan lovage and white peony). The result was a notable increase in conception rates compared to women who had IUI without such therapies. This success may have been due to increased blood flow to the uterus and better hormonal balance.

Promoting fertility naturally

Here are some suggestions for natural treatments that may help to boost fertility in some cases. But be sure to discuss these remedies with your doctor before using them, and stop at once if you experience any side effects. If you still fail to conceive, seek a specialist's advice.

Royal Jelly is said to have many health benefits besides enhancing fertility.

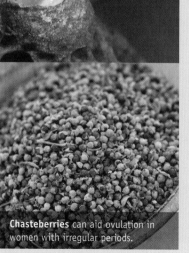

Chasteberries can aid ovulation in women with irregular periods.

Royal jelly In bee colonies the queen is fed royal jelly, which is rich in vitamins, minerals, amino acids, and estrogen-like hormones to boost her egg production. Royal jelly is an ancient Chinese remedy that may improve fertility in humans—of both sexes.

Zinc and folic acid Zinc is vital to the production of testosterone and sperm, and its effect is boosted by folic acid. A Dutch study found that men who took 66mg of zinc and 5mg of folic acid a day for 26 weeks increased their sperm count by 74 percent. Zinc is present in oysters, lean beef, dark turkey meat, eggs, and lentils. Leafy green vegetables and whole grains are rich in folic acid.

Siberian ginseng For more than 2,000 years, the Chinese have used Siberian ginseng to aid fertility. A supplement made from the plant's root is often used to treat infertility brought on by the stress of failing to conceive. This can affect both sexes. The remedy also helps to regulate the menstrual cycle and promotes implantation of the embryo.

Chasteberry The fruit of the chaste tree (*Vitex agnus-castus*) is an ancient fertility enhancer used in the Mediterranean region. Studies in Germany and the Czech Republic have found that taking the berries helps to regulate the menstrual cycle, balancing the amounts of estrogen and progesterone a woman produces, and stimulating ovulation.

Seeds and nuts Chinese medicine uses sunflower and pumpkin seeds to deliver arginine—an amino acid essential to sperm production—to men with low sperm counts. Other sources of arginine include peanuts and nuts, especially Brazil nuts, which also contain the mineral selenium, which is known to promote the production of healthy sperm.

Vitamins Vitamin C raises progesterone levels in women and can stimulate ovulation, but high doses can suppress it.

Trials suggest that vitamin E may improve sperm motility (ability to move)—this effect is said to be enhanced if coenzyme Q10 is also taken. Vitamin B12 may increase sperm count and boost motility.

Raspberry leaf tea Women in Europe, China, and the Americas have traditionally drunk raspberry leaf tea during pregnancy. It is reputed to strengthen the uterus and boost blood flow to its lining, helping the embryo to implant and lowering the risk of miscarriage.

Ayurvedic approaches The Hindu system of medicine uses yoga, diet, and herbal supplements in its fertility treatment. Yoga is said to strengthen the pelvic region and improve circulation to the uterus. Foods used to increase sperm production and promote conception include organic fruit and vegetables (especially asparagus and broccoli), milk, rice pudding, mangoes, dates, cumin, and turmeric. The herb gotu kola is used to improve blood circulation to the sex organs.

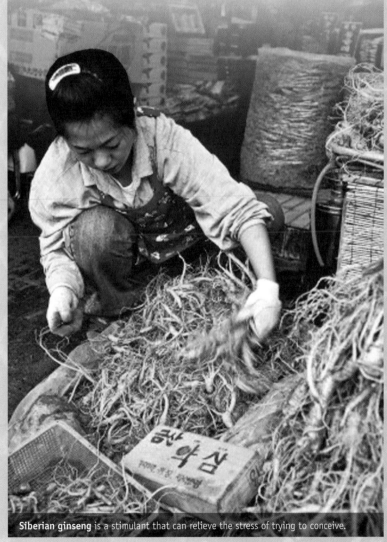

Siberian ginseng is a stimulant that can relieve the stress of trying to conceive.

Becoming
A MOTHER

Even before you conceive, you can plan for a healthy pregnancy by making changes to your diet and lifestyle. A combination of traditional and innovative modern approaches can support you through the minor inconveniences of pregnancy and help you give your new baby the very best start in life.

● **Take folic acid ...** It's essential for the healthy growth of the fetus to have adequate amounts of this B vitamin, also known as folate, before conception and during the first months of pregnancy. Doctors recommend that women take a supplement of 400mcg a day (double the normal adult requirement) for a month before conception and for the first 12 weeks of pregnancy. Folic acid is vital in these early weeks to guard against defects of the neural tube (the embryo spine), which can result in spina bifida, and also against anencephaly, a malformation of the brain. Here are some common food sources:

★ **Avocados**
★ **Broccoli, spinach, and other leafy green vegetables**
★ **Beans and legumes**
★ **Fortified breakfast cereals**
★ **Whole grains**
★ **Orange juice.**

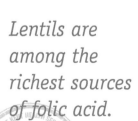

Lentils are among the richest sources of folic acid.

● **... then stop it** There's no need to take folic acid supplements after the 12th week of pregnancy, although you should continue to eat a folate-rich diet. When taken later in pregnancy, some studies have suggested that excess folic acid increases the risk of children developing asthma.

● **Take vitamin D** The demands of your growing baby could reduce the density of your bones. Add oily fish and fortified cereals to your diet. Prenatal vitamins in the US provide 400 IU of vitamin D daily, but high-risk women may benefit from higher amounts according to the Mayo Clinic.

● **Eat well, but not too well**
A nutrient-rich diet is essential for a healthy pregnancy, but never be tempted to "eat for two." Piling on the pounds is bad for your health and increases the risk of complications in pregnancy and labor. Women of normal weight should gain no more than 35 lb (16kg). If you're already overweight or obese, the amount of weight you should gain is considerably less. Ask your doctor or midwife to advise you.

● **Stay trim, protect your child from heart disease** Gaining too much weight could raise the risk of your child suffering from heart disease in later life. British researchers looked at the levels of "bad"

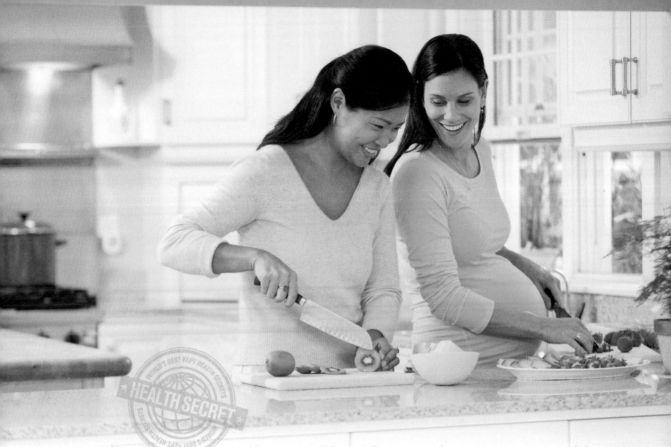

Eating more fresh fruit and vegetables when you're pregnant could protect your child from future obesity.

(LDL) cholesterol—the substance implicated in heart and vessel disease—in the blood of nine year olds and the pregnancy weight gains of their mothers. The children of overweight mothers had significantly higher levels of LDL than those with trim mothers, as well as being heavier than average by 2¼ lb (1kg). Their waists were also about ¾in (2cm) larger.

● **Admit to the cravings** Hankering foods such as ice cream, chocolate, or hot curries when you're pregnant is normal, but you need to worry if you want to eat coal, chalk, paint, earth, or some other inedible substance. No one knows why some women develop odd cravings, but they may indicate mineral deficiencies. If you're affected, it's important to talk to your doctor however embarrassing it may seem. Blood tests and,

if necessary, mineral supplements may be offered. Psychological counseling and behavioral therapy can sometimes help.

● **Get more fruit and veggies** Studies indicate that antioxidants in these foods during pregnancy help to reduce the risk of a child becoming obese by limiting the baby's ability to form fatty tissue. What's more, increasing the amounts of fresh fruit and vegetables in your diet during pregnancy will help to keep your weight gain within the healthy range.

● **Take ginger to beat morning sickness** Fresh ginger is a time-honored remedy for feelings of nausea during pregnancy. For many women, morning sickness can make the first few months of pregnancy miserable and for a few, the

Birthing stool

All around the world, and for centuries before the invention of anesthetics or high-tech labor rooms, women gave birth sitting on a low birthing stool—and for good reason. Not only does sitting or squatting allow gravity to help the baby descend down the birth canal, but it is much easier for the pelvis to move freely—something that is virtually impossible lying down. This also allows the uterus to contract more efficiently and helps to reduce the perception of pain. In some modern versions of the chair, women are also provided with bars to hold onto as they squat, making it easier for them to push when necessary.

misery lasts the full nine months. Ginger contains gingerols, which are pungent substances that act to calm nausea. Here are some ideas for using this root:

★ **Tea** You can make tea by infusing a teaspoon of grated ginger root or the same amount of powdered ginger in a mug of hot water. Strain the liquid and add lemon juice and a little honey to taste, if needed, to make the drink more palatable.

★ **Crystallized form** Try chewing small quantities of crystallized ginger.

★ **Capsules** Dried ginger is available in capsule form from health food stores.

It's wise to consult your doctor before using ginger products to relieve your morning sickness, and to stop if this approach seems to be making the problem worse—it doesn't work for everyone.

● **Apply pressure** Acupressure bands, originally designed to combat seasickness, can also relieve the unpleasantness of morning sickness. Each elasticized band incorporates a button that is worn against an acupuncture point in the wrist. To locate

this point, put the fingers of one hand on the inside of your other wrist, measuring three fingerwidths from the crease of your wrist, between the tendons at the end of your arm. Where your third finger falls, feel lightly for a slight dip. The button on the band should fit over the dip. When you experience a wave of nausea, press on the button 20 to 30 times at one-second intervals, to give a stimulating boost. Repeat on the other wrist. If you forget your wristbands, simply press alternately on the two points with your fingers, or ask someone to do it on both wrists together.

● **Sleep on your left side** It can be difficult to find a comfortable sleeping position in the later stages of pregnancy, and sleeping on your back can cause backache and raise blood pressure. Sleeping on your side is best, and if you choose the left side it will boost the blood flow to the placenta. Put one pillow under your head, another between bent knees to ease pressure on your hips and to help support your weight, and a third in the small of your back to stop you rolling onto your back.

● **Ask for a safer test** Until now, women undergoing amniocentesis, a test for Down's syndrome and other chromosomal abnormalities, have had to face a risk of miscarriage as high as one in 100. The old test used a needle to take a sample from the placenta or the amniotic fluid. Now there is a new test that doesn't entail any risk of miscarriage. It is known as noninvasive prenatal diagnosis technique or NIPD—performed on a blood sample taken at between 11 and 14 weeks of pregnancy. In the laboratory, fetal DNA found in the mother's blood is examined for signs of chromosomal disorders. Ask your doctor if this test is available in your area.

Making light
OF LIFE CHANGES

One of the major milestones in a woman's life is the cessation of monthly periods—menopause. This involves hormonal turmoil that can cause a range of symptoms over several years. Men also go through a parallel change of life. Read on to discover the strategies that can help to lessen the impact of these changes.

● **Switch to soy** A "superfood" for women in their middle years, soy contains isoflavones, which act like natural estrogen and ease symptoms such as hot flashes and fluid retention. Easy to add to your diet, soy has many other benefits:

★**Heart health** Soy proteins and isoflavones reduce blood levels of cholesterol and make the blood less likely to clot.

★**Bone density** By helping to maintain both estrogen and calcium levels, soy helps to keep bones strong.

★ **Immune system boost** Antioxidants in soy help protect against infections. Soy also contains genistin, a substance that may inhibit breast and colon cancers.

Build more soy into your diet by switching to soy milk and yogurts, using tofu in stir-fries, dips, and spreads, or adding soy flour to your baking (try mixing it half and half with wheat flour). Look for edamame (young soybeans), which are delicious eaten hot in their pods sprinkled with a little sea salt. Miso, a fermented soybean paste, makes a tasty broth, but don't have too much if you have high blood pressure as it is high in sodium.

● **Beat hot flashes with antidepressants** If you're having problems with hot flashes, and if HRT is not an option for you, ask your doctor about the latest antidepressant treatments. Studies in the USA on an SSRI (selective serotonin reuptake inhibitor) antidepressant, drugs that work by increasing levels of the "feel-good" hormone serotonin in the brain, found that hot flashes were reduced by more

As well as lifting your spirits, antidepressants can reduce hot flashes.

Miracle magnet

A discreet plastic magnet not much bigger than a large coin could ease the symptoms of menopause. Available in pharmacies under the brand name Ladycare, this device may raise levels of female sex hormones. In one study, 508 women who were going through menopause were asked to attach one of these magnets to their underwear, day and night, for three months. All the women noticed some benefits, with anxiety, mood swings, fatigue, sleeping problems, incontinence, and breast tenderness being reduced by up to 70 percent. Hot flashes, night sweats, and irritability improved by 30 percent, as did reduced libido and concentration. In addition, one in every five of the women lost weight.

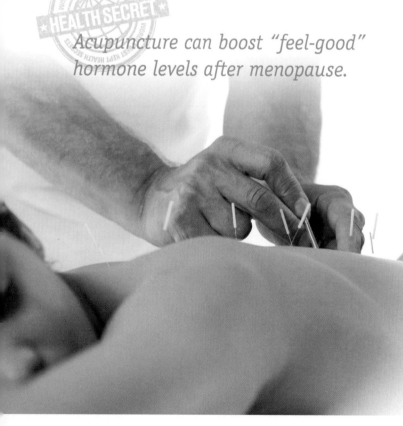

Acupuncture can boost "feel-good" hormone levels after menopause.

than 20 percent in those taking it. Serotonin appears to produce this effect by altering the way in which the walls of the body's blood vessels expand and contract.

● **Ease them with "E"** Vitamin E is the most helpful vitamin for easing hot flashes. And when taken for four months or longer, a daily dose of as little as 400IU has been found to relieve vaginal dryness. You can also get these benefits in the form of a vaginal pessary. Before you take a vitamin E supplement, check with your doctor to make sure it is safe for you. Good food sources include leafy green vegetables, almonds, and sunflower seeds.

● **Deal with dryness** The hormonal changes following menopause inevitably cause vaginal dryness, making sexual intercourse uncomfortable and sometimes painful, but you can ask your doctor for a vaginal cream that contains estrogen to ease the problem. Alternatively, you may be prescribed an estrogen ring, which is about the size of a contraceptive diaphragm; this is left in place for three months. With both these treatments you may need an additional water-based lubricant. Experiment to find out what feels most comfortable for you.

● **Try acupuncture** Consider tackling troublesome menopausal symptoms with acupuncture. This traditional Chinese technique has been shown to increase the levels of estradiol, a specific type of estrogen, circulating in the bloodstream, which is important for maintaining healthy bone structure and guarding against mood swings and depression. Acupuncture also boosts the levels of endorphins, the "feel-good" hormones that lift and stabilize mood, and steady the body's temperature.

● Don't ignore male menopause

There has long been controversy about whether "male menopause" (or andropause) exists, but thanks to studies of the male hormone testosterone, scientists are now sure that it does occur. From the age of about 40 the production of testosterone, which is responsible for the male sex drive, gradually falls, and between the ages of 40 and 60 men can suffer symptoms that may creep up slowly. These are similar to those of the female menopause including lowered libido, lethargy, and depression. There may be some loss of bone mass, making the bones more susceptible to fracture. Lower levels of testosterone also put heart health at risk, making the coronary arteries more prone to the spasms that are a major cause of angina. Here are some tips to help men stay healthy through the andropause:

★ **Seek support** Find new ways to relieve stress, such as taking part in support group activities and seeking one-to-one support from a partner or friend.

★ **Get exercise** which produces mood-lifting endorphins as well as helping to keep bones and muscles strong and healthy.

★ **Adjust your diet** A low-fat, high-fiber diet, with plenty of protein will help boost hormone production.

★ **Maximize minerals** A diet rich in zinc—pork, cashew nuts, and seafood, particularly oysters—will all help to keep testosterone levels high.

★ **Try Ginkgo biloba** to help maintain healthy circulation and to prevent erectile dysfunction. Ask your doctor's advice first.

★ **Cut out grapefruit** This fruit contains a substance that may convert testosterone into estrogen. Avoiding grapefruit could help to maintain testosterone levels.

★ **Avoid excess alcohol** which adds to the problems of andropause by further lowering testosterone levels.

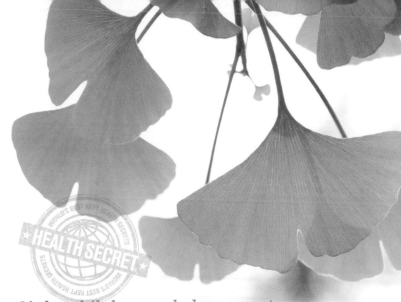

Ginkgo biloba can help prevent erectile dysfunction.

BELIEVE IT OR NOT!

Menopause boosts creativity

Following menopause, a woman's brain undergoes changes—both positive and negative—due to the reduced estrogen in the bloodstream. Modern research techniques, which make it possible to map the functions of the brain, suggest that menopause may limit the actions of the left side of the brain, producing an increase in "fuzzy" thinking and a reduction in precise mental skills, such as mathematical ability. But the good news for older women is that the activity of the right side of the brain increases, bringing a surge in creativity. This knowledge can empower women and encourage them to make the most of new-found creative skills in art, music, and writing.

★ **Consider male HRT** Hormone replacement therapy (HRT) for men is increasingly available and for severe symptoms it could be the best route to physical and mental health. Discuss the possibilities with your doctor.

10
Fighting
INVADERS

The immune system, which includes germ-fighting cells and the substances that determine the body's response to invaders, rogue cells, and allergens, protects us from infection and cancerous cell changes. Medical research is revealing more and more about its workings and scientists are also turning their attention to traditional remedies to provide new insights.

Boosting
RESISTANCE

The battle against infection never ends—each day, your immune system fights off any number of would-be invaders. Here you'll find out why what you eat, how you feel, and the amount of exercise you take can all play a part in strengthening your defenses.

● **Have a giggle** Laughter can boost your immunity as well as your mood. It raises the levels of antibodies in the blood and those of the white blood cells that attack and kill bacteria and viruses. It also increases the number of antibodies in the mucus made in the nose and respiratory passages, the entry points for many germs. So find ways to laugh with your family and friends, and boost everyone's health.

● **Sing your way to health** A study of a German choir revealed that singing activates the spleen, helping to increase the blood concentrations of antibodies. If you don't want to join a choir, sing in the shower.

● **Choose friendly fats** Some fats are essential for building cells and for the production of prostaglandins. These hormone-like compounds help to regulate the immune system's response to infection, such as the way it reacts by making the white blood cells that combat invaders. Italian athletes on very low-fat diets were found to be significantly short of these cells. The secret is to choose your fats with care:
★ **Go unsaturated** Opt for unsaturated vegetable fats rather than saturated ones from animal foods, which reduce the ability of the white blood cells to zap bacteria and increase the risk of cancers.
★ **Avoid trans fats**, the manufactured fats labeled as "hydrogenated" or "partially

| BELIEVE IT OR NOT! |

You can overdose on vitamins
Vitamins are good for your immune system—but not if you overdose on them. Try to get as many vitamins as possible from fresh food, and choose and use supplements sensibly. Take special care with vitamins E and A, which are stored in the body if taken in excess, rather than simply being excreted in the urine. In doses above 250mg a day, vitamin E can impair, rather than enhance, the day-to-day renewal of body cells, increasing the risk of prostate and other cancers. You need vitamin A to help build immune cells, but supplement doses above 1,000mcg a day put you at risk of serious liver disease.

hydrogenated." Often found in processed foods and baked goods, these fats can also interfere with the immune system.

● **No sugar, thanks** Just 2½oz (75g) of sugar—10 teaspoons, or the amount in two 12oz (330ml) cans of cola or carbonated lemonade—impairs the ability of the white blood cells to deactivate or kill bacteria. Opt instead for a natural sweetener, such as one made from the stevia plant, and avoid calorie-free alternatives such as aspartame.

● **Feast on fish** Oily fish such as sardines, herring, and mackerel contain protein—essential for building the cells that fight off invaders—and the fatty acids called

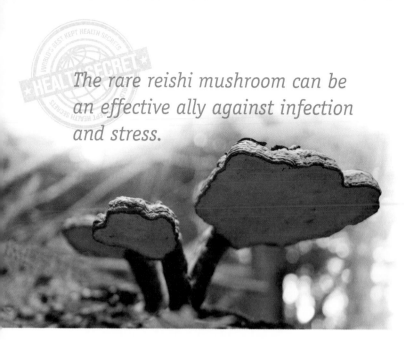

The rare reishi mushroom can be an effective ally against infection and stress.

omega-3s, which regulate the function of the immune system. When the body is attacked, acute inflammation is the body's first response. But omega-3s lower the production of inflammatory compounds and increase the production of anti-inflammatory ones, thus aiding recovery and even suppressing the growth of cancer cells. In clinical trials, omega-3s have also been found to activate parts of the immune system that switch off the activities of attack cells once their job is done.

❄ MIND POWER

Lift mood, boost immune function

Depression is bad for the immune system. When you're depressed, the body produces too much of the stress hormones cortisol and adrenaline, delaying antibody production and suppressing the activity of specialist cells that are involved in the body's immune response. These hormones also hamper the manufacture of interferon, a protein key to the fight against viral infection. In addition, depression can cause overproduction of interleukin-6, an inflammatory substance that has a role in immune-system related conditions such as arthritis, gum disease, and even cancers. So as well as making you feel good about yourself, treatment for depression can significantly boost your physical health.

● **Get some mushroom magic** The rare reishi mushroom has been valued in the Far East for over 2,000 years and it has now been found to have the following actions that benefit the immune system. It:

★ **Stimulates** the production of T-cells—white blood cells involved in protecting the body from infection

★ **Increases** levels of substances that strengthen the immune response

★ **Promotes** sleep and reduces stress by suppressing the production of the stimulant hormone adrenaline.

Reishi essence—a convenient way to get the benefits—is available in health food stores.

● **Have more citrus fruit** Vitamin C, found in high concentrations in oranges, lemons, limes, and grapefruit, boosts the activity of phagocytes (cells that engulf and digest bacteria) in the blood. The body can't store vitamin C, so you need to have some every day.

● **Exercise your immune system ...** Your immune system responds to exercise by producing more of the blood cells that attack bacterial invaders. And the more regularly you exercise, the more long lasting the changes become. US research shows that people who exercise moderately on five or six days a week have half as many colds and sore throats than those who don't.

● **... but get rest, too** Moderation is the key, when it comes to boosting your immune system through exercise. If you work out intensively for 90 minutes, production of germ-fighting cells called macrophages dips temporarily, increasing the risk of infection. So always include plenty of recovery days in your training schedule to preserve immune system health.

Combating INFECTION

From healthy eating to keeping yourself and your home clean, there's plenty you can do to hold off would-be invaders. Even when they breach your defenses, you can call on a range of powerful substances in food to help your body stop germs in their tracks.

● **Toughen up with almonds** To help ward off viral infections, make 3oz (85g) of almonds part of your daily diet—but keep the skins on. Italian researchers studying the herpes viruses that cause cold sores have found that a chemical in almond skins improves the ability of white blood cells to detect viruses; they found that the chemical could also help to prevent a virus from spreading throughout the body. So add a handful of almonds to your morning muesli to keep viruses at bay.

● **Keep warm, stay well** You're more likely to catch an infection if you—and especially your extremities—are cold. In one study, 90 people kept their feet in a bowl of cold water for 20 minutes and the same number just put their feet in an empty bowl for a similar length of time. Five days later, 20 percent of the people with chilled feet had developed colds compared with 9 percent of those whose feet stayed warm. Having cold extremities seems to reduce the supply of white blood cells, the immune system's first defense against invaders.

● **Guard against Giardia with soy** *Giardia* is a type of protozoan that can cause diarrhea and vomiting, and children are particularly susceptible. *Giardia* is common in tropical countries, but it also occurs in

Bundling up in winter really can keep germs at bay.

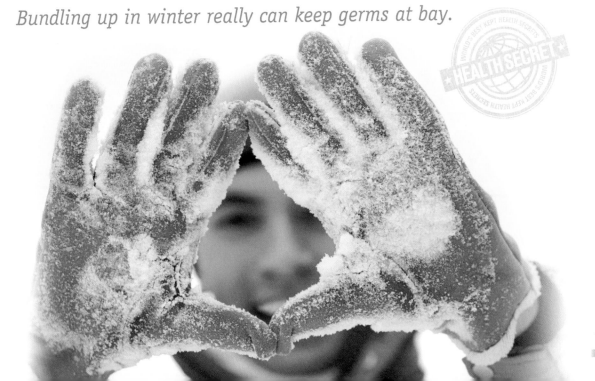

Feed a cold, starve a fever

Granny was right when she uttered those wise words. When you eat a meal containing around 1,000 calories, the body increases its production of gamma interferon, the substance it uses to fight viruses such as those that cause colds and flu. By contrast, fasting for 12 hours increases levels of a substance called interleucin-4, made by the body to help combat life-threatening infections that cause high fevers, such as typhoid.

temperate regions in streams, lakes, and rivers, or anywhere that has poor sanitation. Research has shown that substances called saponins in soy kill many disease-producing protozoa. If you live in a high-risk area, increasing your intake of soy-based foods, such as soy milk or tofu, could help to

Running your empty washing machine on a hot cycle will help to keep it germ-free.

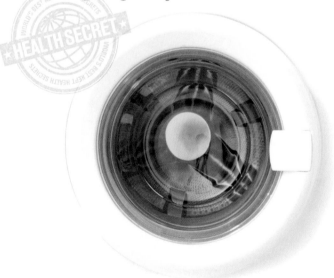

protect you against this unpleasant and sometimes debilitating infection of the gastrointestinal tract.

● Resist infection with vegetables

Garlic and onions in soup, stews, and other dishes are both sources of potent antiviral substances that can boost your resistance to infections. And plenty of other vegetables can add to your infection-fighting armory, including carrots and sweet potatoes that are rich in beta carotene, which has an anti-inflammatory action and raises the rate at which white blood cells are produced. Other powerful allies include:

★ **Chile peppers** work quickly to thin nasal mucus.

★ **Shiitake mushrooms** aid white blood cell manufacture.

★ **Ginger** counteracts inflammation.

★ **Goji berries** (available in dried form) also boost white cell production.

● Don't stop when you're winning

Every year, bacteria become increasingly resistant to antibiotics. This is why if you don't finish an entire course of antibiotics, because you think you're better, the infection may not be completely wiped out, leaving a potentially resistant bacteria strain free to multiply. And this is also why the use of antibiotics should be kept to a minimum. The more antibiotics are used, the more chance the bacteria have to fight them by changing their DNA.

● Run your washer on a hot cycle

Your clothes may look clean, but they may not be germ-free. Many bacteria can survive in a washing machine at up to 179°F (82°C) and flu viruses can tolerate temperatures up to 212°F (100°C). For maximum hygiene, run your empty machine on a complete hot cycle with bleach added.

The most effective way to kill bacteria and viruses on your hands is to wash with old-fashioned soap and water.

● **Careful cleaning** With all the new cleansing products that are on the market, it may come as a surprise to learn that washing with old-fashioned soap and water is still the most effective way of getting bacteria and viruses off your hands. Follow these simple guidelines:

★ **Soap your hands** on both sides.

★ **Open your fingers** wide and interlock your hands and rub them together for 20 seconds so they are thoroughly cleansed all over. Take note: Right-handed people tend to wash their left hand more thoroughly than the right.

★ **Scrub under and around** your nails with soap and a small brush, and remove jewelery before washing, as bacteria can linger under rings.

● **Get the right gel** If you choose to use an alcohol-based hand-cleansing gel—perhaps because you're on the move and away from hand-washing facilities—check the contents: It must contain at least 60 percent alcohol to be effective against germs. So read the label carefully.

● **Wash more—if you're a woman**
Women need to take particular care with hand washing. Studies have found that, although they often wash more, women carry different bacteria from men and a greater number of different types—usually over 150. The reason for this is that men's skin appears to be more acidic, which deters bacterial growth. So if you're a woman, be sure to pay particular attention to the advice on hand washing given above.

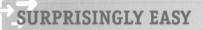

SURPRISINGLY EASY

Protection for gardeners
If you tend a garden or enjoy outdoor hobbies, make sure you're protected against tetanus. The bacteria that cause this potentially fatal infection, live naturally in the soil and can easily enter the body via puncture wounds in the skin made, for example, by nails or rose thorns. Five doses of the vaccine should give you long-term protection. But if you're not sure how many doses you've received over the years, you may need a booster dose after a puncture wound. Always get medical attention for any serious wound acquired outdoors or one that causes muscle stiffness near the injury or that is slow to heal.

Secrets of nature's
ANTIBIOTICS

Centuries before the 1928 discovery of penicillin by Scottish scientist Alexander Fleming, people around the world used natural remedies to beat infections. Now researchers are investigating and rediscovering their curative powers, despite the many modern antibiotics available. Here's why.

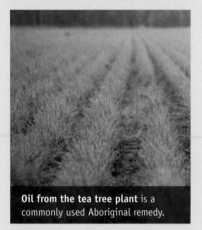

Oil from the tea tree plant is a commonly used Aboriginal remedy.

The development of antibiotics in the 20th century transformed the treatment of infectious diseases, including tuberculosis, syphilis, and meningitis. But the scientists who discovered them did not predict that various strains of bacteria would become resistant to these drugs, and that new antibiotics would be needed to keep up with the mutations that bacteria undergo. The impact of antibiotics on the digestive system, and other side effects, has also become a concern. In the search for new drugs, scientists are looking to traditional remedies and their findings suggest that plants and other natural substances may have effective infection-beating powers.

Turning back to nature

Here's a selection of remedies from around the world, which scientific analysis shows can either kill unwelcome bacteria or prevent them from multiplying. However, if you are ill, you may also need prescription drugs. Always consult your doctor if you notice any unusual symptoms and discuss any natural remedies you plan to use.

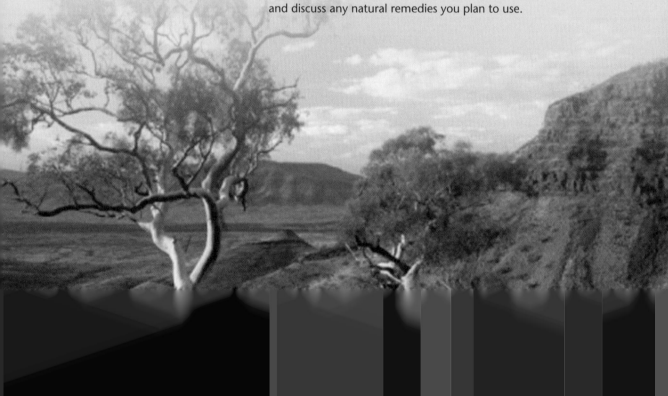

Allspice This spice can help to keep bacteria from multiplying in food. It is excellent in Caribbean and Asian dishes.

Asparagus Asparagus extract boosts the numbers and activity of white blood cells to protect against a range of bacteria, including *E. coli* and *Staphylococcus aureus*.

Basil The leaves and seeds of this aromatic herb, which reached the West from India over 2,000 years ago, have antibacterial properties. Use it in cooking or apply basil ointment to wounds.

Bearberry *Arctostaphylos uva ursi*, a plant that grows in Europe, Asia, and North America, contains a compound that combats urinary and intestinal infections. It is available as capsules and tincture.

Blueberries contain compounds that counter *E. coli* infections. Their tannins inhibit bacterial growth and prevent bacteria from sticking to the cells lining the urinary tract. The highest concentrations of tannins are found in blueberry juice.

Cherries Black cherry juice blocks the bacterial activity that leads to the formation of dental plaque, helping to prevent gum disease.

Cranberries Native to North America, these berries contain compounds that prevent *E. coli* bacteria from taking hold in the urinary tract. Concentrated extract or undiluted juice is most effective.

Echinacea This American Indian remedy derived from the purple coneflower plant stimulates the process by which bacteria are destroyed by white blood cells. It is usually taken as a tincture.

Eucalyptus Aromatic leaves from this common Australian tree are rich in eucalyptol. This powerful antibacterial is used in the form of an inhalation to treat respiratory infections or applied externally to prevent infection in wounds.

Garlic Rich in the antibacterial compound allicin, garlic has been used since ancient times to treat potentially fatal diseases and ward off sepsis in wounds. Use raw or in cooking or take garlic capsules.

Goldenseal Long used by American Indians to treat infections, this plant contains the alkaloid berberine, which attacks bacteria and boosts the immune system.

Green tea contains polyphenols, key antimicrobial agents that disrupt the metabolism of bacteria, preventing them from multiplying.

Honey has antibacterial properties that help to prevent wound infection. The most potent type is manuka honey, traditionally used by New Zealand's Maori people. It can even combat the antibiotic-resistant *Staphylococcus aureus* (MRSA).

Oregano This easy-to-grow herb is rich in essential oils that possess antibacterial properties. Over-the-

Pomegranate fruit is packed with antibacterial and anticancer compounds.

Bearberries have been used medicinally for almost 2,000 years.

counter ointments that contain oregano extract are available to treat wound infection.

Pomegranate When mixed with vitamin C and iron salts to make an ointment, pomegranate rind kills *Staphylococcus aureus* (MRSA) microbes. The juice, as the ancient Chinese knew, helps prevent infection of the mouth and gums.

Tea tree Used externally, oil from this native Australian plant, an ancient remedy for skin and wound infections, has strong antimicrobial properties.

Yogurt The "good" bacteria in live yogurt stimulate the production of white blood cells, which then attack invading micro-organisms.

Keeping
CANCER AT BAY

Medical treatments for cancer—when rogue cells grow and reproduce uncontrolledly, destroying healthy organs and tissues—are becoming increasingly successful. But there is plenty we can do in terms of our diet and lifestyle to reduce our risk of developing this disease.

● **Shoot it down** The cancer-fighting abilities of broccoli are well known, but broccoli sprouts, which taste like a peppery alfalfa, work even better. US researchers found that compared with fully grown heads, 3-day-old broccoli shoots contained between 20 and 50 percent more of the protective chemical sulforaphane, which helps to neutralize cancer-causing chemicals before they have a chance to take hold. The shoots are easy to grow in a jar or in a custom-made sprouter, but be sure to rinse them thoroughly twice a day.

Tasty broccoli sprouts contain surprising amounts of cancer-fighting chemicals.

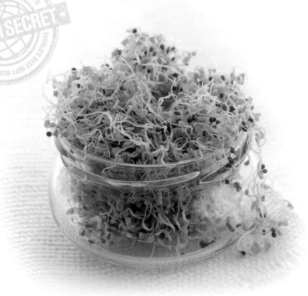

BELIEVE IT OR NOT!

It's in the blood
A blood test has been developed that can save lives by detecting lung cancer up to five years before symptoms appear, and in 2012 it was being tested on 10,000 smokers in Scotland. When cancer cells first form they emit proteins known as antigens. These are detected by the body's immune system, which responds by making large numbers of auto-antibodies. Scientists are now designing a range of proteins to which auto-antibodies will bind if they are present in the blood, thus revealing the presence of cancer cells. A similar test for breast cancer is expected to be available by the end of 2012.

● **Go for citrus** Not only are they an excellent source of vitamin C, but oranges and grapefruit are also packed with naringenin, a compound that can inhibit the growth of cancers. What's more, studies show that it can fight infection and reduce levels of blood cholesterol.

● **Get the aspirin advantage**
Researchers at Oxford University in the UK think that a 75mg daily dose of aspirin could be invaluable in the fight against cancer. Some of the ways in which aspirin could protect include:

★ **Halting the spread** Aspirin stops blood platelets from sticking together, which helps prevent cancer cells from spreading around the body to different organs. It is also thought to be able to help repair damaged DNA and to make faulty cells self-destruct before they can become cancerous.

★ **Protecting the bowel** Aspirin is particularly effective for people with the hereditary condition Lynch syndrome, often called hereditary nonpolyposis colorectal cancer, or HNPCC. The researchers discovered that people who took 75mg of aspirin daily, whether they had Lynch syndrome or not, were 25 percent less likely to develop bowel cancer.

★ **Limiting tumors** A daily aspirin dose may help to prevent the growth of tumors in the breast, prostate, and esophagus. It may also provide some protection against the spread of some types of lung cancer.

A word of caution: Although this medicine is available over the counter, be sure to consult your doctor before taking aspirin regularly, as it can cause internal bleeding.

● **Cut cancer risk with legumes**
Legumes (beans, peas, and lentils) all contain powerful anticancer chemicals. High on the list of these fighters are:

★ **Saponins,** which can stop cancer cells from reproducing and slow tumor growth

★ **Protease inhibitors,** which can slow cancer-cell division and stop tumor cells from destroying their healthy neighbors

★ **Phytic acid,** which can slow the growth of tumors.

Legumes are also rich in fiber and because of this, they provide added benefit in helping to reduce the risk of bowel cancer, as well as cancers of the esophagus, stomach, breast, and prostate.

SUPRISINGLY EASY

Salad power
Improve your body's cancer-fighting ability by enjoying a herb-enhanced salad, prepared using ingredients long renowned for their powers to prevent tumors. Mix watercress or shredded spinach with finely divided cauliflower florets, red pepper, onion, mint, and cilantro. Add to the protective effects with a dressing of flaxseed (linseed) oil and lemon juice, plus a little garlic.

● **Back off the booze** Not everyone who drinks alcohol develops cancer, but researchers agree that alcohol may cause cancer if drunk in excess. Common alcohol-related cancers are those of the throat, esophagus, larynx, and liver, but alcohol also increases the risk of colon and breast cancer. The body converts alcohol into acetaldehyde, which can damage DNA. It also makes liver cells multiply faster than normal which, in turn, can lead to cancer. The recommended limits are:

★ **Men** 14 drinks a week; no more than 4 drinks at one time.

★ **Women** 7 drinks a week; no more than 3 drinks at one time.

A "drink" is defined as: A mixed drink, 1.5oz (44ml) of 80-proof hard liquor, such as gin, whiskey, or rum; a 5oz (148ml) glass of wine; a 12oz (355ml) bottle of beer. Both men and women should have at least two alcohol-free days each week.

● **Female? Take the soft option** It's not just a question of size. Women need to be especially careful about their alcohol consumption, because their bodies contain more fat, a tissue in which alcohol can become concentrated. And alcohol can

Tumor genes predict best treatment

By looking at the genes in the cells of breast and colon cancer tissues, doctors are now able to decide whether or not chemotherapy—which can lead to hair loss, infertility, and weakened immune system—is going to have long-term, positive effects. In a test known as Oncotype DX, genetic material from a sample of the tumor is analyzed. From the results, doctors can estimate the chances of the cancer returning in the future. If the chances are low, then chemotherapy and its unpleasant side effects can be avoided.

Cooked tomatoes contain high concentrations of lycopene, which can reduce your cancer risk.

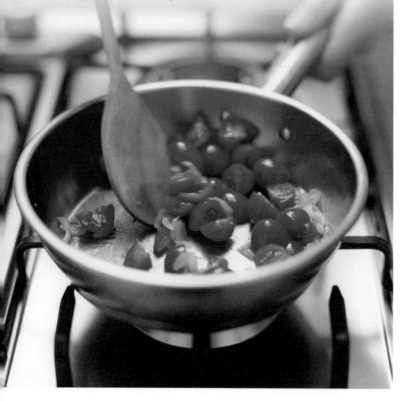

increase the level of estrogen, a hormone implicated in breast cancer. Make a soft drink your usual choice.

● **Use the power of tomatoes** Eat plenty of tomatoes—they top the list when it comes to fighting cancer. Their most potent ingredient is lycopene, a powerful antioxidant able to defend the body against cancer. Tomatoes also contain the flavonoids quercetin and kaempferol, as well as beta carotene, all of which inhibit cancer cell growth. Studies show that men who eat dishes such as pasta with tomato sauce at least twice a week may cut their risk of prostate cancer by up to a third. Similarly, women with high lycopene levels in their blood have a reduced risk of breast cancer. Try these tips to get the most benefit:

★ **Cook** your tomatoes to increase their lycopene content.

★ **Use** olive oil for cooking. Because lycopene is fat soluble, it becomes more readily available to body tissues when tomatoes are cooked with a little fat.

● **Treat yourself** Chocolate is good for you, as long as you don't overindulge. It is rich in flavonoids—antioxidants that stop cells from being damaged by free radicals, thus preventing them from turning into fast-dividing cancer cells. Dark chocolate is best, since it is lower in sugar and fat than milk chocolate and contains eight times the level of antioxidants found in fruits such as strawberries and blueberries.

● **Don't double your trouble** If you drink alcohol as well as smoke, you multiply your cancer risk because alcohol makes it easier for cancer-causing chemicals in smoke to be absorbed into mouth and throat tissues. So consider giving up smoking as well as drinking less.

❋ MIND POWER

Stress-busting techniques

The link isn't fully understood yet, but there's no doubt that stress lowers the body's ability to prevent cancer cells from developing, repair faulty DNA, and produce killer cells, such as T-cells. To help relieve stress and calm your mind:

● Put your hands on your stomach and slowly breathe in through your nose, then slowly breathe out. Do this for between 10 and 20 minutes each day.

● Try meditation. Sit in a quiet room and choose a word or phrase to say to yourself in coordination with your breathing. Use it as you breathe in and again as you breathe out. Do this for 20 minutes, while imagining a scene that will relax and soothe you.

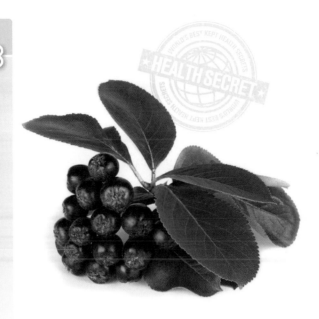

The aronia berry contains more cancer-protective flavonoids than any other fruit.

● **Benefit from berry power** The aronia berry, also known as chokeberry, contains more protective flavonoids than any other fruit. This berry was used by Native Americans, who appreciated its health-giving properties and also used it as an aphrodisiac. For a great start to the day or a cancer-fighting snack, have a handful of berries, blended with honey, yogurt, and banana to make them palatable. Aronia juice can be drunk on its own or mixed with apple juice if you prefer.

● **Barbecue less often** If you barbecue on several nights a week, cut down to reduce your cancer risk. Studies in France showed that a 2-hour barbecue can release high levels of dioxins—substances that may encourage cancer formation. High temperatures from grilling also produce cancer-causing heterocyclic amines (HCAs); the longer food is heated, the more HCAs

are produced. And during grilling over charcoal, polycyclic aromatic hydrocarbons from flare-ups may splatter onto the meat, raising the risk of stomach cancer. Here are some useful pointers to help you make your barbecues healthier:

★ **Use** low-fat meat.

★ **Choose** smaller portion sizes that cook more quickly.

★ **Partially precook** meats such as chicken or other cuts of meat on the bone, that take a long time to cook.

● **Eat Brazil nuts** To ward off cancer, increase your intake of selenium. Brazil nuts are the best natural source of this mineral: One nut contains about 75mcg. In one study, cancer death rates were found to be halved among people who took 200mcg of selenium a day for 7 years. Selenium activates an enzyme that makes cancer cells break apart and die.

Allergies and
INTOLERANCES

An allergic reaction occurs when a usually harmless substance—such as a specific food or pollen—produces an abnormal response in the body. Prevention of allergic reactions involves avoiding the "trigger" substance and keeping your immune system at the top of its game.

● **Eat yogurt** to combat lactose intolerance. If, for no apparent reason or following a bout of gastroenteritis, you suffer from bloating, loose stools, or diarrhea, you may have become temporarily intolerant to lactose in milk. If you suspect this may be your problem, consult your doctor. Meanwhile, it will do no harm—and may do some good—to add live yogurt to your diet. The "good" bacteria in live yogurt can help to restore the healthy bacteria in your intestines. It's safe to eat because most of the lactose in live yogurt has already been converted into lactic acid, which doesn't cause a reaction.

● **Combat mold** If you have a cough, itchy eyes and throat and a runny nose all year round, or if your symptoms get worse in damp weather, then it's possible that you're allergic to the spores produced by molds. Every home has them, but they are difficult to see at a glance. The worst culprit is black mold, which thrives in dark, damp places, such as under shower mats, in kitchen crevices, in washing machines, and even in the rubber seals of fridges. Mold also appears as orange, green, or brown stains in wet areas. Problems with a home's damp basement or leaks from water pipes will exacerbate the condition. Try the following tips for combating mold.

★ **Scrub it** Use soap and water and a stiff brush to scour all mold-prone surfaces. Powerful sprays are available for removing stubborn mold.

★ **Clean your carpets** thoroughly.

★ **Fix structural causes** of dampness and improve ventilation.

★ **Consider a dehumidifier** This may help, as long as you also keep its water reservoir scrupulously clean.

★ **Test the air** If your allergy persists, it may be worth getting your air tested for mold spores with a kit that can be bought or rented.

● **Don't worry about baby ailments** If you have a baby or young child, don't be overly concerned if they catch a cough or cold. Studies suggest that getting these infections early in life may give a child greater resistance to asthma later on. One

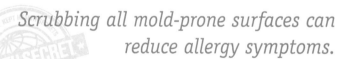

Scrubbing all mold-prone surfaces can reduce allergy symptoms.

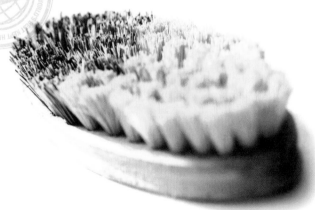

FOOD ALLERGY, SENSITIVITY, OR INTOLERANCE?

There's a great deal of confusion about the difference between food allergies, sensitivities, and intolerances to certain foods. The surest way to distinguish between these different adverse reactions is the timing of the response. The role of the immune system in bringing them about also differs.

Allergy

A truly allergic reaction happens fast. When a food such as a nut is eaten, or when the body responds adversely to an insect bite or medication, the immune system releases histamine and other chemicals such as immunoglobulin E (IgE). The result is usually the almost instant development of a rash or flushing of the skin, plus a quick, severe swelling, especially in the mouth and throat, which can restrict breathing. This potentially fatal condition, called anaphylactic shock, requires emergency medical attention.

Sensitivity

A sensitivity or delayed allergy to a food or medicine (often wrongly called an intolerance) comes on more slowly, taking from 45 minutes to 3 days to develop. The effects can vary widely, from swelling or a rash to headache, bloating, severe indigestion, or diarrhea. The immune system is involved in the reaction through the overproduction of a different set of immunoglobulins— IgG and IgM—and the release of inflammatory "complement proteins." The best way of detecting a food sensitivity is with an elimination diet, which involves removing specific foods from your diet for at least six weeks, plus blood tests to assess your immune system's reactions. Keeping a food diary is often helpful.

Intolerance

A true food intolerance doesn't involve the immune system but occurs when the digestive system is unable to process a particular type of food. For example, in lactose intolerance, the body doesn't produce enough of the enzyme lactase, which is essential to the digestion of lactose— the natural sugar in milk. Intolerances may be genetic in origin.

theory is that the infection stimulates the production and action of protective T-cells, which are made in the thymus—a gland most active during the first years of life.

● **Find the right balance** When it comes to allergy prevention for your children, balancing the risks of poor hygiene against the benefits of healthy exposure to potential allergens is the best approach. Dr. Marc McMorris, paediatric allergist at the University of Michigan Health System, advises parents to let their children get dirty through healthy play outside to give their immune systems the right stimulus—as long as you make sure they get clean afterward.

● **Get a fiber boost** Australian research reveals that fiber-rich foods strengthen the immune system. In the gut, fiber is broken down by bacteria into short-chain fatty acids—molecules that are essential to the working of the immune system and that also help to prevent autoimmune disorders. Without these fatty acids, the cells of the immune system go awry, causing diseases as diverse as asthma, inflammatory bowel disease, and multiple sclerosis. The average adult needs to eat a minimum of ¾oz (18g) of fiber a day from fresh fruit and vegetables, whole grains, legumes, nuts, and seeds. As a guide, a slice of whole-grain bread contains 4g of fiber and an apple has nearly 2g.

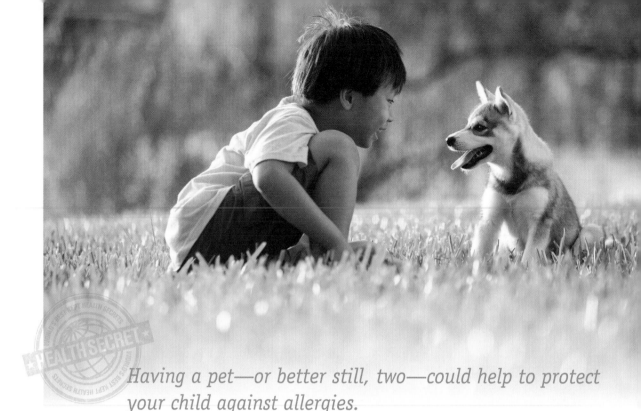

Having a pet—or better still, two—could help to protect your child against allergies.

● Give your children pet protection

Children who live with at least two pets in early life are less likely to develop allergies. The evidence suggests that contact with animals strengthens a child's immune system. US studies found that exposure to two or more cats and dogs in their first 12 months made children less susceptible to allergy-inducing substances, such as dander from dust mites, by the age of seven. Some scientists believe that homes with pets contain more endotoxins, the bacterial components that may steer children's immune systems away from allergic responses. While owning a pet isn't an option for all, there seems to be a health bonus for children if you do.

SECRETS OF SUCCESS

Hay fever shots

If you get hay fever, take comfort from the fact that immunization is arriving at last. Until now, available injections have been far from patient-friendly, involving weekly shots for six months, followed by shots every two weeks or monthly for another three years. The new vaccine does the job in a single shot by staying in the body tissues and "training" the immune system not to react to airborne pollen. When tested in Europe, the USA, and Canada, it showed significant results in eliminating or reducing the symptoms. Researchers hope that this type of vaccine may also soon help to prevent asthma and other allergies.

● Go for probiotics in pregnancy

If you're a mother-to-be, adding probiotic yogurt to your diet may help to keep your baby free from allergy-based diseases such as asthma and eczema—or at least minimize their impact. One German study showed that probiotics reduced the cases of eczema in children up to two years old by 40 percent, and those children who did have eczema suffered less severely. Probiotic yogurt, as long as it's made with pasteurized milk, is perfectly safe to eat during pregnancy— but, if you are concerned, check with your doctor first.

● **Good reason to push** A "natural" birth may give babies significant protection from allergic conditions such as asthma. Evidence is growing that helpful bacteria acquired during passage through the mother's vagina enter the baby's intestines and "prime" the immune system against allergies early in life. The effect is thought to be even stronger in breastfed babies, since breast milk boosts these protective bacteria.

● **Beware of hidden histamines** This group of allergy-provoking substances are present in a wide range of common foods and can cause a variety of symptoms from severe headaches to rashes and asthma, and in severe cases even anaphylactic shock, a life-threatening allergic reaction. Foods that are high in histamine include:
★ **Fermented drinks and foods** such as red wine, aged cheese, and foods that contain yeast
★ **Spinach**
★ **Tomatoes**
★ **Citrus fruit** These don't contain histamine, but can trigger its release.

If you suspect you are allergic to any of these foods, consult your doctor.

● **Kitchen remedies** For mild allergies, when overproduction of histamines leads to a runny nose, watery eyes, and itchy skin, go to the kitchen, not the medicine cupboard. Here are suggestions for foods with antihistamine properties you can try:
★ **Pineapples,** whose main active ingredient is the enzyme bromelain which stops histamine from being released by cells.

★ **Apples** and other fruits contain plenty of the natural antihistamines quercetin and vitamin C. Have some fruit every day.
★ **Hot spices** Capsaicinoids—chemicals that help give cayenne pepper its fiery taste—and the isothiocyanates of the hot Japanese spice wasabi are also excellent for combating allergic reactions of all kinds.

● **Watch out for sulphites** These sulphur-containing preservatives are often added to packaged foods such as dried fruits, canned vegetables, cakes and pastries, jams, pickles, and bottled sauces. They are also added to, but sometimes occur naturally in wine and beer. Sulphites can trigger asthma attacks in susceptible people and in rare cases may even cause anaphylactic shock. The presence of sulphites is usually noted on the labels of drinks that contain them and are therefore easy to avoid if you think you may be sensitive to them.

● **Choose gluten-free beer** If you like beer but cannot tolerate gluten, which is present in many beers, try some of the new sorghum-based beers instead, or other beers made from buckwheat, corn, or rice. Wine is gluten free, as are many spirits, but always check the label carefully.

Sorghum-based beer may be an option for those who cannot tolerate gluten.

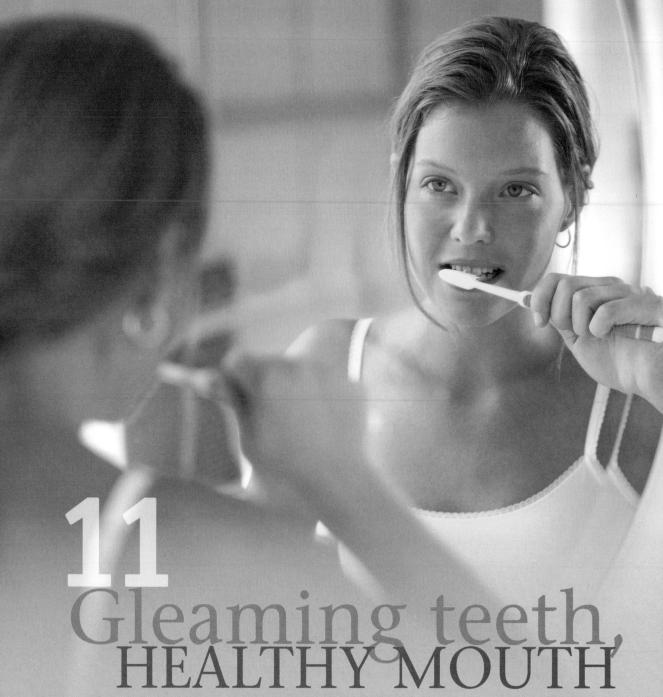

11
Gleaming teeth,
HEALTHY MOUTH

Keeping your mouth infection-free will do far more than give you a sparkling smile and sweet-smelling breath. It could help to ensure that you're protected from other serious disorders, including heart problems. Read on to discover the traditional know-how and up-to-date dental knowledge that will help to keep every part of your mouth in top condition throughout life.

Caring for TEETH AND GUMS

Many of the best disease-fighting foods are crunchy (think fruit, vegetables, whole grains, and nuts), so we need a good set of teeth to eat them. Having healthy gums guards against major health problems too, including clogged arteries and even some types of cancer.

● **Don't rush to brush** Always wait at least 20 minutes—ideally an hour—after you've eaten before brushing your teeth. During this time the mouth is still producing saliva, the body's own mouthwash, which helps to to keep the mouth free from germs. If you clean your teeth immediately after a meal, you risk losing these important benefits.

● **Clean with salt** This traditional tooth-brushing method works because salt is highly effective for killing the plaque-forming bacteria that cause gum disease. Just mix the salt into a paste with a little water, dip in your brush, and get to work. Follow up by brushing with regular toothpaste. An alternative way of giving your mouth the antibacterial benefits of salt is to dissolve a teaspoon of salt in a small glass of warm water and use this mixture as a daily mouthwash.

● **Try lemon and sage** Mix the mashed flesh of a lemon with 1 teaspoon of chopped sage leaves. Add ½ teaspoon of cinnamon oil and 1 teaspoon of orris root powder, then stir in 1 tablespoon of distilled water to make a thick paste. Rub this mixture onto the teeth and gums to help to remove brown stains from teeth and to discourage oral bacteria, which inflame and weaken the gums. Any unused paste will keep for up to 12 months if sealed in a sterilized jar.

BELIEVE IT OR NOT!

Plaque-beating formula
Tomorrow's toothpaste may contain a hefty dose of cranberry extract. US researchers have discovered that cranberries make the teeth slippery, stopping plaque-forming bacteria from getting a hold. They also inhibit the enzymes that the bacteria use to build plaque. Because it is sweetened and diluted, ordinary cranberry juice won't do the trick. So scientists are working on other ways to deliver cranberry, such as using it as a toothpaste ingredient.

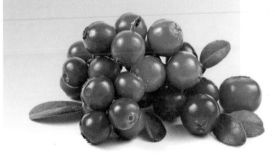

● **Blast with water and air** Even efficient brushing reaches only 60 percent of the tooth surface, which is why flossing (or interdental brushing) is essential. There's nothing new about flossing—evidence exists of it in human remains over 2,000 years old. The latest device for cleaning between the teeth fires bursts of air and water, removing nearly 100 percent more plaque than brushing alone.

● **Set a timer** You need to brush your teeth for 2 minutes to ensure that your mouth is properly clean. But one UK survey estimated that the average brushing time is just 45 seconds. Using an electric toothbrush cleans up to 50 percent more efficiently than manual brushing. Look for an electric toothbrush that makes 40,000 brush strokes a minute and has a built-in 2-minute timer. "Sonic" brushes provide additional cleaning by agitating the mucus around the teeth, which dislodges more dental plaque.

● **Chew gum to combat infection**
Chewing gum, especially after a meal, helps oral health by increasing saliva production. It's most effective if the gum contains xylitol or birch sugar, which can be safely ingested by children. Xylitol suppresses the action of *Streptococcus mutans*, one of the chief bacterial culprits causing tooth decay, and helps to repair damaged tooth enamel.

● **Wipe your baby's teeth** To give your baby's teeth the best possible start, clean them by rubbing with xylitol wipes. This has been shown to significantly reduce the levels of bacteria in a baby's mouth.

● **Sip a daily mug of green tea** and improve your oral health. Researchers in Japan studying men between the ages of 49 and 59 found that those who drank the most green tea showed the fewest symptoms of gum disease. The benefit of green tea is thought to be due to the action of an antioxidant it contains called catechin, which has been shown to reduce the inflammatory effects of oral bacteria.

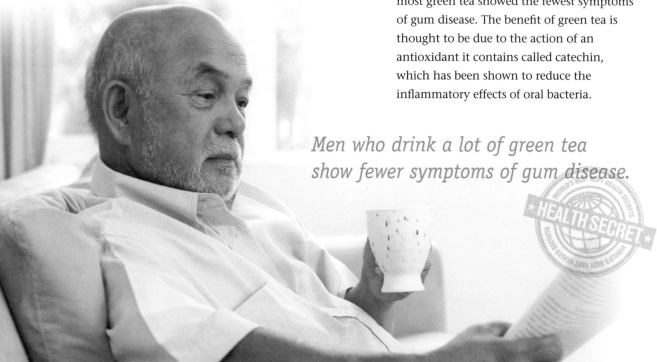

Men who drink a lot of green tea show fewer symptoms of gum disease.

HEALTH SECRET

WHY MOUTH BACTERIA CAN DAMAGE YOUR HEALTH

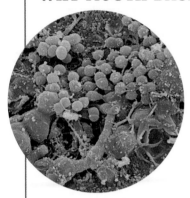

Few people realize why neglecting your teeth can have such a devastating impact on general health. Studies reveal that when streptococcus bacteria, which cause both dental plaque (pictured) and gum disease, enter the bloodstream, they create a protein that makes blood platelets stick together. This can lead to the formation of blood clots, growths on the heart valves that hinder their action, or inflammation of blood vessels, which swell up and block the passage of blood to the heart and brain. *Streptococcus tigurinus*, has been discovered in people suffering from endocarditis (inflammation of the lining of the heart), and from meningitis and spinal inflammation. The bacteria are thought to enter the bloodstream when infected gums bleed.

In a 2011 study, US scientists analyzing tissue samples from people with bowel cancer found that some contain high levels of *Fusobacterium nucleatum*— a strain of bacteria often present in dental plaque. It is thought that this germ may play a part in the growth of the cancer.

What's more, the low-grade inflammation that results from bacterial infection of the gums can contribute to the development of type 2 diabetes, osteoporosis, and when it affects a woman who is pregnant, low birth weight in the baby.

● **Drink licorice** The roots of licorice plants contain the compounds licoricidin and licorisoflavan A, both of which are effective in killing the bacteria responsible for causing dental cavities and gum disease. You can get the benefits of this natural treatment by having a cup of licorice infusion twice a day. Put 1–2 teaspoons of the powdered root in boiling water. Let brew for 10 minutes, then strain and drink. If you have high blood pressure, you should check with your doctor before drinking this infusion regularly.

● **Choose fruit at mealtime** Fruit is an essential part of everyone's diet because it provides vital nutrients and fiber—but you should try to eat it mainly at mealtimes and avoid it between meals. Although the "intrinsic" sugars found in fruit are less directly harmful to your teeth than the refined sugars found in processed foods, they still provide food for the acid-producing bacteria that cause plaque and gum disease. And fruit also contains acid, which can start to wear away tooth enamel if too much is eaten between meals.

● **Tackle teething trouble naturally**
Take the pain out of your baby's teething with one of these natural remedies:
★ **Mix** two drops of clove essential oil with at least 1 tablespoon of vegetable oil and rub this into the gums (test it on yourself first to make sure it is not too strong).
★ **Rub** the gums with one or two drops of chamomile oil up to twice a day, using a wet cotton swab.

● **Check the peroxide level** If you decide to whiten your teeth with a home kit, make sure you check the level of hydrogen

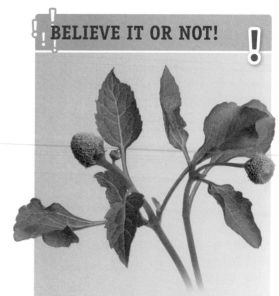

No more needles

An ointment made from the South American plant *Acmella oleracea*, which the ancient Incas used to treat toothache could put an end to painful dental injections. The plant contains the chemical spilanthol. When absorbed through the tissues of the gums, spilanthol can block the pain receptors in the nerves. In 2012, a Cambridge University team in the UK successfully produced a gel from the plant, and the gel is currently undergoing clinical trials.

peroxide carefully—it shouldn't be more than 0.1 percent. Levels higher than this can aggravate gum disease, make the teeth ultra sensitive to heat and cold and, at high levels, even cause chemical burns in the mouth. Always get professional advice from a dentist before using any home treatment for tooth whitening.

● **Guard against grinding** If you grind your teeth at night, you may be doing more than interrupting your partner's sleep. Tooth grinding, or bruxism, can wear down and fracture teeth, bring on headaches, migraines, and tinnitus, and may even cause

disorders of the jaw joints. The most common causes are stress, anxiety, smoking, and alcohol, but grinding can also result from an abnormal alignment of the teeth and jaw, all of which need expert attention. Your dentist may advise you to wear a night guard to protect your teeth or a mandibular advancement device, which holds the lower jaw and tongue forward. Behavioral therapy and hypnosis to combat stress and anxiety have also proved successful in helping to cure the problem.

● **Get help from the kitchen cupboard** To relieve toothache while waiting to see a dentist, apply one of the following tried and trusted home remedies:

★ **Cloves** Apply clove oil or, if this is not available, use whole cloves. Put a few in your mouth, allow them to soften and then bruise them between your back teeth to release their oil. Hold the softened cloves against the painful tooth for up to 30 minutes or until the pain has eased.

★ **Ginger and cayenne** Mix powdered ginger and cayenne pepper with a little water to form a paste. Dab this it on with a cotton ball or swab.

★ **Cabbage leaves** Make a compress from bruised savoy cabbage leaves (from which the tough center stems have been removed) wrapped in a linen bag. Hold this against the cheek over the area of the painful tooth for as long as you like.

● **Get a tonsil check** if your child grinds his or her teeth at night. The problem affects at least one in five children under 11, disturbing sleep and making behavioral problems worse. For reasons that are not fully understood, enlarged tonsils and/or adenoids often occur alongside tooth-grinding, so be sure to bring this problem to the attention of your doctor.

Protect your
MOUTH, LIPS, AND TONGUE

Bad breath, or halitosis, is not just an embarrassing condition—it may also indicate a more serious health problem. Looking after your mouth and tongue will keep halitosis at bay. And don't forget your lips—you never know when you'll need to pucker up.

● **Stimulate saliva** Chewing sugar-free gum can be a quick fix for bad breath if you're unable to brush your teeth. It stimulates the production of saliva, which prevents the mouth from drying out, acting as a natural breath sweetener.

● **Know the drink dangers** For a healthier mouth, cut down on alcohol. When alcohol breaks down in the body it produces acetaldehyde. This chemical reacts with proteins in the mouth to create substances that can block repair of DNA in the protective mucus-producing cells lining the mouth and throat, causing mutations that can result in cancer.

● **Choose alcohol-free mouthwash** It's not just a question of the alcohol you drink—your mouthwash may contain as much as 26 percent alcohol. As well as posing a risk to cells lining the mouth, alcohol-containing mouthwashes dry the mouth, slowing saliva production and creating an environment likely to cause bad breath and exacerbate gum disease.

● **Attack food odors with aniseed** Gargle with an aniseed mouthwash to counteract bad breath caused by foods such as garlic and onions. Put 2 tablespoons of aniseed in a bowl and pour in 3½oz (140ml) of boiling mineral or purified water. Let cool, then strain off the liquid and mix

An aniseed mouthwash can banish pungent food odors.

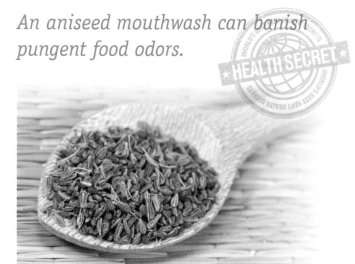

it with 2oz (50ml) of rosewater. Pour the liquid into a dark glass bottle and shake it vigorously. After brushing your teeth, dilute a small amount of the mouthwash in a glass of water and swish it thoroughly around in your mouth for a minute before spitting it out. Do not swallow the mixture.

SUPRISINGLY EASY

Fresh-breath check
Test the freshness of your breath with this simple action. Lick your palm and smell it while it is still wet. If you detect bad odor, then you need to freshen your breath.

An ancient remedy, aloe vera is not just for skin conditions; it can soothe lip sores, too.

● **Track down the cause** It may seem trivial, but bad breath can be the symptom of one of a range of medical conditions—including sinusitis, bronchitis, and tonsillitis. Even the common cold can cause halitosis. Some odors are specific to underlying problems: gallbladder problems produce a heavy, pungent smell, while chronic kidney problems are linked to a fetid, fishy odor. The breath of diabetic people when they need insulin smells like nail-polish remover (acetone), a condition called ketohalitosis. This odor also occurs in people who follow high-protein, low-carbohydrate slimming plans, such as the Atkins Diet. If you have recurrent bad breath with no obvious cause, see your doctor.

● **Scrape your tongue** Use a tongue scraper to keep your breath sweet. Starting at the base of your tongue, place the scraper flush against the surface and make slow, sweeping strokes from the back to the front and from side to side. Pay special attention to the middle and back, where bacteria are most likely to accumulate. Then dab toothpaste on the scraper and carefully coat the tongue with it, reaching as far back as you can without gagging. Leave it on for about 90 seconds, then rinse off with water.

● **Kick the habit** Giving up smoking won't just benefit your heart and lungs—it'll bring big benefits for your mouth. Recent research shows that the mouths of smokers are home to "ecosystems" of unhealthy bacteria that cause high levels of gum disease and destroy healthy oral bacteria. Smoking also increases the risk of mouth cancer. In 2010, a UK study estimated that about 70 percent of cancers of the mouth and throat suffered by men and 55 percent of those suffered by women were due to smoking. Even living with a smoker puts oral health at risk. If you never smoked but are persistently exposed to second-hand smoke at home, in a car, or at work, your risk of oral cancer increases by over 60 percent and rises to more than 80 percent after a period of 15 years or more.

● **Soothe gums with ancient aloe** For more than 2,000 years, the juice of the aloe vera plant has been used to soothe skin conditions, and it's now being recommended by experts in dental health as a treatment for oral problems including cold sores, gum disease, and the uncomfortable rash inside the mouth typical of the condition known as oral lichen planus. Studies in the US found that drinking about ¼ cup (60ml) of aloe vera juice daily or applying aloe vera lip balm to the lips provided effective relief.

● **Herpes 1 or 2? Know the difference** The virus that usually causes cold sores, herpes simplex-1 or HSV-1, is not the same as HSV-2, the usual cause of genital herpes, but both are contagious and can affect both the mouth and the genital area. You can contract genital herpes if HSV-1 when a mouth sore comes into contact with your genital area. Likewise, if HSV-2 comes into contact with your mouth, you can get cold sores, though this is less likely because HSV-2 is fussier about where it lives. What's more, you're most likely to spread the virus to your sexual partner in the first few days when the blisters are forming. The risk of herpes transmission is a clear reason for caution—and condom use.

● **Don't forget your lips** When you're out in the sun, don't forget to apply sunscreen to your lips. Sudden exposure to the sun (or the wind) can quickly reactivate dormant cold sore viruses, resulting in the appearance of a sore that could spoil your vacation fun.

● **Steer clear of foam to avoid cold sores** It's pleasant to have a toothpaste that makes a foam as you brush, but if you're prone to cold sores, check toothpaste ingredients before you buy. Sodium lauryl sulphate (SLS), the ingredient that creates

MIND POWER

Stress causes bad breath
Anxiety can increase your risk of mouth problems. The hormones released when you're anxious dry the mouth by inhibiting the production of saliva. The enzymes in saliva that aid digestion also combat the growth of bacteria in the mouth and so help to keep your breath sweet. If stress is interrupting your sleep, this can exacerbate the problem by interfering with the activity of the immune system.

the bubbles, can also trigger cold sores by causing microscopic damage to the tissues of the mouth. Danish researchers found that people suffering from cold sores who stopped using toothpaste containing SLS for three months saw a 60 to 70 percent improvement in their condition. Since it dries the mouth, SLS can also contribute to gum problems and bad breath.

Sun or wind can reactivate cold sores so protect your lips with sunscreen.

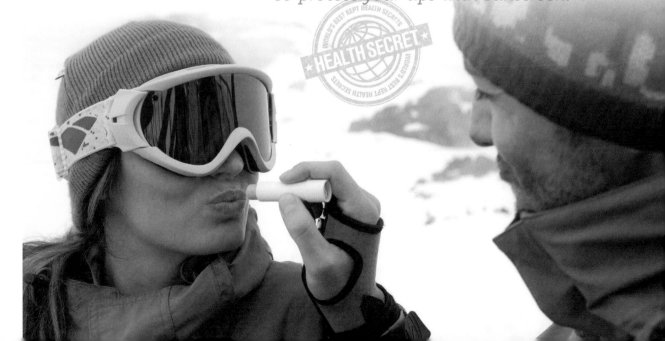

Secrets of HEALTHY TEETH

You might expect the world's wealthiest countries, where good dental health is encouraged, to have the healthiest teeth. But global statistics reveal a surprising truth. Dental health in many of the poorest countries of the world—in parts of Africa and Asia—is much better than that of many populations in the West. The question is why?

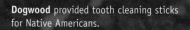

Bundles of neem sticks are displayed in the markets of India and Pakistan.

Dr. Weston A. Price, a dentist from Cleveland, Ohio, traveled the world in the early 20th century, visiting isolated communities, from Indians in South America and the Polynesians of the South Sea Islands to African tribes. He was on a mission to discover why these people had such fine teeth compared with city dwellers. Weston found that these communities had certain things in common: Their diets had several times the amount of minerals—such as calcium, phosphorus, iron, and magnesium—than those in the industrial West. They also contained more than 10 times the amount of fat-soluble vitamins (A, D, E, and K), most of which came from animal sources such as butter, fish, eggs, shellfish, and meat, including offal.

Patterns of decay

Weston was on to something, as data compiled by the World Health Organization (WHO) shows. The WHO has been tracking the dental health of 12-year-olds and adults around the world for 40 years, and definite trends have emerged. Developed countries have higher rates of DMFT (Decayed, Missing, and Filled Teeth) than do developing countries among both 12-year-olds and 35 to 44-year-olds. In the adult group the difference is pronounced, and the Americas, Western Europe, and Australia are clearly the worst affected. However, over recent decades the rate of DMFT has been falling among children in developed countries due to improved dental self-care, lifestyle, and public health measures, such as water fluoridation.

Dogwood provided tooth cleaning sticks for Native Americans.

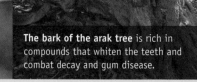

The bark of the arak tree is rich in compounds that whiten the teeth and combat decay and gum disease.

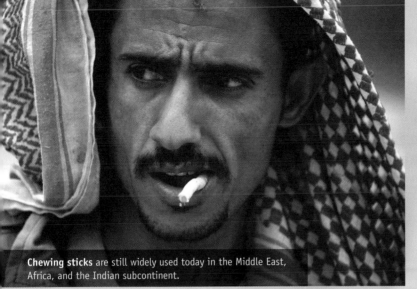

Chewing sticks are still widely used today in the Middle East, Africa, and the Indian subcontinent.

Tooth and gum health without dentistry

Many people in developing countries do not use any of the manufactured dental care products common in the West. Instead, they take care of their teeth and gums with natural cleaning methods—chewing sticks and plant-based mouthwashes—and by following a traditional diet. Yet in some developing countries, DMFT rates have been slowly but steadily rising among 12-year-olds, a trend that the WHO attributes to changes in diet and expects to continue, "particularly as a result of a growing consumption of sugars and inadequate exposure to fluorides."

Learning from traditional dental care

The *miswak*, or chewing stick, is a traditional way to keep teeth and gums clean and healthy throughout Africa, the Middle East, and parts of Asia. It is made from the roots, twigs, or bark of trees or plants that have properties beneficial to dental health—in fact, modern toothbrushes and interdental brushes employ similar principles for cleaning teeth and gums, and keeping decay and infection at bay. Here you will learn how to make and use chewing sticks along with other tips for tooth and gum care:

Natural toothbrush To make a natural toothbrush as used in traditional societies, buy chewing sticks of one of the different types described below from an African, Asian, or Arab food shop. Chew a piece of your chosen twig until the end becomes frayed, and use this to clean around and between your teeth, and to massage the gums.

● **Arak** This is the Arabic name for *Salvadora persica*, also known as the toothbrush tree in English and the *mswaki* in Swahili. It is common throughout the Middle East and in several African countries. Research suggests that the tree contains substances that benefit dental health, including: silica and sodium bicarbonate, which whiten the teeth; tannic acid, which removes plaque and protects against gum disease; antibacterial sulphur compounds; fluoride, which counters decay; and calcium, which benefits tooth enamel. Arak chewing sticks are so effective that their use is advocated by the WHO.

● **Licorice root** The licorice plant, *Glycyrrhiza glabra,* became popular as a chewing stick in Europe during the 15th century and is used in India today. It has been shown to reduce plaque and has an antibacterial effect.

● **The neem tree** The people of rural India and Pakistan chew neem sticks throughout the day. As it is chewed, the wood of this tropical evergreen tree, *Azadirachta indica*, releases an oil that is highly effective in killing the *Staphylococcus mutans* bacteria responsible for plaque and tooth decay. At the same time, the chewing action stimulates the production of saliva, which also helps to keeps the mouth healthy.

Natural mouthwash Infuse hawthorn berry (dried or tincture), licorice, or cinnamon bark with warm water to create a natural herbal mouthwash.

Eat healthy Eating lots of fresh fruit and vegetables, along with protein obtained from meat, fish, and dairy products, should provide you with enough minerals and vitamins to promote healthy gums and teeth. Avoid snacking on fruit, fruit juice, or smoothies between meals—eat them as part of a main meal to minimize the impact of fruit acids on your tooth enamel. And minimize the amount of processed foods you eat.

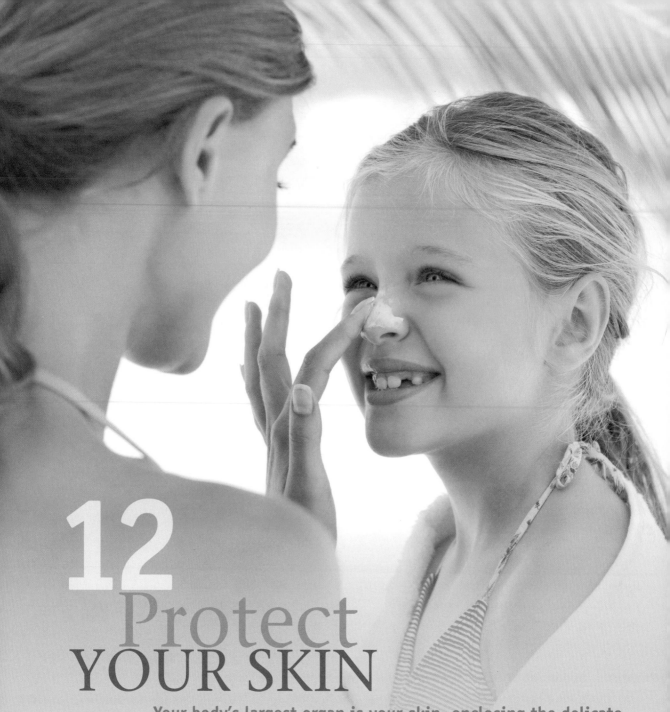

12
Protect
YOUR SKIN

Your body's largest organ is your skin, enclosing the delicate tissues beneath and shielding you from the elements. It is also the first line of defense against germs and damaging substances in the environment. Yet doctors may treat a specific problem but rarely advise on general skin care. Read on to discover top tips that will help you keep your skin healthy throughout life.

Essential
SKIN CARE

Your skin is protected against everyday damage by natural oils and constantly renews and repairs itself throughout your life. You can help these natural processes by taking a variety of simple measures while being alert for signs of disease.

● **Get sweaty** It may have a bad reputation, but sweat is actually essential for healthy skin. Sweating is nature's way of eliminating toxic chemicals that build up under the skin. So don't avoid exercise on a hot day, and make sure you work up a sweat with a regular run, bike ride, or a stint of strenuous gardening. Saunas and steam treatments can provide similar sweat-stimulating skincare benefits.

● **Avoid sunburn, not sun** Many of us fear exposing our skin to the sun at all, in case we damage it—but sunshine is essential to health. The latest medical advice is to expose as much of your body as possible to sunlight, without sunscreen, for about 10 minutes a day when it's sunny—less if you're very fair-skinned and more if your skin is darker. Even this short exposure will boost the body's production of vitamin D, which protects against some forms of cancer and strengthens bones.

But if you're out in the sun for longer periods, take the following precautions:

★ **Use sunscreen** with a sun protection factor (SPF) of 15 or more.

★ **Choose a broad-spectrum sunscreen** to protect against both UVA and UVB rays.

★ **Use at least two tablespoons** of sunscreen to cover the whole body.

★ **Re-apply sunscreen** at least every 2 hours and after going in the water, even if it's labelled waterproof.

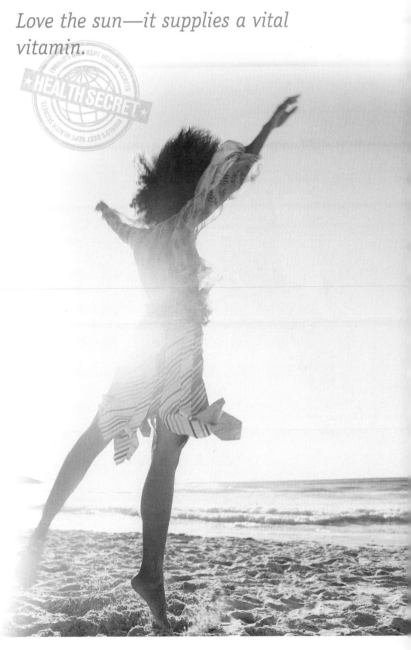

Love the sun—it supplies a vital vitamin.

HEALTH SECRET

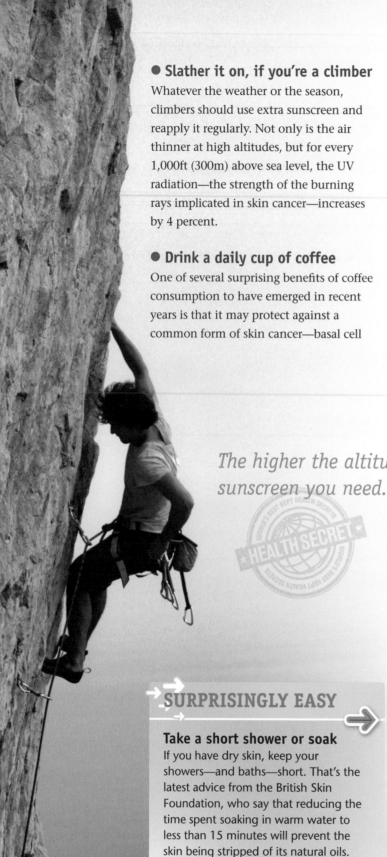

● Slather it on, if you're a climber

Whatever the weather or the season, climbers should use extra sunscreen and reapply it regularly. Not only is the air thinner at high altitudes, but for every 1,000ft (300m) above sea level, the UV radiation—the strength of the burning rays implicated in skin cancer—increases by 4 percent.

● Drink a daily cup of coffee

One of several surprising benefits of coffee consumption to have emerged in recent years is that it may protect against a common form of skin cancer—basal cell carcinoma (BCC). Around 30 percent of Caucasians develop this type of skin tumor at some time in their lives. The most common area to be affected is the face. US research suggests that just one cup of coffee a day reduces the risk of developing BCC by 20 percent.

● Consider the skin benefits of HRT

The estrogen component of hormone replacement therapy (HRT) for menopausal symptoms counteracts the slowdown of oil-producing glands that normally follows menopause, helping keep skin thicker and more supple longer. If you are already having HRT, you may want to extend the duration of the therapy to benefit your skin. Current UK guidelines recommend that HRT should be taken in the lowest possible dose

The higher the altitude, the more sunscreen you need.

for the shortest possible time—but in light of studies showing that estrogen also reduces the risk of breast cancer, many gynecologists now believe that the treatment can be taken for longer. Ask your doctor if an extended period of HRT may be suitable for you, but remember, this drug treatment will not be prescribed for cosmetic reasons alone.

● Save on skincare products

Don't spend too much on over-the-counter anti-aging creams. Some do have an effect on wrinkles: They stimulate the production of fibrillin-1, a protein that makes the skin more elastic. In one small study carried out by Manchester University in the UK, 70 percent of those tested with one cream had significantly fewer wrinkles compared with

→ SURPRISINGLY EASY

Take a short shower or soak
If you have dry skin, keep your showers—and baths—short. That's the latest advice from the British Skin Foundation, who say that reducing the time spent soaking in warm water to less than 15 minutes will prevent the skin being stripped of its natural oils.

those who used a placebo. But when a team from the UK consumer organization Which? tested 12 antiwrinkle eye creams, the difference between the cheapest and most expensive was found to be minimal.

● Use sunscreen, not face cream

If you want to keep those wrinkles at bay, the best anti-aging remedy is a good sunscreen. Modern sunscreens are widely acknowledged by dermatologists as the best way of preventing skin aging. They limit deep collagen and elastin damage by protecting against both UVA and UVB rays.

● Get plant protection Plants add

moisture to the air in your home in two ways: First, as the plant's leaves transpire, releasing water into the air; and second, as water evaporates from the damp soil in which they grow. By boosting the humidity of the air in your home, houseplants help to keep your skin moist—and also enhance your home.

● Lift baggy eyes with exercise

If you're tired, your eyes are baggy and your skin isn't looking great, get some gentle exercise in the evening. This will improve your skin condition by boosting circulation

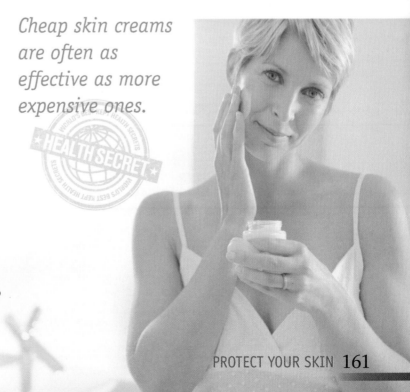

Cheap skin creams are often as effective as more expensive ones.

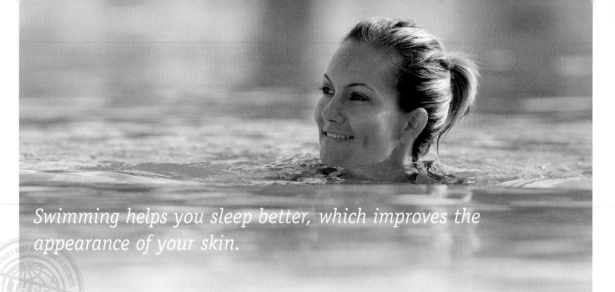

Swimming helps you sleep better, which improves the appearance of your skin.

and reducing stress-related blotchiness, redness, or itching. But perhaps the most effective way in which exercise benefits the skin is by promoting sleep. Try gentle exercise, such as swimming or yoga, to induce healthy tiredness, thereby breaking the skin-damaging cycle of lack of sleep, irritability, anxiety, and depression.

● **Moisturize when it's cold** Take special care of your skin in winter—cold air outside and central heating inside result in drier skin. If you have oily skin, the cold dry air may mean fewer spots or blemishes. But normal or dry skin is more likely to become flaky, itchy, cracked, or rough, which can lead to premature wrinkling over time. Here are some simple steps you can take to reduce the effects of winter weather on your skin:

★ **Keep an eye** on your skin's moisture level. From time to time, scratch a small area with a fingernail; if it turns white, the skin needs extra moisture and exfoliation.

★ **Use cleansing cream**, not soap, especially on your face, since soap removes the protective oils from your skin.

★ **Use a heavier than usual**, oil-based facial moisturizing cream to finish your cleansing routine. Don't ignore the delicate thin skin on your hands, neck, and chest.

★ **Smooth a couple of drops** of olive oil over your face, elbows, knees, and the backs of your arms every evening, if it feels soothing. The monosaturated fat in olive oil refreshes and hydrates the skin without leaving a greasy residue.

● **Avoid aftershave,** especially alcohol-based products, if you have skin that tends to become inflamed after shaving. To prevent an outbreak of irritated skin, the Mayo Clinic also recommends that you always soak your face in warm water first, use a clean, sharp razor blade, shave in the direction of hair growth, and rinse well afterward. Try using a soothing moisturizer as an alternative to aftershave to complete your shaving routine.

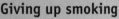

SECRETS OF SUCCESS

Giving up smoking

"Smoker's face" is a medical term for the lines and wrinkles—typically radiating at right angles from the upper and lower lips—that develop on the faces of people who smoke. But it's not just the wrinkled face that characterizes the persistent smoker. US researchers recently found that loss of skin elasticity on the upper arms was "significantly" linked to the number of cigarettes smoked per day. And studies on identical twins, only one of whom smoked, revealed that the smoker's skin was up to 40 percent thinner than that of the nonsmoking twin.

Treating
SKIN PROBLEMS

Numerous conditions—from acne to allergies and, more seriously, cancer—can affect the skin. On the following pages you'll find a wide range of topical treatments, diet suggestions, and home remedies that can help to improve your skin's health.

● **Give up milk to beat acne** A study at the Harvard School of Public Health found a clear link between teenage acne and drinking milk. And those who drank skim milk were found to be just as likely to develop acne as those who opted for the full-fat variety. The researchers speculate that the high hormone content of milk may be to blame. Whether that's true or not, if you have acne, try cutting out milk and milk products, but be sure to eat plenty of calcium-rich foods of other types, such as sardines, soybeans, and figs.

● **Laser your pimples** Ground-breaking laser therapy developed as a cosmetic treatment to smooth wrinkles and sun damage is now being used to treat severe acne. Laser therapy can reach the deeper layers of skin and halt the overproduction of sebum, preventing acne from developing. It also seems to promote the formation of new collagen below and around the affected areas, smoothing and improving the skin condition. If you suffer from severe acne, ask your doctor about laser treatment.

● **Treat dry skin with aloe vera**
Cleopatra insisted that aloe vera was the best beauty treatment; if she suffered from dry skin, then she was right, according to the Mayo Clinic. Studies have confirmed the moisturizing value of the gel that accumulates inside the large fleshy leaves of

---

BELIEVE IT OR NOT!

Nature's antibiotic
A special type of honey is proving effective at treating stubborn wounds that don't respond to normal antibiotics. In fact, honey was a common wound treatment right up until World War II, when antibiotics took over as the main weapon against infection. Today, researchers at Cardiff Metropolitan University say that honey—made by bees foraging in the manuka trees of New Zealand and Australia—is more effective than antibiotics at treating wounds that won't heal. It seems that manuka honey can also kill wound-associated bacteria that have become resistant to antibiotics, such as MRSA (methicillin-resistant *Staphylococcus aureus*). Scientists are currently seeking ways to include manuka honey in new antibacterial agents that can be applied directly to stubborn skin wounds as a supplementary therapy to antibiotics.

---

this desert-loving plant. You can grow the plant indoors and make your own aloe vera gel—or you can buy it from a natural health store.

● **Soothe your sunburn** In summer be prepared to treat mild sunburn with a natural skin cooler made from plants you can grow at home—aloe and marigolds.

Blend the gel from two mature fresh aloe leaves with four fresh marigold flowerheads and 16 drops of lavender essential oil. Freeze the mixture in an ice cube tray. Keep the cubes in the freezer and apply them as required to sun-reddened skin. They'll melt quickly to produce masses of soothing gel that will cool and moisturize your skin and limit the damage. But be sure to consult your doctor if the sunburn seems severe.

● **Have some ice cream** As with a burn anywhere else on your body, the best thing you can do to a scalded mouth is cool it down. Rinsing and gargling with cold water for 5 or 10 minutes until the pain eases is one way. An even faster method, particularly popular with children, is to dig into ice cream as quickly as possible. A scoop (or three) eaten soon after the burn is deliciously soothing.

● **Hasten burn healing with food**

If you've suffered a burn, you can help your skin to repair itself more quickly with a few changes to your diet. The healing process makes extra demands on your reserves, and after a burn, fluids, minerals, and essential fatty acids can be depleted. So it makes sense to adjust your intake of key nutrients.

★ **Drink water** and avoid alcohol and diuretics (fluid depleting substances) such as tea, coffee, and cola.

★ **Go for vitamins A, C, and E** to boost collagen production, the tough protein found in the dermis, which is particularly important for speeding the healing of wounds and burns.

★ **Get potassium** from bananas, grapes, and vegetable soups.

★ **Top off your calcium** from milk and other dairy products, tahini (sesame seed paste), and tofu (soybean curd).

Ice cream quickly soothes a scalded mouth.

● **Take fish oil to protect your baby** from eczema. This was the conclusion of an Australian study of more than 700 pregnant women with an inherited tendency to allergies. The results suggested that these essential fatty acids, found in fish oil, could pass across the placenta to the unborn baby and provide protection against allergic skin reactions in the first few months of life. If you have a family history of childhood eczema or other allergic conditions, consider taking fish oil during pregnancy, but be sure to ask your doctor's advice first.

● **Don't install a water softener** if your only reason for doing this is to prevent or alleviate eczema in your child. A UK study concluded that, contrary to a widely held belief, softened water provided no added reduction in eczema symptoms in children over that provided by standard treatments alone.

● **Avoid the soft touch** If you suffer from eczema, don't add fabric softener to the final rinse when washing your clothes or bed linens. You might think that such products, which make fabrics more pleasant to the touch, would be good for you. In fact, the reverse is true, and highly perfumed

softeners are often the worst offenders. The products leave residues that can irritate the skin. Try doing without them and see if your eczema improves.

● **Tape it** To get rid of troublesome warts and verrucas (plantar warts), cover them with duct tape, after soaking the affected area in warm water and gently rubbing it with a pumice stone. Renew the tape each week. Studies show that in seven out of ten cases, the wart will disappear within four weeks, avoiding the need for pricey over-the-counter treatments. If the wart or verruca is not causing a problem, you can safely leave it alone—most disappear within ten weeks and the rest within two years.

MIND POWER

Laugh away your eczema

A really good giggle reduces levels of the body chemicals that are involved in the allergic responses that produce some types of eczema. When Japanese allergy specialist Hajime Kimata assessed 26 eczema patients who had just watched Charlie Chaplin's *Modern Times*, there was a significant reduction in the skin disorder— a result not replicated when the same group watched a factual program, in this case, a weather forecast.

Fabric softener leaves irritant residues that can provoke eczema.

Secrets of
THE BEST SKIN FOODS

What you eat contributes more to skin health than many people realize. Eating healthily will show directly in your skin's appearance —as will eating unhealthily. Some nutrients also enhance the skin when applied externally, as women across history and throughout the world have known.

Modern science has revealed strong evidence for the benefits of particular nutrients and exactly how they improve the condition of skin. Fruit, vegetables and fish have all been found to be vital for skin health. And it's not just a question of what you eat. Throughout history, women have also applied food ingredients directly to their skin to enhance their complexions.

Food for your face

The following nutrients have been proven to maintain and improve the health and appearance of skin. They are all present in foods you can easily include in your daily diet. To keep your skin well hydrated, which helps to prevent lines and wrinkles, it is also important to drink plenty of fluids.

Antioxidants in foods rich in vitamins A, C, and E are essential for the production of collagen, a group of fibrous proteins present throughout the body. Sometimes referred to as the body's glue, collagen plays a vital role in maintaining the firmness and elasticity of skin. Antioxidants tone the skin as well as strengthening the tiny blood vessels in its surface and boosting its healing process. To obtain a range of antioxidants, eat rainbow-colored fruit and vegetables, from carrots and pumpkins to broccoli, avocados and peppers. Add berries such as strawberries and black currants to get the best of everything.

Lycopene A phytonutrient found in red fruit and vegetables, such as tomatoes, pomegranates, and peppers, lycopene protects against premature aging of the skin and, in particular, from the harmful effects of sunburn. In one study, eating lycopene-rich tomato paste daily was found to reduce skin damage caused by exposure to the sun by 40 percent.

Omega-3s These fatty acids found in high concentrations in oily fish such as salmon, mackerel, and sardines are vital to the health of skin cells. Skin experts recommend that you eat oily fish at least twice a week. If you don't

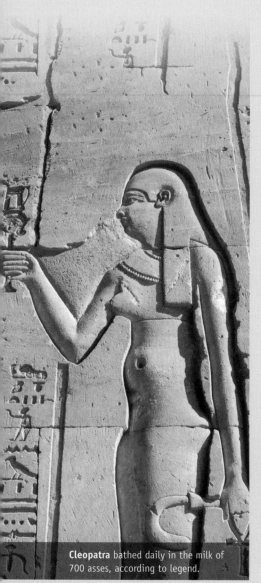

Cleopatra bathed daily in the milk of 700 asses, according to legend.

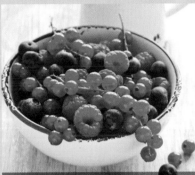

Currants and berries are rich in skin-healing antioxidants.

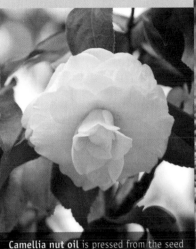

Camellia nut oil is pressed from the seed pods of the white Japanese camellia.

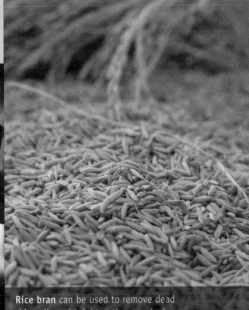

Rice bran can be used to remove dead skin cells and brighten the complexion.

eat fish, you can obtain omega-3s from flaxseed (linseed) oil or from supplements.

B vitamins, especially B12, are vital for the growth and division of cells. Remember that your skin is constantly replacing dead cells with new ones, and it needs plenty of nutritious support. Any protein from an animal source is rich in B vitamins—especially eggs, white fish, seafood, lean meat, and dairy products. Non-animal sources include green vegetables, seeds, and dried fruit.

Zinc is a mineral found mainly in shellfish but also in legumes, pumpkin seeds, whole-wheat bread, and other whole grains. It boosts the skin's ability to heal and helps prevent skin infections.

Fluids Keeping your body hydrated is essential for your skin's health. Drink plenty of non-alcoholic liquids, including herbal teas and juices, but go easy on caffeinated teas, coffee, or cola. Green tea, rich in antioxidants, is especially good for the skin.

Edible cosmetics

Here are some ideas from around the world for nourishing your skin by applying food ingredients from your pantry.

Fruit face mask Mash the flesh of a soft fruit to a pulp and rub it gently into your skin. Leave it to absorb for a few minutes before rinsing it off. Indonesian women say that mango flesh is best for unblocking pores and toning skin; French women prefer to use freshly cut grapes.

Olive oil skin soother Italian women have traditionally used olive oil as a lip balm, while Greek women massage it into dry or sunburned skin. In Asia, women use white camellia nut oil to moisturize and soften skin and also to reduce stretch marks.

Carbohydrate eye firmers A traditional beauty tip from Spain is to apply thin slices of potato beneath the eyes for 10 minutes to make dark circles fade after a night of partying. Japanese women splash the water used to rinse rice on their faces, which is said to smooth the skin.

Oatmeal skin relief Finely ground oatmeal added to a warm bath is a European folk remedy that works for soothing itchy and irritated skin. Also used in face masks, oats seem to have moisturizing properties and protect the skin against irritants.

Grainy exfoliator Japanese women have used grains to gently exfoliate their skin for centuries. Rice bran and adzuki beans are the most widely used. Rice bran is made from the brown outer layer of the rice kernel. It's rich in oil and contains phytic acid, a substance that stimulates the exfoliation process, which helps your skin to replace dead cells. Indian women also use rice as a facial scrub.

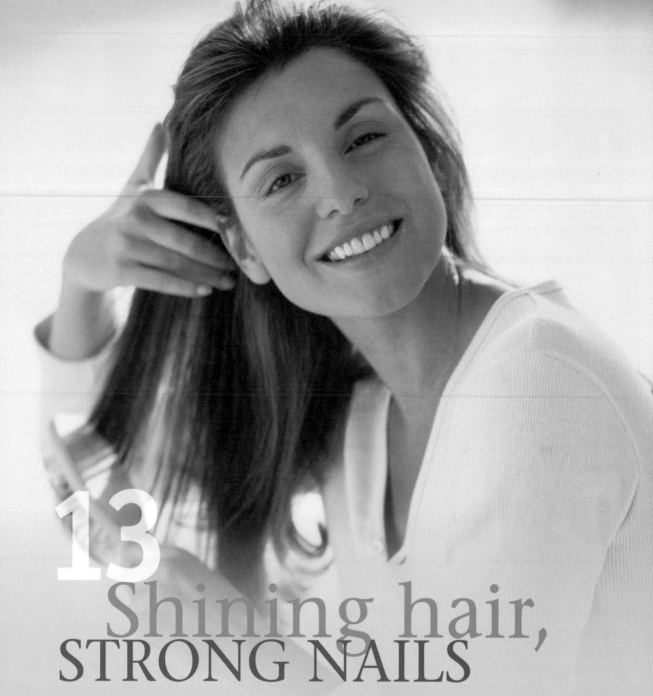

13
Shining hair,
STRONG NAILS

When it comes to looking and feeling good, healthy hair and nails have an important role to play. But caring for them is not just about looks and self-confidence. Their condition is also a barometer of your overall health, so it would be foolish to ignore them. In this chapter you'll find lots of tips to keep hair and nails in good shape.

Caring for YOUR HAIR

We can all have bad hair days and styling is not the only problem. Hair can become greasy, dandruff may take a hold, and hairlines may recede. But there's a lot you can do to keep your hair and scalp in top condition and counter hair loss. Here are some tips.

● **Don't brush your hair** or at least don't brush it too vigorously or for too long. Following the traditional advice of "a hundred strokes before bedtime" is now known to risk damaging the hair. Brushing pulls out hair that isn't ready to fall out, often breaks healthy hairs, and scratches the scalp. Brush gently for styling only—not to stimulate the scalp.

● **Dye naturally** If you want to color or lighten your hair without resorting to the chemicals of commercial hair dyes, why not choose herbal preparations such as henna for a shining brown or chamomile to lift mousey to blonde. But be warned, while natural dyes are better for you, they can be messy to apply and the results are not always totally reliable. If you decide to use a commercial hair dye, choose a temporary or semipermanent one, simply because there is a very small increased risk of breast and bladder cancer associated with the long-term use of permanent dyes. Whatever dye you choose, test a little on an unobtrusive patch before treating your whole head.

● **Rinse with herbs** Calm over-greasy hair with this leave-in herbal conditioner treatment, which can help to reduce the amount of oily sebum produced by the sebaceous glands in hair follicles. Mix a teaspoon each of dried rosemary leaves, dried chamomile flowers, and dried stinging nettle leaves in a bowl and pour on ½ cup (about 100ml) of water and a tablespoon of fruit vinegar. Leave for 10 minutes then strain. Apply this liquid to damp hair after washing and leave it in without rinsing.

Using natural products eliminates the slight risk of cancer associated with permanent dyes.

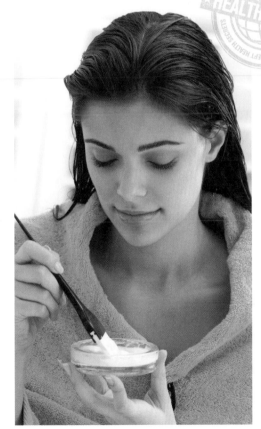

● **Combat dandruff with coal tar**
For hard-to-treat dandruff, often associated with infection by the yeast-like organism *Malassezia globosa*, try shampoos containing coal tar. It has natural antifungal properties. Products that contain salicylic acid, which helps to dissolve away dead cells that accumulate on the scalp, are also effective. Tea tree oil, now included in many shampoos, is another effective antifungal agent. Make sure to change the type of product you use every few months, because the micro-organisms that cause dandruff quickly build up resistance.

● **Try flaxseed oil for an itchy scalp** whether caused by dandruff or seborrhoeic eczema (a more severe condition that results in thick, greasy, yellow-colored scales on the scalp). A tablespoon of flaxseed oil twice each day may help counter irritation by reducing inflammation. For best effect, take the supplement with food to maximize absorption. Be patient—it can take up to three months before you notice a significant difference. If you prefer, you can massage the oil into the scalp.

● **Make the most of minerals** To keep hair strong and healthy, make sure you're getting enough zinc and iron, but ask your doctor before using supplements if you're taking prescription drugs:

★ **Zinc** This mineral helps hair to grow strongly and prevents it from becoming fragile or falling out. Meat, seafood, and dairy foods are the best dietary sources. If taking a supplement, be careful not to exceed the recommended dose—too much zinc can impair the immune system.

★ **Iron** A key ingredient of hemoglobin, the oxygen-carrying component of red blood cells, iron is vital for healthy hair. In one study, 72 percent of women with thinning hair were found to be deficient in iron. Take it as part of a multivitamin supplement or get it from foods such as leafy green vegetables and red meat.

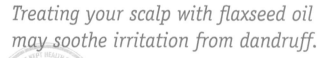

Treating your scalp with flaxseed oil may soothe irritation from dandruff.

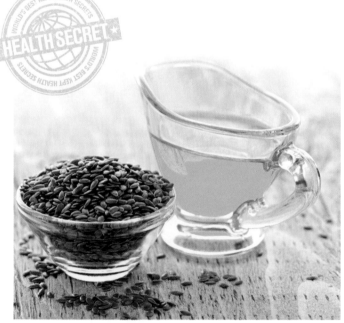

● **Kill head lice with fragrant oil**
Avoid or reduce chemical treatments for
head lice by combing essential oil of
lavender or ylang ylang through the hair
daily using a fine comb designed for the
purpose. The oil will make the hair slippery
and prevent the eggs (nits) from sticking
and adult lice from gripping the hairs. It will
also kill the adult lice by clogging up their
breathing pores. Before you comb, wet the
hair. Use the oils carefully and stop at once
if the scalp stings, burns, or becomes itchy.
You can use standard hair conditioner as
an alternative.

● **Banish with a pill** If you or a member
of your family is plagued by recurrent head
lice infestations, it may be encouraging to
know that tests with a drug, invermectin,
are proving very successful. Taken orally,
invermectin can work in a single dose,
saving repeated applications of unpleasant
chemicals. The drug is available only with a
prescription, so ask your doctor if this might
be suitable for you or your child.

● **Get your hormones checked** If bald
patches develop on your head, or if your
hair starts to falls out for no apparent
reason, you may have a hormone problem.
Consult your doctor, in case treatment is
needed to restore your hormone balance to

*Head lice can be eliminated by daily
combing with essential oils.*

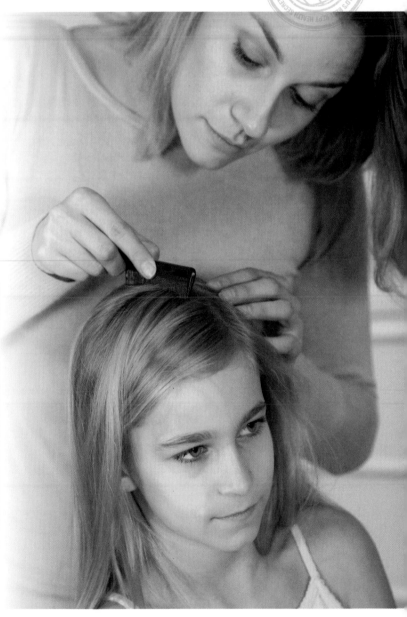

❄ MIND POWER

Worry can make your hair fall out

Severe stress—which can be caused by
any of the traumatic events that occur
during life—can cause hair to fall out. All
hair follicles normally undergo periodic
"rest" periods and sudden stress can
cause them to enter this resting phase
prematurely, making the hair fall out in
the three months following the event.
Normally hair growth restores itself
naturally, but it is important to deal with
stress and to seek medical advice to rule
out any underlying illness, hormonal
imbalance, or drug side effects.

Nettles may help to slow male pattern baldness.

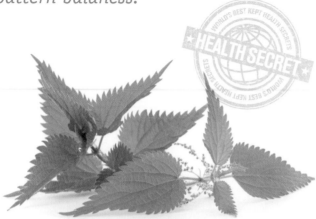

normal. An under or overactive thyroid gland can cause hair loss or thinning, as can an imbalance of androgens and estrogens—the male and female sex hormones.

● **Put egg on your hair**—at least if it's dry. This is a traditional, but effective treatment for dry, brittle, and lifeless hair. Mix one whipped egg white with two egg yolks, a teaspoon of honey, a tablespoon of olive oil, and the juice of a lemon. Apply the mixture to your hair and scalp and massage thoroughly, then leave for a few minutes before rinsing. The condition of your hair should improve within a few weeks with regular applications.

● **Cool solution** A process called scalp cooling may prevent hair loss in people undergoing chemotherapy. It involves wearing a cap that is filled with a chilled gel or liquid coolant for 30 to 40 minutes prior to chemotherapy. Cooling restricts the blood flow to the scalp. This reduces the amount of the drug that reaches the follicles, making it less likely that they will be damaged. It does not work with all cancer types and treatments. Your oncologist will advise you.

● **Keep your hair** Male pattern baldness, a hereditary condition, is the usual reason why men (and some women) lose their hair as they age. If you want to try to stimulate regrowth, here are some options:

★ **Massage with nettles** Preparations made from the stinging nettle plant (*Urtica dioica*) may prevent testosterone from being converted into dihydrotestosterone (DHT)—a reaction believed to be key in causing hair to fall out. You can buy nettle supplements and nettle-extract shampoos.

★ **Apply nasturtium and thyme lotion** Nasturtium contains sulphur which can help to combat hair loss. Soak ¼ cup (55g) dried nasturtium seeds and leaves and ¼ cup (55g) dried thyme in 4 cups (1L) of vodka for 10 days. Strain and massage the lotion into your scalp daily.

★ **Topical treatment** Available in pharmacies as a solution called Rogaine, minoxidil is a drug that was originally used to treat high blood pressure, but which has proved effective in stimulating limited regrowth of hair lost as a result of male pattern baldness.

★ **By mouth** Finasteride (Propecia), a drug also used to treat benign enlargement of the prostate gland, has an 80 percent success rate in restoring hair growth in men suffering from male pattern baldness. You will need to get a prescription from your doctor for this drug and check with your health plan to see if the cost is covered.

★ **Brew up** The antioxidants found in green tea can stimulate follicles and promote stronger, thicker hair growth. Steep two green tea bags in a cup of boiling water and apply the tea to the scalp while it is still warm (but not hot). Leave it in place for an hour before rinsing it off.

★ **Eat a variety** of brightly colored fruit and vegetables, which will add antioxidants to your diet, to boost hair growth.

Looking after
YOUR NAILS

Made of a hard protein called keratin, our nails protect the tips of the fingers and toes, and enhance our sense of touch and fine motor skills. When they become brittle, discolored, or infected, they need attention. Try these tips for keeping your nails healthy and strong.

● **Fight fungus with tea tree** Fungal infections can be treated by brushing tea tree oil on affected nails and cuticles twice a day. The oil, from the leaves of the tree *Melaleuca alternifolia*, has been used for centuries by indigenous Australians to combat infections of the skin and nails. For best results, use the pure oil. Rub in plenty of moisturizer before applying it, since hard, dry tissues around the nail can form an impenetrable barrier to the oil.

● **Wear cotton socks** Fungal infections flourish in moist conditions. Keep your feet dry by wearing 100 percent cotton socks, which are best at absorbing moisture, and

change them daily. Other tips for turning your feet into a fungus-unfriendly environment include:

★ **Dry your toes** thoroughly for at least 2 minutes after swimming or showering.

★ **Air out sneakers and work shoes** overnight after you've worn them. Ideally, have an extra pair of each, so that you don't wear the same shoes two days in a row.

● **Drink filtered water** You need to drink plenty of water to keep the nail bed hydrated and nail growth healthy, but chlorine in tap water can weaken the nail. If possible, drink water with the chlorine filtered out—a standard water filter will do

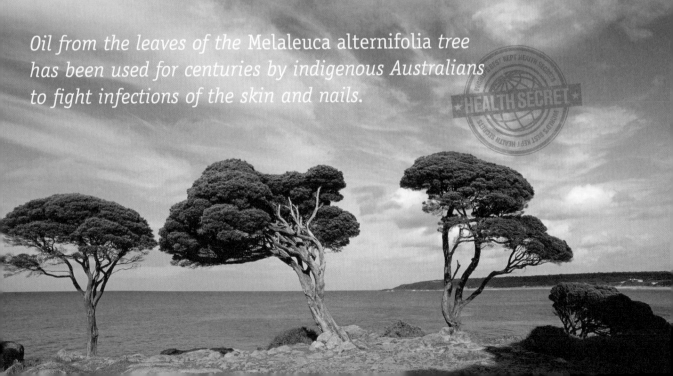

Oil from the leaves of the Melaleuca alternifolia *tree has been used for centuries by indigenous Australians to fight infections of the skin and nails.*

HEALTH SECRET

Fungal fix

To help prevent fungal infections of the feet, kick off your socks and shoes—and go barefoot whenever it's warm enough. The more fresh air you can get to your feet, the better fungal growth will be inhibited.

the job. Maintaining adequate hydration is especially important during menopause, when reduced levels of estrogen can contribute to brittle nails.

● **Strengthen your nails with silica**
This mineral promotes strong nails, so if your nails are thin and brittle, increase your silica levels with an infusion of the horsetail plant. This silica-rich plant was used by the English 17th-century herbalist Nicolas Culpepper and by native Americans to promote wound healing. You can buy ready-made horsetail preparations or make your own by infusing 2–4g of the dried plant in 7oz (200ml) of boiling water for 10 to 15 minutes. Drink a cup of the cooled infusion daily. Other ways of getting more silica from your diet include eating leafy green vegetables, oats, and soy products. Taking a flaxseed (linseed) supplement can also provide the silica you need.

● **Cover up** Paradoxically, immersing your hands in water while washing up or other chores can weaken your nails by robbing them of moisture, so make sure you protect them with rubber gloves.

● **Stay well oiled** Keep nails hydrated by rubbing castor oil into your cuticles and the skin around your nails every night before bed. As a bonus, you'll also be adding vitamin E, which is excellent for keeping the cuticles in good condition, softening them, and preventing them from cracking.

● **Maximize nail strength with minerals** Make sure you get the right minerals in your diet to maintain the strength of your nails. These include:
★ **Calcium** is an essential component of nails. It is found in milk and dairy products, and in green leafy vegetables, and its absorption is boosted by vitamin D (made by the body in response to sunlight) and L-lysine (an amino acid found in soybeans, legumes, and Parmesan cheese).
★ **Zinc** is particularly important for the prevention of white spots in the nails. This mineral is present in meat, shellfish, whole-grain cereals, and dairy products.

● **Benefit from biotin** Also known as vitamin H, biotin can combat thin, brittle nails. In US studies, women receiving a daily 2.5mg biotin supplement for six months experienced improvements in nail thickness of up to 25 percent and a reduction in splitting. Biotin appears to work by being absorbed into the core of the nail, where new cells are generated. To include natural

An infusion of the horsetail plant may strengthen your nails.

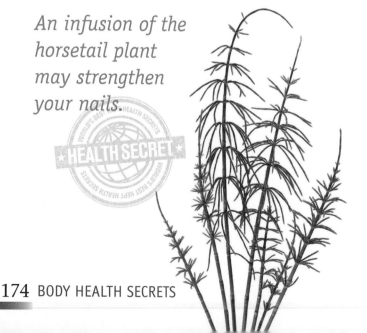

TELLTALE NAIL CHANGES

The condition of your nails can say a lot about your health.
Be alert to any changes and discuss them with your doctor.

Type of change	What it may indicate
Pits in the nails	Can indicate the skin conditions psoriasis and eczema, alopecia areata (patchy baldness), or reactive arthritis—a condition in which the immune system attacks the joints and muscles.
Horizontal ridges or depressions	Known as Beau's lines, these often appear after serious infections and following chemotherapy. People with circulatory problems can also develop these ridges.
Half white, half brown nails	May signify kidney failure. This causes a chemical change in the blood, which in turn releases the pigment melanin. If your nails develop this condition, get urgent medical attention.
Dark vertical stripes	Common in people with dark skin and can be perfectly normal. But because they can also be a sign of a type of skin cancer that originates beneath the nail bed, you should always bring them to your doctor's attention.
Red or brown streaks under the nails	These are usually caused by damage to small blood vessels, but they can also indicate infection of the heart valves—so don't ignore them.
Downward-curving nails	May indicate a heart or lung disease that causes reduction in the oxygen supply to the nails.
Upward-curving nails Spoon-shaped nails	Can be a sign of anemia, caused by deficiency of iron or vitamin B12.

sources of biotin in your diet, choose foods that contain nuts, oatmeal, legumes, brown rice, and barley.

● **Buff your nails** Not only will you smooth any ridges but you will also improve the circulation around the base of the nail, promoting growth. Be sure your nails are clean and dry, and buff in one direction only. Stop as soon as your nails feel warm or you may damage them.

● **Eat liver**, which is a highly concentrated source of vitamin A, to prevent white flecks in the nails. Other foods rich in vitamin A include oily fish, egg yolks, and cheese. But be careful not to have too much of this vitamin, because it can build up in the body over time and may weaken bones. Pregnant women are advised not to eat liver or liver products (such as liver pâté). For everyone else, the maximum recommended intake of liver is one serving a week.

Secrets and myths
OF HAIR AND NAILS

Throughout history, hair has mattered to humans—not just as an important part of our self-image. It also has a strong symbolic and cultural significance, playing a major role in fairytales, myths, legends, and religions. As a result, hair and also nails are the subject of many popular beliefs and sayings—some true, some false ...

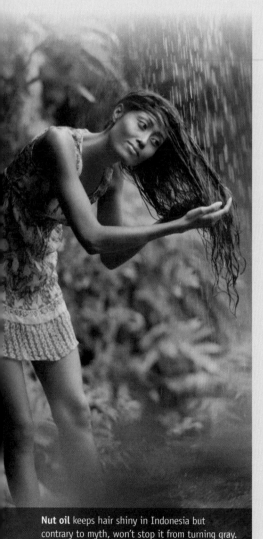

Nut oil keeps hair shiny in Indonesia but contrary to myth, won't stop it from turning gray.

For thousands of years we have cut, colored, and shaped our hair according to convention and fashion. Growing at about ¼in (6mm a month, it is the part of the body that most noticeably changes with time, despite being made entirely of dead cells. For individuals, hair can express sexuality and personality. In human societies, its style has denoted anything from power and dominance to marital status. Its loss, voluntary or imposed, may symbolize the adoption of a spiritual life (in monastic communities), military defeat, or loss of identity (prisoners). Small wonder that so many myths have grown up about it. And the style of nails—from the hugely long famously cultivated by the nobility in ancient China to the carefully manicured and lacquered talons of today's supermodels—can also convey cultural messages.

Nailing down the truth

Here's a guide to some of the most common myths and truths about hair and nails:

✘ Black hair is stronger than blonde hair Despite this widespread belief, particularly among African Americans, black hair is one of the most fragile. Nor is it true that braiding and beading the hair makes it grow more quickly. Tight braids and beads can damage hair.

✔ Worry brings gray hair Research suggests that this might be true. It seems that the stress hormone adrenaline may damage DNA in the genes responsible for the production of melanin, the pigment that gives hair its color.

✔ Bald men have higher testosterone levels They do, and their baldness is caused by the exposure of the hair follicles to excessive amounts of the chemical dihydrotestosterone (DHT), which is produced by the male sex hormone testosterone.

✔ Hair grows faster in summer When it's cold, blood is diverted to internal organs to maintain body temperature, decreasing blood flow to the scalp. In warm weather, enhanced

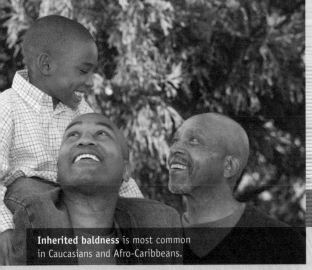

Inherited baldness is most common in Caucasians and Afro-Caribbeans.

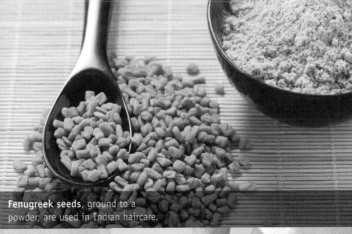

Fenugreek seeds, ground to a powder, are used in Indian haircare.

circulation to the skin boosts follicle activity and therefore increases the rate of hair growth. Hair grows 10–15 percent faster during summer than in winter.

✔ **... as do nails** In summer, more sunlight falls on your skin, producing more vitamin D, which enhances nail growth. Nails grow faster in warm climates and men's nails grow more quickly than women's. Interestingly, fingernails grow faster on your dominant hand because that hand receives the greater blood flow. The nail on the middle finger grows fastest; the thumbnail slowest. And fingernails grow five times faster than toenails.

✘ **Hair can turn white from fright** New York dermatologist, Dr. David Orentreich says no. You can't lose pigment in your hair because hair is dead when it leaves your scalp. But a severe shock can trigger alopecia areata, an autoimmune condition that causes pigmented hair (black, brown, red, or blonde) to drop out, leaving only gray and white hair behind.

✘ **White flecks on nails mean lack of calcium** This myth may arise from the fact that calcium is white. While calcium is vital for forming strong bones and teeth, nails, like skin and hair, are made of the fibrous protein keratin, which contains only a small amount of calcium. White spots, known medically as *leukonychia punctata*, are usually the signs of minor injuries, but may indicate zinc deficiency.

✔ **Cut toenails straight across** If you cut into the sides of a big toenail, the skin around the nail may swell up at the nail edge, eventually leading to an ingrown nail. Cutting straight across is the best way to prevent this.

✘ **Shaving the head of a newborn prevents baldness** There is no truth in this Indian myth. Most male baldness is inherited. If a father has a tendency to early hair loss, any sons he has are very likely to inherit the same tendency (the American Medical Association puts the chance of inheriting the baldness gene at

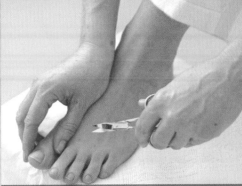

Cutting toenails straight across will help prevent painful ingrown nails.

4 in 7). If a baby boy's grandfather (his mother's father) and his own father both had this characteristic, then the boy will always inherit it.

✘ **Fenugreek strengthens hair** A powder made with fenugreek is widely used in India but, while it keeps hair soft and shining, and also prevents dandruff, there is no evidence that it strengthens it.

✘ **Cutting hair by the moon speeds its growth** One Brazilian myth is that hair cut between a full and quarter moon grows more strongly; in Asia that cutting hair under a waxing moon promotes growth. Neither are true. Hair does not grow back more strongly after it's cut—at any time.

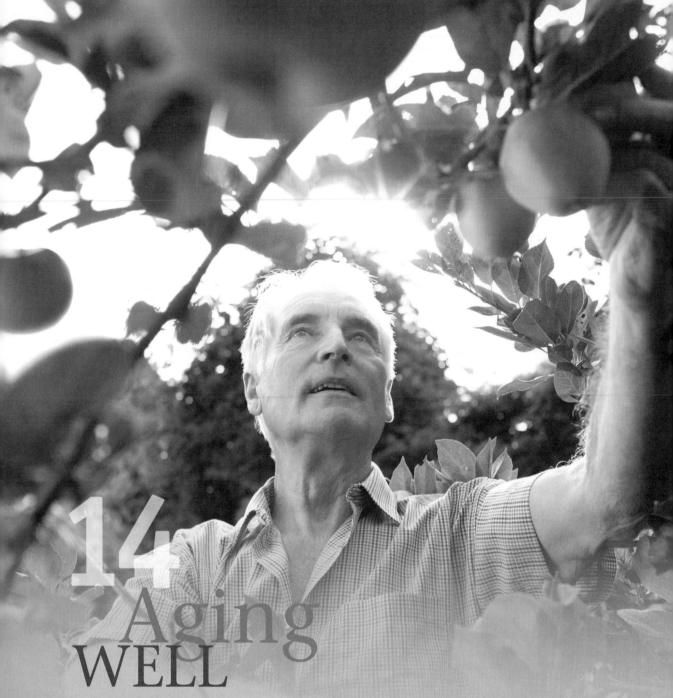

14 Aging
WELL

Our understanding of the aging process has taken huge strides
forward in recent years. It is becoming ever clearer that,
although you can't stop the clock, you can certainly influence
how well you age. Diet, exercise, and stress are just some of
the factors that can affect your health in later years. Read on
to find out what researchers have discovered.

Lifestyle MATTERS

How we work, sleep, and spend our leisure time, our range of social contacts and even how we think about ourselves and about life can all play a role in keeping us as young as possible. Here you'll find a wealth of effective tips for maintaining your vigor through the years.

● **Don't focus on stereotypes** Just thinking about the clock ticking away can make you age more quickly, say American researchers who studied people aged 74 and over. They found that accepting negative stereotypes of older people from the media can send you on a downward spiral. Stay-young secrets involve focusing on the positive aspects of getting older, such as spending more time on enjoyable activities, relaxing with family and friends, and trying out new things.

● **Choose warmth over passion**
Emotional and physical closeness to your partner can be just as satisfying as steamy nights of passion as you grow older. It's true that keeping up a sex life as you age brings many benefits to your health, but when researchers assessed sexual activity and satisfaction levels among women with an average age of 67, they found that closeness to the partner was more important than orgasm. If you don't feel as frisky between the sheets as you once did, don't let this prevent you from getting plenty of cuddles.

● **Sing together** A US study carried out on 168 healthy older adults revealed that those who joined a choir were in better health, used less medication, were less lonely, and had fewer falls after a year than a similar group of nonsingers. This could in part be due to the impact that singing has

on breathing, but the emotional benefits of giving voice in a crowd may be just as important. So if you enjoy it, whatever the quality of your voice, try to find the chance to sing communally, whether in a formal choir, at a family singalong, in church, or in a crowd of thousands at a football game.

● **Love your age** Think positively about your time of life and you'll live longer. One US study asked people aged 50 and over how they felt about a range of statements

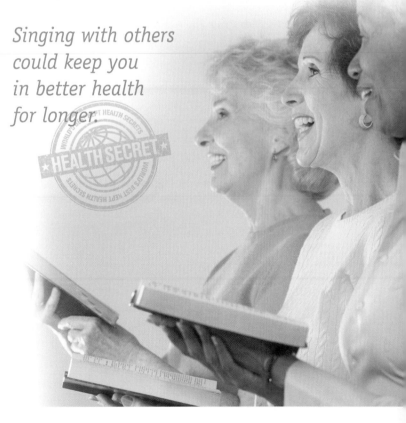

Singing with others could keep you in better health for longer.

HEALTH SECRET

designed to assess their outlook on the future. Almost three decades later, follow-up research found that those who viewed aging in a hopeful light had lived an average of seven and a half years longer than those with a more pessimistic outlook. You're likely to have better coping strategies and be more likely to seek support when you have problems if you try to see your cup as half full, rather than half empty.

● **Care for others** Kindness may help you to live longer, according to a new theory called "survival of the nicest." The theory suggests that humans have prospered as a species because we are compassionate. When US researchers analyzed ancient societies, they found that kindness was key to the survival of communities and that we all have an built-in capacity for helping others, especially those close to us. Showing kindness and compassion to others will help you thrive, too.

● **Get tough** Those who can weather what Shakespeare called "the slings and arrows of outrageous fortune" are more likely to live to a ripe old age, suggest studies from Harvard University. Psychological hardiness (mental resilience in the face of stress, anxiety, and depression) is crucial for survival, especially as we get older. The

secret is to adopt an accepting attitude and go with the flow, so that you can cope with whatever life throws at you.

● **Don't think you need less sleep** It's a common myth that we need fewer hours of sleep as we age, but evidence suggests that this is not true. Sleep disorder experts have found that having less than 6 hours sleep a night can adversely affect your mood. If you have trouble dozing off or can't go back to sleep when you wake up, try getting into a good sleep routine:

★ **Go to bed** and get up at more or less the same time each day.

★ **Avoid exercising** or eating too close to your bedtime.

★ **Keep your bedroom** for two activities only: sleep and sex.

★ **Ban late-night googling**, online shopping, or TV watching.

● **Invest in relationships** Good relationships—whether with a loving partner or warm, supportive friends—are vital to health and longevity. Research shows that we benefit mentally and physically when we have someone to love and care for. In a study of women aged 61 to 90, US psychologist Elliot M. Friedman found a link between having good friends and low blood levels of an inflammatory chemical called interleukin-6. High levels of interleukin-6 are associated with a range of illnesses, including heart disease, cancer, and dementia. Studies have shown that:

★ **Happily married people** live longer than those who are single or divorced.

★ **Those who feel needed** are less likely to suffer from chronic illness.

And the converse is also true. A US study found that those who considered themselves lonely were more likely to develop cognitive problems and Alzheimer's disease. Make the effort to invest in your relationships and reap the rewards in health and happiness.

● **Have faith** Research shows that positive emotions associated with attending religious services—such as hope, faith, forgiveness, joy, compassion, and gratitude—can help to reduce stress and regulate the body chemicals that protect us against it. US researchers have found that regular church attendance can add two to three years to your life. This may be due to the power of faith or linked to the advantages of belonging to a community or having a sense of purpose. No one knows for sure. But whether as a part of a faith or secular group, it could benefit your health to take time out every week to reflect on life alongside others of a like mind.

● **Get organized** People who live well-organized lives tend to live longer than less careful types, perhaps because they look after their health better and avoid risky behavior, concludes the US-based Longevity Project, a landmark eight-decade study. If you want to introduce more order into your life, start with small changes, such as filing your correspondence. Then gradually extend this approach which could help to set you on the path to longevity.

● **Work hard** Yes, you may think retirement beckons but staying on the treadmill could extend your life, say researchers on the Longevity Project. They found that many long-lived, successful professionals worked (at least part-time) well after retirement age. We're conditioned to think that working hard can inflict unhealthy levels of stress. But this research suggests that success, even in a demanding job, can enhance well-being. So, if you're in

good health, you may not want to give up work entirely. You may find it possible to reduce the hours or days you work—or even continue to work full time for a few more years.

● **Surf for your brain's sake** Search the internet to keep your brain active, say US scientists. In one US study people age 55 to 76 who carried out a series of web searches all showed increased activity in the regions of the brain that control language, reading, memory, and visual ability. Those who already surfed regularly showed a significant boost in the areas that deal with decision-making and complex reasoning. And using the internet has many other benefits for

Older people can improve their mental agility by surfing the internet.

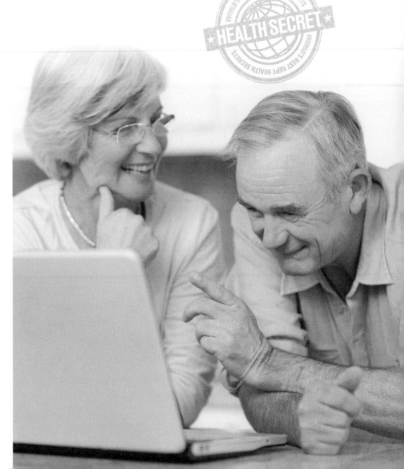

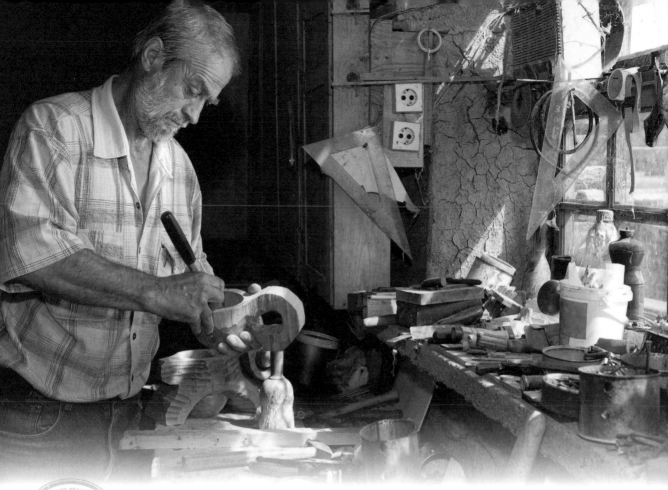

Learning a new skill can boost your powers of concentration.

older people such keeping up with trends in a favorite field of interest or discovering new ones. Do your brain a favor and get online today—after only one week of surfing for an hour a day, your decision-making centers will benefit.

BELIEVE IT OR NOT!

Parental divorce affects longevity

Broken families can have devastating effects on a child's long-term health. Parental divorce during childhood emerged as the single strongest predictor of early death in adulthood in the Longevity Project, a US research study. Of course, you can't rewrite your parents' past. But if this applies to you, it can provide an added incentive to reduce the impact of the health risks that are within your control.

● **Learn to paint** Taking up a creative hobby will boost concentration, give yourself a focus, and distract you from everyday pressures. A UK study of older women found that quilting improved mental health in ways that physical or outdoor activities could not. It concluded that creative pursuits offer valuable alternatives for people who find outdoor activities difficult or uninteresting. Choose from knitting, crochet, carpentry, painting, sculpture … or whatever appeals to you. And you could make new friends.

● **Reward yourself** If acquiring a new skill seems daunting, take heart from a US study that found that older people learn just as well as younger people, provided they have an incentive. The study found that younger and older adults were both much more likely to achieve their aims if promised a financial reward. So set up a savings account and reward yourself each time you reach a learning goal.

● **Challenge your mind** The benefits of keeping mentally active as you age are well known—your mental health in general will be better: You will be less likely to suffer from depression, retain your problem-solving abilities, and be better able to keep at bay the symptoms of degenerative illnesses such as dementia. Ways to keep your mind alert and agile include:

★ **Solving crossword puzzles**
★ **Taking a course or class**
★ **Learning a language**
★ **Playing online games,** especially multiplayer strategy games.

● **Walk the dog** Dog ownership can provide a physical and emotional boost. Walking the dog will improve your fitness and protect against feelings of loneliness, according to a UK study of dog walkers. They reported that the regular daily exercise improved their sense of well-being, and that while walking their dog they often met and chatted with others, which made them feel happier. If you're not able to keep a dog, try dog-walking with a friend.

● **Look forward to an age of contentment** Forget the notion of grumpy old people. Growing older is a happier time than most of us imagine. UK researchers looked at attitudes to life and found older people to be just as happy as the young. This may be because after clocking up six decades or more, most are resilient and have developed a battery of strategies for dealing with life's ups and downs. So don't dread old age—unexpected joy could lie ahead, whether from developing

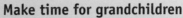
relationships with younger members of your family, making new friends, having time to pursue your hobbies, or traveling to places you've always wanted to visit.

● **Help in your local hospital** If you're retired with time on your hands, consider taking up volunteer work. Countless studies show the health dividends of giving your time and skills to benefit others. Not only does it help to keep you in touch with life and meet new people, but you will also feel that you are contributing to society—a vital aspect of good mental health. Volunteering could even help you live longer. US research suggests that it helps to:

★ **Reduce** stress
★ **Boost** levels of "happy" brain chemicals
★ **Relieve** chronic pain
★ **Improve** cardiovascular health.

There are many ways to get involved, such as asking your local hospital friends group, nearby charity shop, or community

People with high blood pressure who practice Transcendental Meditation live longer.

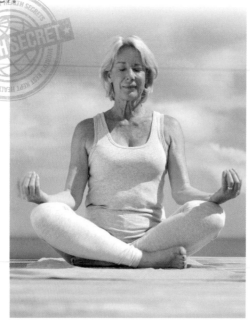

gardening project if they need help. You can investigate a wide range of possibilities on the website www.volunteermatch.org.

● **Shop till you drop** Shop regularly and you may live longer—that's the conclusion of a 10-year study of around 2,000 over-65s in Taiwan. The researchers found that men who shopped daily had a 28 percent lower risk of dying early than those who shopped less often; among women, the risk reduction was 23 percent. Social contact, better physical fitness, and greater mental agility are the key factors. If you want an excuse for a bit of retail therapy, look no further.

● **Say "ohm"** If you have mildly elevated blood pressure, regular Transcendental Meditation (TM) can lengthen your life, says a US study published in the *American Journal of Cardiology*. The researchers followed people with an average age of 71 who had slightly elevated blood pressure. Some followed a TM program; others used behavioral techniques, such as mindfulness or progressive muscle relaxation; and others had health education. The study tracked subjects for up to 18 years and found that the TM program was highly effective, reducing death rates by 23 percent compared to the other techniques.

● **Follow the rule of seven** There's more than luck to aging successfully say researchers. A study carried out at Harvard University, which followed 569 young people into old age, pinpointed seven key lifestyle factors that can determine how well you will age if you adopt them before the age of 50:

★ **Not drinking alcohol** excessively
★ **Not smoking**
★ **Having** a stable and happy marriage
★ **Exercising** regularly
★ **Maintaining** a healthy weight
★ **Developing** good coping mechanisms
★ **Pursuing** education.

Of course, some things you cannot control, such as your genes and your background—but these have less influence as life goes on. Focus on changing the things you can.

❋ MIND POWER ❋

Feed your nostalgia

Foods from your childhood can ease loneliness. A US study on day-to-day things that alleviate stress and isolation as we age found that we associate certain foods with close friends and family, and that thinking about these foods or eating them triggers warm memories of happy moments spent together. It will do no harm and could provide a mood boost to indulge yourself now and then with "nursery foods" such as mac'n'cheese or Mom's rice pudding.

Eating for a
HEALTHIER OLD AGE

Choosing appropriate foods can sustain your body at its maximum potential, even into old age. The right diet will help preserve your mental abilities, keep you mobile, ward off disease, and even delay the aging process.

● **Have some curry** Curry may boost your mental ability, say researchers in Singapore. They looked at the diet of more than 1,000 Indian villagers aged 60 to 93 and found that those who ate curry even just twice a year scored better on cognitive performance tests than people who didn't. The key ingredient seems to be turmeric, the yellow spice used in most curries. It contains the plant chemical curcumin, which has antioxidant, anti-inflammatory, anticancer, and cholesterol-lowering properties. Or you can try a curcumin supplement of 400–600mg three times a day.

● **Put on some weight** As you get older, you can afford to become a bit cuddlier. A healthy body mass index (BMI) is normally considered to be between 18.5 and 24.9. But a BMI of around 27—overweight according to this measure—is linked to a greater chance of living longer once you hit 70, according to Dutch research. But a BMI of over 31 or under 21 was linked to a higher risk of dying early. For more information on BMI, see page 80.

● **Become a flexitarian** Vegetarians live longer, the evidence suggests. But if you don't want to give up meat entirely, become a flexitarian and eat red meat only occasionally. Recent US research shows that swapping just one serving a day of red meat for alternative foods (fish, poultry, nuts,

> **SUPRISINGLY EASY**

Nibble on veggies
Sliced-up carrots, broccoli, celery, and peppers not only make a satisfying snack but can also help you live longer. Just ¼ cup (60g) a day of vegetables can add two years to your life, say Italian scientists.

legumes, low-fat dairy, and whole grains) reduces the risk of dying early by 7–19 percent. Try making one day a week vegetarian day. Go veggie all day or take the meat out of your main meal.

Turmeric, a key curry ingredient, could help to keep you mentally active.

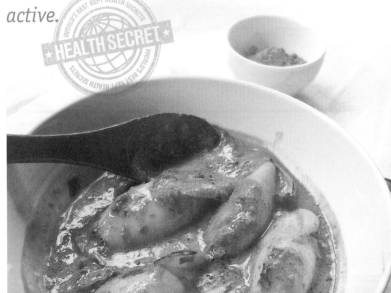

● **Eat apples, stay young** Apples contain antioxidants called polyphenols, which are thought to help mop up free radicals, the damaging rogue molecules that contribute to age-related changes and a range of diseases. Carry apples in your bag to snack on, cut them up into fruit salads, or make them a breakfast regular.

● **Go extra virgin** Spanish research suggests that extra-virgin olive oil is worth the extra cost, since it may add years to your life. Researchers found that this oil, extracted from the first cold pressing of the olives without any further refining, interfered with some of the key processes involved in both aging and cancer. The active ingredients appear to be a group of bitter plant chemicals called polyphenols.

● **Get fishy** Omega-3 fatty acids, from oily fish such as salmon, mackerel, and sardines, can help your cells to stay young. A US study of people with heart problems found that those with a high omega-3 intake from oily fish had longer telomeres—the tips on the end of strands of DNA, whose length is associated with cell-aging and how long you live. So be sure to eat oily fish regularly or take a fish oil supplement.

● **Say "no" to a second glass** when it comes to alcoholic drinks. The Royal College of Psychiatrists advises those over 65 drink no more than 1.5 alcoholic drinks a day or 11 drinks a week. This is half the recommended adult limits, which are too high for older people, due to the physical changes that occur with age. The body does not break down the alcohol as efficiently and the liver is more suceptible to alcohol-related damage. Aim for no more than a small glass of wine or half a pint of beer per night. To help you to make your drink last longer, add seltzer water to wine or lemonade to beer.

● **Remember your weight at 21**
If you're in your middle years, make sure your weight now does not exceed the amount you weighed at the age of 21 by more than 10 lb (4.5kg). Compared with those who gained no more than 5 lb (2.25kg) between the age of 20 and middle age, men and women who put on 11–22 lb (5–10kg) tripled their risk of diabetes, high blood pressure, and gallstones.

● **Choose brown over white** Whole grains, such as unrefined wheat, rye, barley, oats, corn, and brown rice, are particularly beneficial for older people. These foods can help to reduce the risk of chronic diseases, such as heart disease, diabetes, and cancer. Whole grains help to prevent constipation and promote a healthy balance between good and bad bacteria in the gut.

● **Drink water** Older people are especially vulnerable to dehydration. Make sure you drink plenty of fluids throughout the day— even though you may not feel thirsty. Remember, nonalcoholic drinks of all types and liquid foods, such as soups and broths, all contribute to your fluid intake.

Move to
STAY YOUNG

There's no need to become locked into a sedentary lifestyle just because you're getting older. Regular exercise and active hobbies not only preserve your muscle mass and keep you nimble, but also offer a host of other health benefits that improve your enjoyment of life.

● **Get active in short bursts** A 2012 study involving a group of healthy but sedentary middle-aged people found that a 30-minute session in which periods of more intense exercise (in this case cycling) were alternated with periods of gentle exercise three times a week reduced insulin sensitivity (a factor in diabetes) by 35 percent within just two weeks. This routine could appeal to those who find it hard to stick to the standard recommendation of 30 minutes of moderate exercise five days a week. Ask your doctor for guidance on a suitable exercise program.

● **Muscle up for a long life** Manohar Aich of Kolkata, India, was Mr. Universe in 1952—he celebrated his 100th birthday in March 2012 and puts his long life down to regular weightlifting. We can't all be world champions, but keeping muscles strong as you age is vital. Scientists say that inactivity, rather than aging, causes age-related muscle loss (sarcopenia). As well as helping to preserve muscle mass, remaining active can help you to look, feel, and behave younger longer. You could try:
★ **Lifting** free weights
★ **Working** with stretchy resistance bands
★ **Using** weights machines in the gym

Exercising with weights can help you to look and feel younger.

★ **Attending** yoga and Pilates classes. These forms of exercise use body weight to help build muscle
★ **Signing up** for a strength-training class that incorporates work with weights.

● **Pick up a can of beans** If you've experienced muscle loss, you can restore lost muscle and regain strength—at any age. Set aside 10–15 minutes for strength training twice a week. You don't have to use weights and machines at the gym—simple household objects like canned goods fit the bill just as well. Start with a weight you can lift easily 8–12 times, and do two sets of repetitions. When you start to find this too easy, just bump up the weight and keep going.

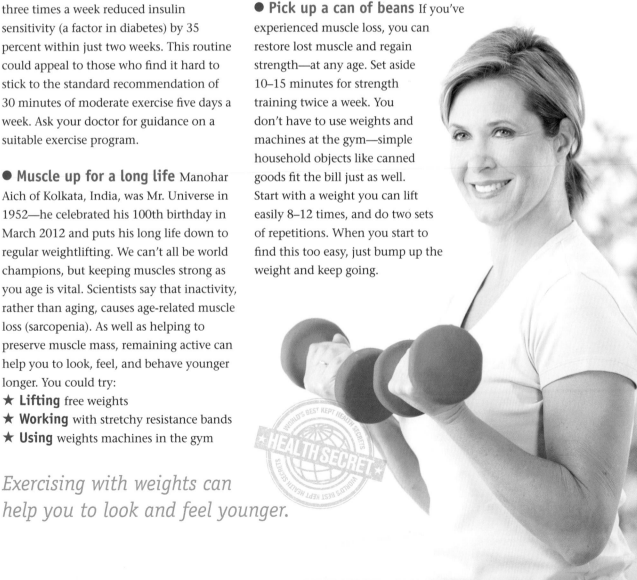

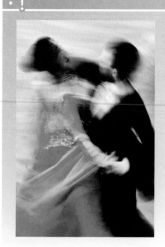

Tango can help Parkinson's

A US study found that twice-weekly tango lessons helped people with Parkinson's disease to improve their balance and move more smoothly. The study supports other research suggesting that tango can help people with the disorder. If you have Parkinson's, consider joining a local tango class.

● **Follow Moshe's method** Poor balance is not inevitable as you get older. Research has shown that the Feldenkrais Method, a gentle program of movement devised by engineer and martial arts teacher Moshe Feldenkrais in 1949, is especially good for balance control as the years roll by. Key principles of the Method include learning more about how you move, think, and feel through a series of gentle exercises. To find a class near you, visit www.feldenkrais.com.

● **Shake it up** Work out on a vibrating platform—a large metal plate that vibrates fast—to fend off osteoporosis. A Belgian study found that vibration training increased bone-mineral density in the hips of women aged 58–74 and improved muscle strength after just six months. It seems that the vibrations activate bone-building cells and reduce the activity of cells that break down bone, which could help to reduce the risk of fractures as you age.

● **Improve your vision with Zumba** Regular working out can protect your sight, says a US study of nearly 4,000 men and

women aged 43–86. The researchers found that those who got hot and sweaty three or more times a week were 70 percent less likely to develop "wet" age-related macular degeneration (AMD), the most common cause of sight loss in people over 60. Choose an activity that you enjoy, as you'll be more likely to stick to it. Good choices include golf, Zumba, tennis, or brisk walking.

● **Stand up straight** with shoulders down and chest expanded—it can make you feel more powerful, in control, and able to tolerate distress. Improving your posture in this way can boost your emotional and mental resilience, even making distressing memories easier to bear. So say US and Canadian researchers who discovered that slouchers tend to be more sensitive to emotional and physical pain. Adopting a powerful, expansive posture may raise levels of the hormone testosterone, which is linked to greater pain tolerance in both men and women, and reduce levels of the stress hormone cortisol.

● **Walk a little faster** for a long life. So say researchers from the University of Sydney, Australia. When they tracked the normal walking speed of more than 1,700 men aged over 70, they found that those who walked faster than about 3mph (5km/h) were 1.23 times less likely to die early than their counterparts who averaged 2mph (3km/h). The message is don't dawdle if you want to keep the years from catching up with you.

● **Dig, plant, prune** If joining a gym doesn't appeal to you, look to your garden for exercise. In a US study, gardeners who averaged 30 hours a week in May and 15 hours in June and July easily passed the recommended daily exercise quota of

30 minutes of moderate-intensity exercise five times a week. Look after your garden to have an enjoyable and ever-changing form of exercise, much of which is weight bearing, which benefits your bones. And being outside exposes you to plenty of mood-boosting sunlight. If you don't have a garden of your own, why not offer to help a friend or neighbor in their garden—you could both benefit.

● **Try tai chi** The Chinese believe that the centuries-old martial art of tai chi can delay aging and prolong life, and now research suggests they could be right. A 2010 review in the *American Journal of Health Promotion* looking at the effects of tai chi on more than 6,400 participants revealed a host of health benefits including:

★ **Better** bone, heart, and lung health
★ **Improved** physical function and balance
★ **Reduced** risk of falls
★ **Enhanced** mood and quality of life.

Ask at your local community center if there are classes in your area or visit the website of the American Tai Chi and Qigong Association at www.americantaichi.org.

Your garden can provide as effective exercise opportunities as a gym.

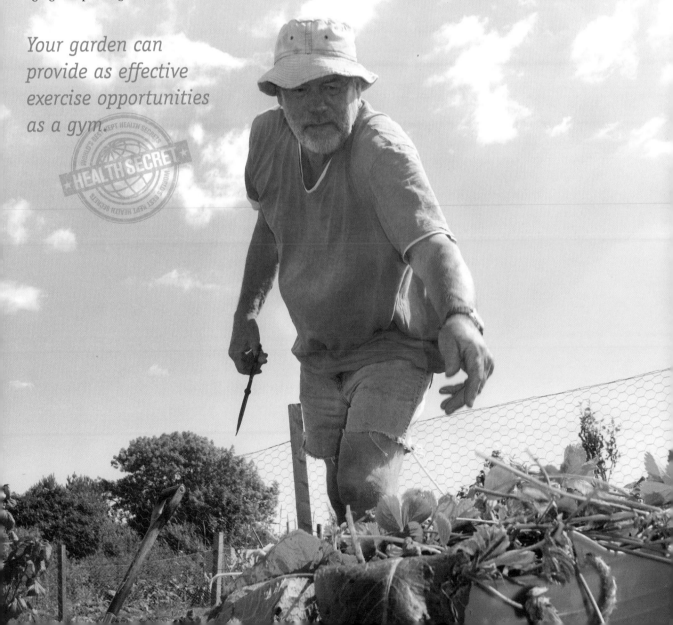

Secrets of
A HEALTHY OLD AGE

In 1999, two experimental gerontologists—Belgian Michel Poulain and Italian Mario Pes—focused their research on a group of villages in Nuoro, a remote and mountainous province of Sardinia. This region, they revealed, boasted the highest concentration of men over 100 in the world. The mystery was how did they do it?

The people of Nuoro were not the first to be hailed as exceptionally long-lived. In the 1960s and 1970s, similar claims had been made about the people of the Caucasus mountains and also the inhabitants of the valley of Vilcabamba in Ecuador. Many of these reports were subsequently found to have been exaggerated. But Poulain and Pes appeared to have found a genuinely super long-lived community.

Longevity hotspots

Since then, other researchers have tracked down more regions where a high proportion of the inhabitants live healthily to 80, 90, and 100 years of age or more.

American writer Dan Buettner has identified several longevity hotspots that he calls Blue Zones. They include:
- The Nuoro province in the Italian island of Sardinia
- The islands of Okinawa off Japan's southern coast
- The Nicoya peninsula in Costa Rica
- The Greek island of Ikaria
- Loma Linda, California in the United States.

Much research has gone into identifying the factors that lead to the long life expectancy in these regions. The secret of the Blue Zones seems to be a remarkable combination of their inhabitants' genes, environment, and lifestyle.

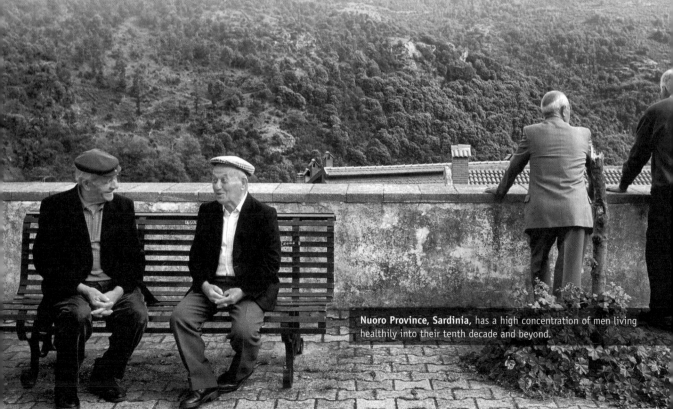

Nuoro Province, Sardinia, has a high concentration of men living healthily into their tenth decade and beyond.

It runs in the family

Studies have found that long-lived people are more likely to have long-lived relatives. They often live in remote locations in mountains, valleys, and islands, and it's thought the genes that predispose others to early death may have been weeded out by natural selection. Another theory is that protective "longevity genes" may have evolved in these populations.

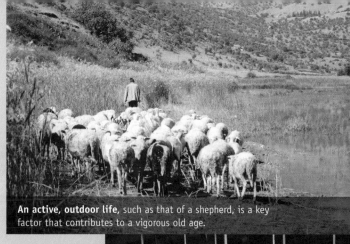
An active, outdoor life, such as that of a shepherd, is a key factor that contributes to a vigorous old age.

The recipe for life

There's not much you can do about your genes, but there are other factors that are thought to contribute to longevity which you can incorporate into your life. Here are some ideas:

Get active Most long-lived people inhabit areas where exercise is part of everyday life. The shepherds of the Nuoro walk long distances up steep paths every day, the Okinawans hunt and fish, and the people of Loma Linda do plenty of walking and sports. This regular activity helps protect against heart disease, cancer, and dementia. There's also evidence that physical activity can extend telomeres—structures on the tips of chromosomes whose length has been linked to longevity.

Have a nap Taking a siesta is another factor that seems to be linked to a longer life. According to the Mediterranean Islands Study (MEDIS), a midday nap is customary among the long-lived people in many of the Greek islands. A noontime nap is thought to reduce the risk of heart disease, possibly by lowering stress levels.

Stay nourished Diet is a key factor, and Blue Zone people eat natural, whole foods, such as

fruit, vegetables, whole grains, nuts, seeds, yogurt, game, and fish. These are low in harmful fats and high in healthy ones, such as omega-3 fatty acids; their protein content is low to moderate; and the fruit and vegetables are rich in phytonutrients. Many foods are picked, farmed, or hunted, so that the diet involves daily exercise.

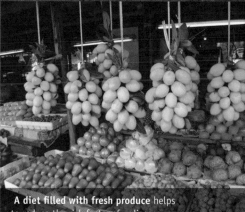
A diet filled with fresh produce helps to reduce the risk factors for disease.

Be involved in your community Research shows that *ikigai* (Japanese for a sense that life is worth living) is one of the factors linked with a long, healthy life. In a study of older people, Japanese researchers found that being productive via work or a hobby, and having friends, frequent conversations, and an interest in life, was linked with a greater sense of *ikigai*. In Loma Linda, where about half of the residents belong to the Seventh-day Adventist Church, faith may also play a role.

Go hungry Another factor uniting the world's longest-lived people is that they tend not to overeat.

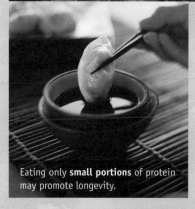
Eating only small portions of protein may promote longevity.

Our bodies evolved to cope with famine, and many aging experts argue that sticking to a relatively low-calorie diet (1,880 calories a day), especially up to middle age, extends lifespan, and research confirms this. Older Okinawans, for example, have a BMI of 18–22. They stay lean by eating mainly vegetables and fruits, foods that have a low calorie density, and by stopping before they feel full.

Medicine
TO THE RESCUE

From gene research to new drugs, scientists are working hard to find weapons to fight the aging process. Check out the latest developments and discover some of the simple things you can do to make sure you're in tip-top shape.

● **Have an eye test** Regular visits to the ophthalmologist will do more than just keep a check on the health of your eyes—they may also help to identify other diseases that can strike as we get older. Disorders that can show up in the eyes include:

★ **Diabetes**
★ **Heart disease**
★ **High blood pressure**
★ **High cholesterol**
★ **Liver problems**
★ **Certain kinds of cancer.**

Regular eye tests offer an opportunity to catch these worrying conditions early and avoid any delay in getting treatment.

BELIEVE IT OR NOT!

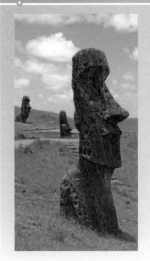

Easter Island may hold an anti-aging secret

A natural antibiotic found in the soil of Easter Island in the Pacific could be key to holding back the years. US scientists have found that rapamycin (after the island's Polynesian name, Rapa Nui) has properties that may extend our average lifespan, and it could pave the way for the development of an anti-aging pill for humans.

● **Fast for a day** Abstaining from food for 24 hours occasionally could reduce your risk of heart disease and diabetes, say researchers from Salt Lake City, Utah. The researchers are unsure of the mechanism underlying this protection but believe it may be linked to lowering of levels of blood glucose and dangerous blood fats called triglycerides during the fast. If you choose to try this strategy, be sure to drink a normal amount of water while you fast. Don't fast if you have type 1 diabetes, and if you have type 2 diabetes or other medical problems, it's essential to consult your doctor first.

● **Don't be macho** If you're a man, do you visit the doctor as often as you should? If the honest answer is "no," think about changing this habit. Men tend to visit the doctor less frequently than women because of the common male tendency to treat symptoms as something to be ignored. The risk of this attitude is that it may allow a treatable condition to progress to a more serious stage before medical help is sought. So if you're a man, it may benefit your health to start thinking like a woman when it comes to unusual or worrying symptoms. If you suffer from anything out of the ordinary, visit your doctor, who will, if necessary, arrange for investigations to find out if there is an underlying problem. And don't forget to get regular checkups and health screenings.

● **See the hygienist to save your bones** Regular visits to your dental hygienist will protect more than your gums and teeth; scientists have established links between gum disease and various illnesses, including heart disease and pneumonia. This is important for older people of both sexes, but postmenopausal women have a particular risk of gum disease due to the natural drop in estrogen that occurs after menopause. A further danger for this age group is that gum disease triggers the production of inflammatory chemicals called cytokines, which research has now linked to osteoporosis. These are all potent reasons to keep up your visits to the hygienist.

A routine eye examination could save your life by identifying a potentially dangerous health problem.

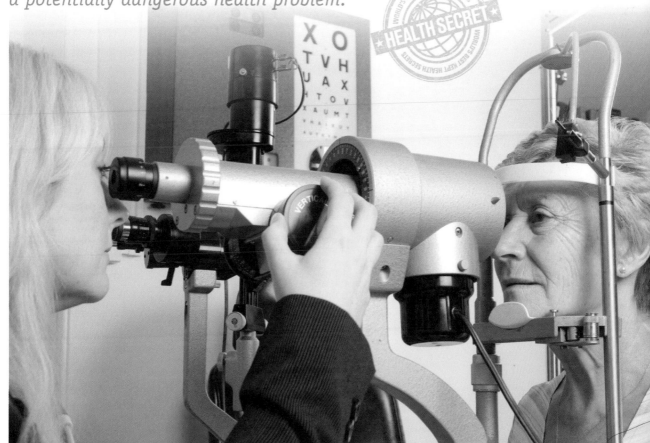

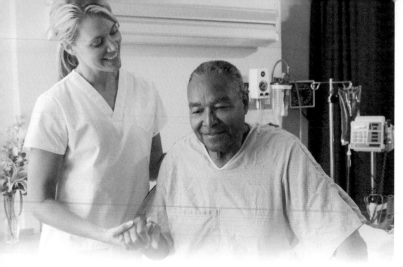

Walking around while in the hospital could shorten your hospital stay by one and a half days.

HEALTH SECRET

● **Get out of bed** The quicker you're back on your feet after an operation or other hospital procedure, the sooner you'll be walking home. When Israeli researchers looked at 485 people aged over 70 who were admitted to hospital for at least 2 days, they discovered that those who walked around while in hospital had a shorter hospital stay—by one and a half days—compared to those who stayed in bed. Older people are particularly vulnerable to the muscle-weakening effects of immobility. So get up

BELIEVE IT OR NOT!

Gene genius
In the not so distant future a gene test could predict your chances of living to a ripe old age. US researchers have discovered 150 gene "hot spots" that are linked to the likelihood of living to be 100. They found that the presence of these hot spots enabled them to predict with 77 percent accuracy whether or not someone was going to be exceptionally long lived.

and get moving as soon as your doctors agree that it's safe. And take advantage of the advice offered by physiotherapists and other health professionals to help you regain strength and balance.

● **Don't look back** Researchers from Canada have found that people who compared themselves unfavorably with more successful friends and neighbors had poorer immunity—and experienced more colds—than people who made comparisons with those who were worse off. Intense life regrets are linked with higher levels of the stress hormone cortisol and with more acute physical symptoms. So learn to let go of "what might have been," and give yourself a pat on the back for what you have achieved during your life.

● **Sun yourself** Spend time in the sun to gain protection against a host of ailments, including autoimmune disorders (when the body turns against itself), cancer, dementia, depression, heart disease, infectious diseases, osteoarthritis, and osteoporosis. As we get older we often lack vitamin D because we tend not to go out as often as we used to or we cover up too much when we do. Some experts suggest that as we age it becomes more difficult for the body to make vitamin D. And obesity, which is more common in middle age, can block vitamin D absorption. To get your vitamin D quota, try the following suggestions:

★ **Stroll in the sunshine** without a sunscreen for 10–15 minutes a day.

★ **Take a vitamin D** supplement, if it's difficult for you to get out—consult your doctor or a nutrition expert.

★ **Eat oily fish**, such as mackerel and sardines, sundried shiitake mushrooms, and sundried tomatoes, which all contain small amounts of vitamin D.

SCREENING TESTS IF YOU'RE OVER 50

As you enter middle age, it becomes increasingly important to watch for signs that all may not be well. Take advantage of screening tests that are available and note that depending on risk factors for a specific condition, more tests may be required. The information below reflects current US guidelines and may be modified based on personal health, family history, and risk factors after consultation with your doctor.

Disease or condition	Who should be screened
Cervical cancer	Women aged 50 to 64 should have a yearly Pap smear; if recent tests have been normal, routine tests are not recommended after age 65, if no other risk factors.
Breast cancer	Recommended that women aged 50 to 74 should have a mammogram every other year; more frequent screening with risk factors. Check with your doctor.
Colonoscopy	Screening for bowel cancer is recommended starting at age 50 for both men and women; then once every 10 years or sooner with risk factors.
Abdominal aortic aneurysm	Abdominal ultrasound recommended for men 65 to 75 who have ever smoked; women 65+ ask your doctor.
Cholesterol	Over 50, every 2 years; over 60, every 2 years or yearly.
Prostate cancer	Average-risk men over 50 should have a digital rectal exam (DRE). Discuss the pros and cons of the prostate specific antigen (PSA) blood test with your doctor.
Osteoporosis	A dual energy X-ray absorptiometry (DXA) which measures bone density is recommended for all women over 65 and men with risk factors such as steroid use. Ask your doctor if you should have this test.
Glaucoma	Men and women should have a baseline eye exam at 40, then every other year; annually after 65, especially if you have a strong family history of this condition.

● **Pop an aspirin** The debate about the pros and cons of an aspirin a day goes on and on. The latest contribution comes from Oxford University in the UK, where researchers have found that a small daily dose of aspirin (75mg) may help to prevent and even treat certain cancers, including bowel cancer. The team says the benefits can start within three to five years—a shorter time than previously throught—which makes this approach more relevant to older people. At present, it's not recommended in the that healthy people take aspirin on a regular basis, but it could be worth asking your doctor whether this medication is advisable in your case.

HEALTHY CONNECTIONS

MANAGING YOUR MOOD

Mind Health Secrets

SAFEGUARD YOUR BRAIN

MAXIMIZING YOUR MEMORY

SHARPEN YOUR SENSES

A BETTER NIGHT'S SLEEP

BREAKING BAD HABITS

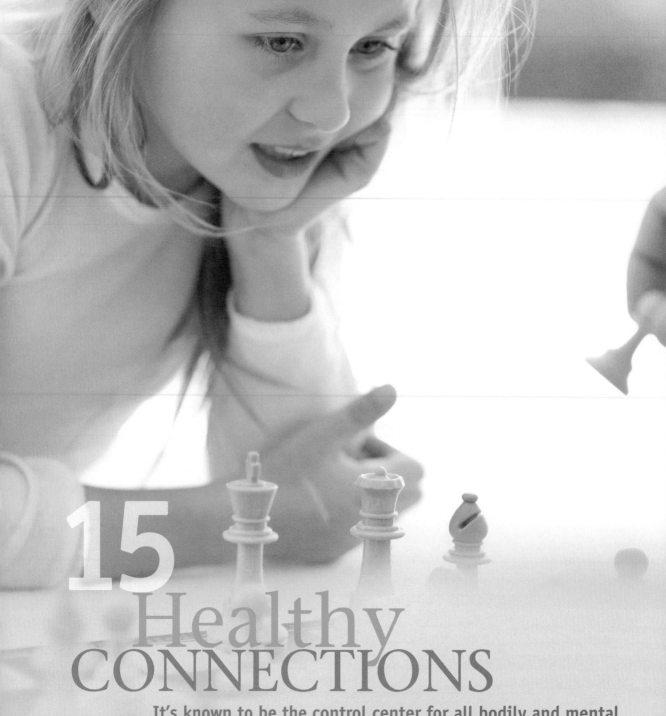

15
Healthy
CONNECTIONS

It's known to be the control center for all bodily and mental functions, but the brain has until recently been the body's most mysterious organ. Thanks to modern medical science, we're now beginning to understand how chemical messengers relay information between brain cells and also to the nerve cells in the rest of the body. As a result, we are also learning many things we can do to promote better brain health.

Boosting THE BRAIN

A constant and plentiful supply of nutrients and oxygen is essential to maintain a healthy brain. And there are many other steps you can take to give your brain the best chance of optimum development and functioning at all stages of life.

● **Ban TV for two years** Watching TV can hinder your toddler's brain development, says the American Academy of Pediatrics. Research has shown that the brains of children under the age of two will develop better if they live in a screen-free environment. This includes staying away from computers and electronic games, and even applies to screens in the background. Resist the temptation to sit your toddler in front of the TV while you're busy making lunch. It's better to encourage play or take your child into the kitchen and stimulate them with talk instead.

● **Wait two years between births**
Spacing additions to your family by two years or more could improve your children's brainpower, say UK researchers. A study involving thousands of children found that a two-year age gap between siblings is the optimum for boosting academic achievement for both children. A shorter gap means that caring for the younger one prevents parents from spending enough time supporting the older child's maths and literacy skills. But an interval longer than two years will not increase the benefit to your children's performance.

● **Learn to juggle** Teaching yourself a new and complex hands-on skill, such as juggling, will boost your brainpower, whether or not you shine at the new

---

BELIEVE IT OR NOT!

Brain-operated artificial limbs
We can learn to ride bikes and drive cars—and now scientists report that we should be able to use the same brain circuits to coordinate the movements of artificial limbs. Thought-controlled prosthetic devices would dramatically improve quality of life for people who have had limbs amputated, which is most frequently as a result of spinal cord injuries or diabetes. The scientists envisage a new generation of prosthetic devices that can be moved using the brain and without people having to concentrate too hard.

Spacing your children by two years or more could improve their brainpower.

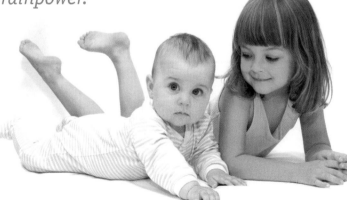

activity, say UK researchers. Learning a skill of this kind promotes the growth of the white matter in the brain that connects what you see to how you move, as well as boosting the amount of gray matter involved in thinking. Your brain develops new nerve connections whether you perform well or not, and the benefits are retained even if you stop practicing the skill. The study looked at juggling, but any hands-on skill, from drawing to motorcycle repair would bring similar results.

● **Get them running** Everyone knows that taking the kids to the park for some fun and exercise benefits them physically, but did you realize it also enhances their classroom performance? The brain soaks up 20 percent of all the oxygen in your body—and getting more of it offers major neurological benefits for children, say Dutch

SECRETS OF SUCCESS

Brain-boosting brown rice

Vitamin B-rich brown rice is widely seen as the brain's superfood. We know that a diet rich in B vitamins is essential to keep the brain and nervous system functioning at its best, and this is especially important for older people. Researchers in the UK are investigating whether taking higher-than-normal levels of B vitamins—specifically folic acid, vitamin B6, and vitamin B12—can prevent cognitive decline by slowing the natural shrinkage of the brain that occurs with age. So far they have found that taking B vitamins can halve brain shrinkage, but further research is needed to ensure that a high intake of these vitamins does not cause unwanted side effects.

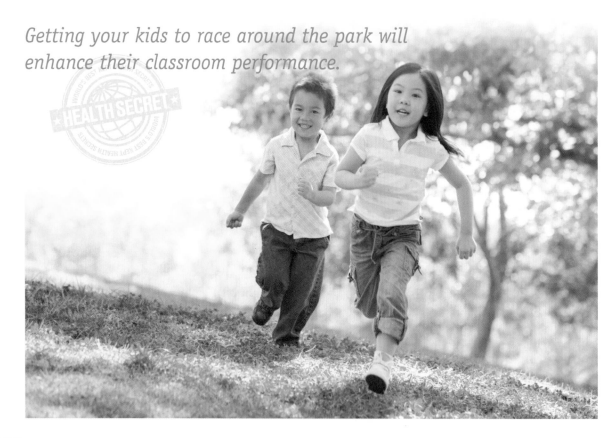

Getting your kids to race around the park will enhance their classroom performance.

scientists. Even children who already perform well academically will do better if they take regular exercise. So encourage your children to walk, swim, cycle, and play sports to get more oxygen into their brains.

● Banish "brain fog" with fruit

You're probably familiar with the experience of brain fog—sensations of dulled awareness and being unable to think clearly. The nervous system requires massive amounts of glucose in order to work efficiently, but, surprisingly, the worst response to brain fog is to eat a sugary treat. It will initially make you feel more alert and better able to function, but will later trigger even greater fogginess, perhaps with emotional swings and low mood. Instead, fuel your brain with the slow-release carbohydrates in fresh or dried fruits, whole-wheat pasta, legumes, or low-sugar, whole-grain breakfast cereal.

● Play war games

If you're older and find that your mental agility is not what it was and that you sometimes have difficulty focusing your thoughts, you could derive great benefit from playing online war games, according to US researchers. These games bring about measurable improvements in cognitive ability in older adults after just a few hours of play. Certain games fit the bill best, say the researchers—those that are cognitively challenging and present players with novel situations in an environment that encourages social interaction. Ask younger family members for advice on the best games—and maybe a couple of lessons.

● Eat oily fish twice a week

Fat is an essential part of your diet, but you may be surprised to hear that it is regarded as the single most important nutrient for protecting and preserving brain function. Avoid saturated fats, which are found in

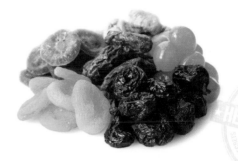

Dried fruits are better than sugary snacks for perking up your brain.

full-fat dairy products and fatty meat, and trans fats, which are widely found in processed foods, such as pies, cookies, cakes, and chips. These fats clog arteries and dull your brain's performance. The brain-boosting healthy fats are omega-3 fatty acids, of which oily fish and fish oil are the best sources.

★ **Eat** oily fish every week, preferably a couple of times.

★ **Cook** with canola, flaxseed (linseed), and olive oils.

★ **Use** these oils to dress salads and drizzle on other dishes.

★ **Snack** on nuts and seeds such as pumpkin seeds and walnuts.

● Add blueberries to yogurt

Eating these tiny but nutrient-packed fruits is one of the best ways to protect and improve your memory. This is thought to be due to their high levels of brain-protective antioxidants. A range of other fruit and vegetables, including apples, bananas, strawberries, pomegranates, oranges, and spinach, will protect your brain's nerve cells in the same way.

● Avoid alcohol binges

We all know that drinking to excess affects the brain, temporarily impairing the senses and interfering with coordination. But regularly binge drinking above the recommended limits is dangerous and the effects may be much more long-lasting. Heavy drinking leads to the death of nerve cells, causing permanent damage to the brain, as well as to the heart and liver. So if you tend to overindulge, cut down and rescue your brain's health.

● **Keep cool, stay alert** As body temperature increases, the number of work-related accidents also goes up. If you're hot and bothered, whatever the reason, have a refreshing drink and take time to cool down before undertaking any activity for which you need to be mentally alert, such as driving or operating dangerous machinery.

● **Harness the power of music** Playing an instrument can increase intelligence. A Canadian study found that children who took music lessons experienced a seven-point rise in their IQ. Another study showed that drumming helps adults reduce levels of the stress hormone cortisol—another plus

for brain health. And singing is also good for your brain. This aerobic activity increases oxygen levels in the bloodstream and reduces stress. If you don't already have a musical activity, try learning an instrument or join a choir to give your brain a boost.

● **Drink more—for the sake of your brain** Quenching a thirst makes you feel much better physically, and it also helps your brain. The loss of more than 2 percent of body fluids can cause as much as a 20 percent reduction in mental ability. So make sure you drink plenty of water and other nonalcoholic drinks throughout the day.

● **Take a power nap** Researchers have found that people who had just had a nap did significantly better in tests of knowledge, vocabulary, eyesight, and hearing than those who drank two cups of coffee halfway through the afternoon (though the coffee drinkers thought they were more alert). So if you find that you sometimes feel sluggish in the afternoons, consider taking a brief nap during your lunch hour.

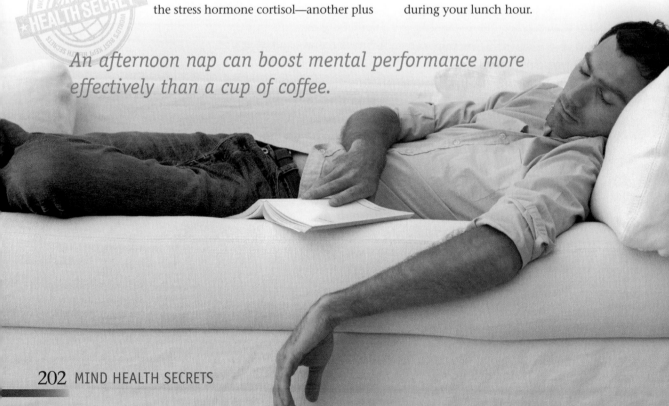

An afternoon nap can boost mental performance more effectively than a cup of coffee.

Headaches
AND MIGRAINES

Dilated blood vessels or tension in the muscles of the head and neck are the most common causes of headache. Migraine—a more severe headache that is accompanied by symptoms such as nausea—can be brought on by a variety of triggers. You'll discover plenty of tips here to deal with both conditions.

● **Warm your feet to cool the pain**
A simple naturopathic headache relief tip is to put your feet in a bowl of warm water. The theory is that this dilates the blood vessels in the feet and draws the blood away from your head, which may ease the pain.

● **Drink strong coffee ...** A strong cup of coffee can provide immediate headache relief because caffeine reduces blood-vessel swelling, a major cause of headaches. This is why some painkillers contain caffeine.

● **... but don't suddenly stop** a caffeine habit if you are a regular coffee drinker; caffeine-withdrawal headaches may result, in which an absence of caffeine

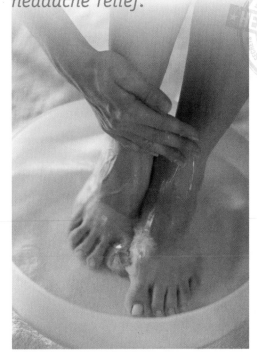

A warm foot bath can provide rapid headache relief.

triggers rebound swelling in blood vessels. The simplest cure is to drink coffee again, but reducing your regular caffeine intake gradually is the best long-term solution.

● **Lose weight to conquer migraines**
If you get migraines and are also carrying excess weight, try losing it—you could end up saying goodbye to your migraines as well. A US study found that seriously overweight people who underwent surgery

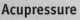

SURPRISINGLY EASY

Acupressure
When painkillers can't banish a headache, acupressure may do the job. With a firm circular motion, massage the web of skin between the base of the thumb and forefinger for several minutes, then switch hands and repeat. Continue until the pain clears up. According to Chinese medicine, the trigger point in this fleshy area is linked to areas of the brain where headaches are said to originate.

Oxygen treatment for migraines

Inhaling oxygen at high pressure is a highly effective treatment for migraines, especially for people who find that drug treatment provides little or no relief, according to a review of research. This therapy brings significant relief from migraine within 45 minutes. The oxygen may alleviate migraine symptoms because it constricts blood vessels—migraine pain is caused by swollen blood vessels—or because it blocks the "chemical pathways" that transmit migraine pain. The treatment is not yet widely available, because it can be delivered only through a hyperbaric chamber—special equipment that is normally used to treat deep-sea divers.

to reduce the size of their stomach in order to lose weight, also noticed a dramatic reduction in the number of migraines they experienced after six months. Research is continuing to discover if less extreme weight loss in people who are not seriously overweight has a similar impact. There's no reason to wait for their results; shedding excess weight has many other benefits, too.

● **Take tablets early** As soon as you notice the first signs of the onset of a migraine, such as nausea or visual disturbances, reach for your medication. Research has shown that the earlier migraine-relief treatments such as sumatriptan (Imigran) are taken, the more effective they will be. And the same is true of other forms of pain relief. So don't try to brave it out or wait for the pain to kick in—take your prescribed medication before the pain of migraine starts.

● **Needle it** If you suffer from either the severe pain of migraines or cluster headaches, which cause sharp, burning pain on one side of the head, try a course of acupuncture. A major review has found

evidence that the ancient Chinese therapy brings more permanent and long-lasting relief than both over-the-counter or prescription drugs. The result is that sufferers have fewer headaches and those they do have are of reduced intensity. To find a practitioner in your area, visit the website of the American Association of Accupuncture and Oriental Medicine at www.aaaomonline.org.

● **Look through tinted lenses** Many migraine sufferers swear that they get fewer headaches when they wear tinted lenses. Research carried out at Michigan State University has now found a scientific basis for the claim. The study used magnetic resonance imaging (MRI) to observe the brains of migraine suffers while wearing lenses tinted to their specific requirements. Those who wore the lenses found that the frequency of migraine attacks was reduced on average by half. The tint color was selected to provide the optimum comfort and reduce "perceptual distortion"—a process called precision ophthalmic tinting (POT). This approach may not work for all migraine sufferers, so ask your doctor if POT lenses might be helpful for you.

● **Drink ginger tea** There is evidence to show that this traditional remedy for migraine headaches works, although the reasons are not fully understood. Ginger has anti-inflammatory properties that may impede the action of prostaglandins, the naturally produced hormone-like chemicals that activate the inflammatory response, contributing to the intense pain of migraines. Make this comforting natural remedy by mixing hot water with a teaspoon of freshly grated gingerroot. Add a little honey if you like, and allow the infusion to cool a litle before drinking.

Relieving pain
AND HEALING NERVES

Pain is a natural reaction to damage caused by disease or injury. It consists of signals relayed from nerves at the site of the problem via the peripheral nervous system and into the central nervous system, where they are interpreted as pain by the brain. Read on to find out what you can do to minimize pain and promote nerve healing.

● **Re-focus your mind** Next time you experience physical pain, try to distract yourself with something absorbing. Researchers have shown that this technique works by testing the ability of people to hold their hands in freezing water while listening to music. Distraction works best, they say, when it fully engages the person's attention: People who were asked questions about the music experienced even less pain. The technique was most effective for people who were the most anxious about the pain. Try focusing on something in which you would normally become completely absorbed— your favorite music or an enthralling book— or better still have someone distract you with conversation or an engaging activity.

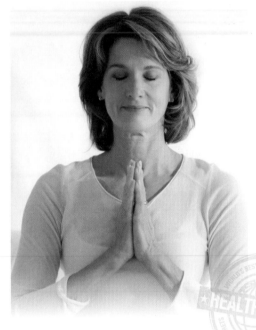

BELIEVE IT OR NOT!

Painkilling placebos
The most effective painkillers of the future could rely heavily on a carefully targeted sugar pill—or placebo—effect. It's no trick. Research has shown that sugar pills are effective at deadening pain. Their action has been pinpointed to cells in the spinal cord that promote pain-linked neural activity. Researchers say that this knowledge could be used to develop new therapies that take better advantage of the role that belief plays in making treatments effective.

Meditation could cut your need for pain-relieving medication.

● **Try meditation** if you have chronic pain. Negative thought patterns mean that people with chronic health problems, such as irritable bowel syndrome, suffer more pain both while anticipating and experiencing it. In other words, if you expect the pain to be bad, it probably will be. Brain scans of people who meditate regularly show that they suffer less pain because they spend less time anticipating it,

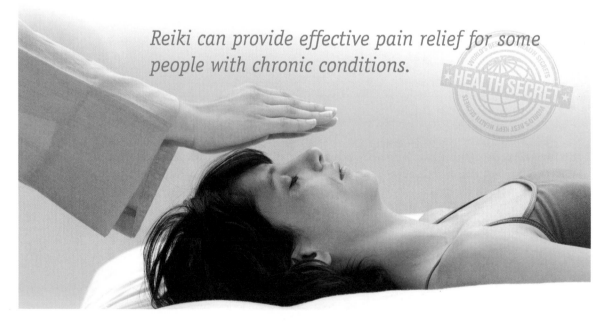

SURPRISINGLY EASY

Warm it

If you suffer from neck pain and stiffness, wrap a flexible heated pad around your neck. You can buy these from suppliers of medical aids. Alternatively, you can improvise with a partially filled and well-covered hot-water bottle.

as meditation trains the brain to focus on the present. One study found that just one hour of meditation cut immediate pain by nearly half—twice the impact of morphine. Ask your doctor or pain clinic for advice on finding a class.

● **Try pyridoxine** Many people who suffer from carpal tunnel syndrome report that vitamin B6, also known as pyridoxine, relieves their wrist and arm pain. The reason why B6 can be of benefit is unclear, but it may be worth trying. Be sure to get your doctor's advice first. The usual dose is 50mg two to three times a day.

● **Cross your arms** According to UK researchers, crossing your hands or arms may ease various types of pain. Placing the hands in an unfamiliar spatial position relative to the body appears to muddle the brain and disrupt the pain message. If you are experiencing pain, try the technique for yourself, experimenting with different positions for your arms.

● **Taking pills? Eat more fruit** You may know that long-term treatment with nonsteroidal anti-inflammatory drugs (NSAIDs) and aspirin can inflame the stomach lining, but you may not be aware that these drugs can also reduce your absorption of vitamin C and another essential nutrient, folate. If you are taking these painkillers on a regular basis, be sure to get plenty of fresh fruit and vegetables in your daily diet. Oranges and kiwis are especially rich in vitamin C, and broccoli and cabbage are excellent sources of folate.

● **Laugh it off** If you're having a bout of pain, try to find something that will make you laugh or look for someone to share a

Reiki can provide effective pain relief for some people with chronic conditions.

HEALTH SECRET

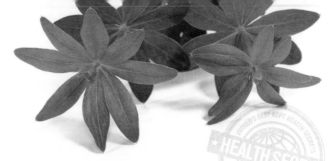

SECRETS OF SUCCESS

Pain-relieving implant

Persistent shoulder pain affects eight out of ten people who have had a stroke. It is frequently resistant to mainstream and alternative therapies, including injections, analgesics, acupuncture, and electrical stimulation delivered through the skin. Now US researchers have developed an electrical implant fitted inside the shoulder muscle, which stimulates the peripheral nerves from the inside to reduce pain. One 76-year-old who suffered agonizing post-stroke shoulder pain for more than ten years has been entirely pain-free since having the implant. Clinical trials are underway to pave the way for a device that could be made widely available in the future.

Sweet woodruff may be the answer to the pain of neuralgia.

been used by healers in many societies throughout history. Although scientific evidence for the efficacy of many hands-on therapies is scant, many people claim to have found benefit from them. A 2008 study singled out Reiki and Healing Touch as the therapies that offer the best results.

● **Drink a cup of sweet woodruff tea**
You may find that traditional herbal remedies may help to relieve neuralgia (nerve pain). Here are some infusions to try:
★ **Sweet woodruff** Add about one tablespoon (10g) of dried herb to 4 cups (1L) of boiling water and allow to infuse for 10 minutes. Drink 2–3 cups a day.
★ **Bitter orange flowers** Add about 2Tbs (20g) to ⅔ cup (150ml) of boiling water and allow to infuse for 10 minutes. Add honey if you like, and drink at bedtime.

You can also get the soothing benefits of plants by soaking in a bath to which you have added an infusion of juniper or essential oil of nutmeg. Or suspend a muslin bag filled with lavender flowers under the hot faucet as you fill the tub. Check with your doctor before using any herbal remedy.

joke with. This is thought to work because a hearty laugh relieves pain, at least temporarily, by releasing physical tension, leaving the muscles relaxed for up to 45 minutes. It also triggers the release of endorphins, the body's feel-good chemicals.

● **Swear to it** Next time you're in need of pain relief, utter a swear word or two. Researchers at Keele University in the UK have shown that letting off steam in this way really does help people bear pain. But save this form of pain relief for when you really need it. The occasional expletive increases people's pain tolerance, but the study shows that it works only if used sparingly. And people who regularly use swear words are much less likely to benefit.

● **Use the power of touch** If you have a chronic painful condition, consider trying a hands-on therapy. The comfort provided by the caring touch of another person has

● **Get enough vitamin B12** If you've suffered nerve damage, be sure to boost your intake of this key nutrient involved in the repair of nerves. Good sources include meat, eggs, fortified soy products, yeast products, and whole-grain cereals and bread.

Secrets of
REPAIRING THE BRAIN

Trepanning—drilling holes into the skull—exorcisms, charms, prayers, and purges were among the many past treatments for brain injuries and disorders. The brain was poorly understood and the dogma long persisted that it was immutable, hard-wired, and unable to change or repair itself. But recent research by neuroscience teams around the world is beginning to reveal a very different picture.

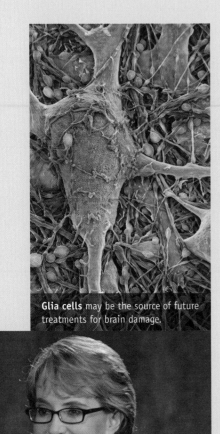

Glia cells may be the source of future treatments for brain damage.

Music therapy helped the recovery of US Congresswoman Gabrielle Giffords from a gunshot wound to the brain.

It's an extraordinarily exciting time for neuroscience. Studies are showing that the brain is capable of remarkable reorganization. Emerging new treatments and other therapies are offering fresh hope to those who have suffered brain damage from illness or injury.

Thinking the way to recovery

From Indian tantras to the rituals of Buddhism, meditation has been practiced for millennia, but research is now proving that it changes the very structure of the brain. Studies at the Massachusetts General Hospital showed that the density of brain cells in the hippocampus—the area associated with learning and memory—was significantly boosted in those who meditated for an average of 27 minutes a day. Other studies at Yale University strongly suggest that meditation can help to correct the faulty neural wiring that is the underlying cause of anxiety and depression—and possibly even schizophrenia. There's even evidence that just imagining that you can perform an activity, such as moving a limb immobilized by a stroke, can stimulate the brain to rewire itself and help to restore movement.

Reprogramming the cells

Packed into the brain alongside its nerve cells are star-shaped glia cells. They were once regarded as no more than a kind of putty holding the brain together (their name means "glue"), but a team at Ludwig Maximilians University, Munich, has discovered that in the human embryo these cells can become brain cells—and that they lose this stem cell ability once the brain is fully formed. But by altering the molecular switches in mature glia cells, scientists can restore this plasticity, allowing the cells to regenerate and opening up the possibility that they could be used to replace dead or damaged brain cells. Even more remarkably, at Columbia University, skin cells from patients with Alzheimer's disease have been reprogrammed and prompted into becoming nerve cells, a result that could have huge potential for treating brain damage and disease.

HEALTH SECRET
WORLD'S BEST KEPT HEALTH SECRETS

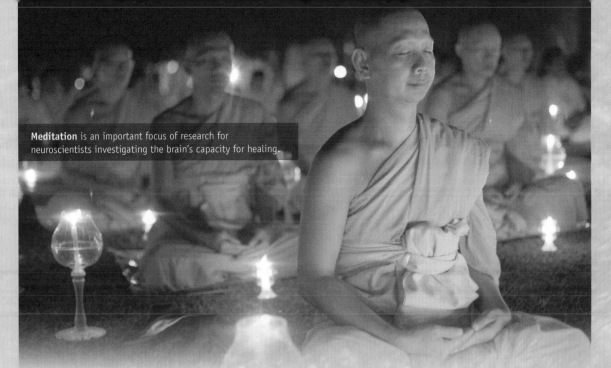

Meditation is an important focus of research for neuroscientists investigating the brain's capacity for healing.

A range of therapies

Treatments that enhance the brain's capacity to recover from illness and trauma are emerging and evolving all the time, from a range of therapeutic areas, not all at the cutting edge of technology.

Brain repair kit Their ability to transform and specialize gives stem cells huge potential for repairing brain injury. At the Institute of Neurological Sciences in Glasgow, six stroke patients who had human stem cells inserted close to the damaged part of their brains recovered significant limb strength. In one patient, the treatment restored the power of speech.

New for old When cells in a specific area of the brain stop making the substance dopamine, the result is Parkinson's disease. Now a team from New York's Sloan-Kettering Institute has successfully converted stem cells into nerve cells able to produce dopamine. Work is underway to create the new cells on a larger scale and graft them into people.

A new role for hormones If administered within 4 hours of brain trauma, the female sex hormone progesterone has been found to cut the risk of death by more than half—and reduce disability, too. The hormone appears to reduce cerebral swelling and brain cell damage.

Coaxing therapy Even after the trauma of injury or a stroke, the brain can alter its wiring and allow the return of movement. Developed at the University of Alabama, constraint-induced movement therapy encourages this by preventing the use of a healthy limb, effectively forcing an affected one into action. The therapy includes 30 hours a week of intensive exercises to improve strength, balance, and stamina.

Technology to the rescue In 2006, Matthew Nagle, a 25-year-old Massachusetts man paralyzed from the neck down due to a severe spinal injury, used thought-control to move a computer cursor, which opened emails and turned on a TV. Matthew was one of the first beneficiaries of the BrainGate Neural Interface System, an electronic implant device that senses electrical signals in the brain, decodes them and translates them into digital instructions, effectively bypassing damaged pathways in the brain and creating new ones.

Musical connections Music therapy—the more rhythmic the better—is proving to be one of the best ways to help establish new nerve connections in a brain damaged by stroke. When patients were encouraged to make their own music by playing the piano or drums, and to sing, restoration of movement improved significantly, and at greater speed.

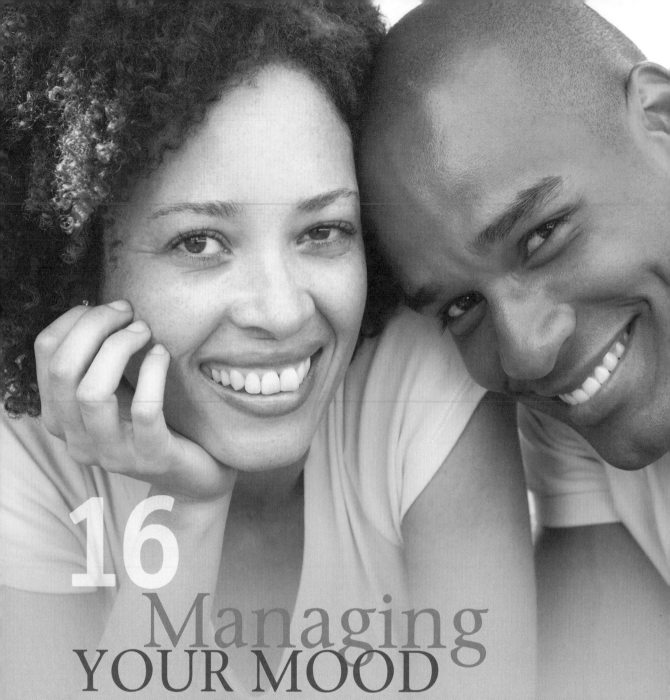

16
Managing
YOUR MOOD

We all expect to experience ups and downs as we pass through
different life phases, each of which can pose special
challenges. But sometimes—and for some people—coping
with stress, loss, life changes, or family worries can seem to
be an insurmountable obstacle, ruining their enjoyment of
life. Your doctor can help in many cases, and in this chapter
you'll learn many additional effective strategies you can use.

Everyday
GOOD SPIRITS

How you feel from day to day depends not only on outside factors, such as your job or family relationships, but also on your general health, built-in attitudes, and the regular activities you undertake—exercise, creative pursuits, and social interaction. Find out here how to bring about positive mood changes through simple measures.

● **Try ice-skating** Stepping outside your personal comfort zone to do something unusual, which makes you feel slightly uncomfortable, is taking a risk—but it can actually bring greater satisfaction, according to German research. There is a whole range of untried experiences that can be uplifting and liberating. You might take a chance by wearing something you've never worn before or trying out a new activity—anything from going to see an opera to taking up a new sport.

● **Listen to music** Poets have described how music "soothes the mind and gives it rest." Now scientists say they have proved that listening to music regularly really is an effective way to enhance your well-being and health—by evoking positive emotions and lowering your stress levels. The study showed that those who listen to their favorite music have lower stress levels than people listening to music that was chosen by someone else or those who listened to no music at all.

● **Just say "no"** You may think being a "yes" person is a sure-fire route to happiness—but you could be wrong. It may be a more effective mood booster to learn to say "no"—at least to people who drain your energy or ask you to do things that are not in your best interests. You can still be a good

SURPRISINGLY EASY

Have sex first thing in the morning

You will start the day in a much better mood than if you had only coffee and a bagel. According to American research scientist Dr. Debby Herbenick, having sex triggers the release of the hormone oxytocin, which makes couples feel loving and bonded all day long. So next time your partner shouts up the stairs, "What do you want for breakfast?"—you know the answer.

You don't have to be good at it to reap the mood-lifting benefits of a new activity.

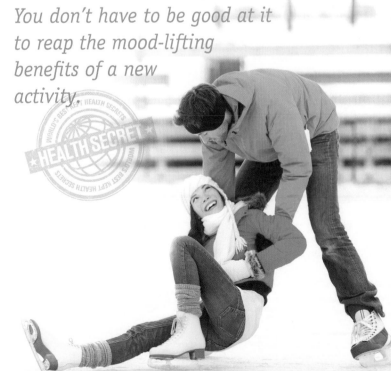

HEALTH SECRET
WORLD'S BEST KEPT HEALTH SECRETS

friend if you refuse a request. And it's likely that others will respect you even more for being true to yourself. If you find yourself in a situation that is no longer life enhancing for you, just say, "no."

● **Use your voice** Think how elated you've felt when singing at the top of your voice in a crowd, whether in a choir or at a sporting event—and how the feeling stayed with you. This is something you can do on your own at home, whether you've got a voice like an angel or are tone deaf—or you could join a choir if you want to put in some real effort. Either way, you're bound to feel your spirits lift.

● **Cherish your goldfish** Time spent with a pet can be more effective at reducing stress than talking problems through with family or friends, say researchers from the University of New York. The simple action of stroking a dog or cat, or even watching fish swimming in a tank, stimulates the body to make endorphins—"feel-good" brain chemicals—and reduces levels of the stress

hormone cortisol. If you're seeking calm, spend quality time with your pet. If you don't have an animal, try stroking a furry toy—surprisingly it can have a similar effect.

● **Beat a bongo** Banging a drum can be an effective and enjoyable way to make negative thoughts fade away and switch on a more positive mood. Researchers speculate that drumming helps to relax the body and the sound vibrations help perk you up. Tapping on your kitchen table may have

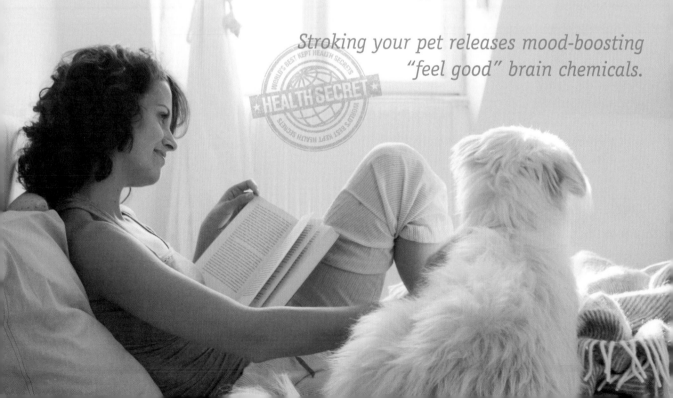

Stroking your pet releases mood-boosting "feel good" brain chemicals.

Beating a drum will relax your body and lift your mood.

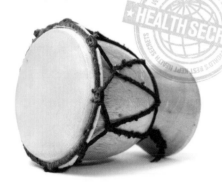

the same effect, but joining a weekly drumming circle could be an even better mood lifter, as the camaraderie will provide an additional boost to your spirits.

● **Down some Adam's ale** Did you know that drinking water can help improve your mood if you're feeling down? It will banish headaches caused by dehydration. And drinking plenty of water each day will also flush out toxins and plump up cells, making you look healthy and helping you feel good. Here are some specific tips:

★ **Aim for** at least eight glasses a day, either still or fizzy, and the chances are that your mood will soon start to sparkle.

★ **Perk up** plain water with a slice of lemon or lime, a sliver of fresh gingerroot or a sprig of mint.

● **Get away from it all** Researchers from the University of Michigan found that people with a heart condition who went on a four-day spiritual retreat had an immediate uplift in mood. Their activities included journal writing, meditation, drumming, guided imagery, and outdoor activities. If you're feeling down, find a free weekend, or even a week, book a retreat, and see what benefits it brings in terms of your mood and outlook.

● **Bump up your Bs** Eating fish and vegetables nourishes your body, and these are also mood superfoods. They are rich in vital B vitamins, which scientists now believe help the body produce the brain chemical serotonin—a proven mood booster. Shellfish, fortified cereal, oatmeal, and wheat germ are all excellent choices. Make sure that shrimp, muesli, yeast extract, and green leafy vegetables feature regularly on your menu.

● **Focus on the present** Focusing on the here and now—being "mindful"—is a way to help you deal with anxiety and depression. The idea is that focusing on sensations and perceptions rooted in the present moment allows you to let go of worries connected to the past or future. Stress levels can plummet if you practice this for half an hour a day, making you better able to cope with life. Learn about mindfulness using books, CDs, classes, or the Internet. Harvard University's helpguide.org website offers mindfulness information and exercises at www.helpguide.org/harvard/benefits-of-mindfulness.htm.

BELIEVE IT OR NOT!

Denmark is the happiest nation
You might not think it if you've seen the gloomy films and TV series gracing our screens, but according to the World Database of Happiness at Erasmus University in the Netherlands, the Danes are the happiest people in the world, followed closely by the Maltese, Swiss, Icelanders, and Canadians.

Savor life's joys

Focus on the freshness of a newly picked flower or the way the sunlight floods the lawn. Psychologists suggest that taking mental photos of pleasurable moments you've experienced helps to lift your spirits in low-mood moments.

● **Give a helping hug** Giving someone a supportive hug can be as rewarding as eating chocolate, having sex, or receiving money, say US researchers. Brain scans showed that when people were giving support to someone else, the areas of their brain associated with reward were more active, suggesting that giving support lifts the mood of the giver as well as the receiver. So next time someone close to you looks like they could use a hug, don't hold back—it will make you feel good, too.

● **Book a massage** Well known for easing aches and pains, a soothing massage session could also help to banish the blues, reveals a Taiwanese review of research. Massage reduces stress and induces relaxation, as well as building a beneficial relationship between the giver and receiver, triggering the release of the bonding hormone oxytocin. Whether you pay a professional masseur or ask a partner or friend to rub your back, the result is the same: a natural mood boost.

● **Ditch the junk** Clearing clutter can help to clear your head as well as your home. If the thought seems daunting, the secret is to start small. Think carefully about the objects that are encroaching on your space. Do you have furniture, equipment or clothes that you simply don't need? Try this formula: If something doesn't lift your mood or if you haven't used or worn it during the past 12 months, it's time to toss it out.

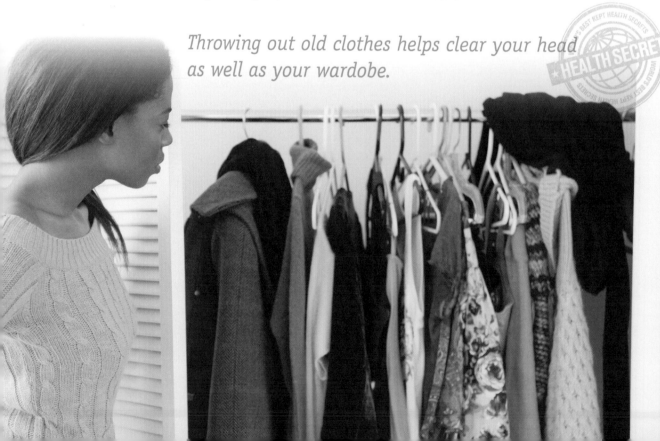

Throwing out old clothes helps clear your head as well as your wardobe.

HEALTH SECRET

SECRETS OF SUCCESS

Daylight lifts mood

Sunshine makes us feel cheerful, and here's why. When light enters the eye, it sends electrical impulses to the brain. These activate the hypothalamus gland in the brain, which helps to regulate mood—the more light, the higher your spirits. Make sure your home and your workplace receive as much daylight as possible. If any place in which you spend a lot of time is on the dark side, try using daylight bulbs or even a light box to ensure you get your daily fix.

Looking at pictures of smiling faces can help brighten your mood.

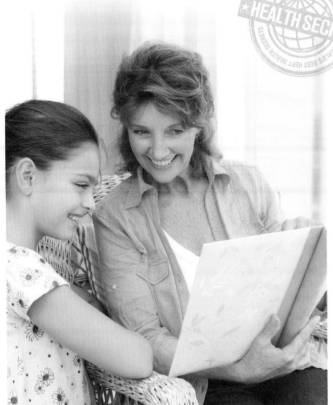

HEALTH SECRET

● **Dig out old snapshots** Why do you tend to be cheerful when surrounded by people having a good time? And why do you feel low when your partner is in a bad mood? The reason is that other people's moods are contagious. Researchers found that even looking at pictures of smiling faces raises levels of brainwaves associated with feeling calm and alert. Next time you're feeling glum, cheer yourself up by browsing through your favorite holiday photos.

● **Treat yourself to chocolate** A little of what you enjoy can do you good, especially if it is a small square of chocolate. According to numerous studies, this tempting treat may help to keep the smile on your face. Cocoa contains a chemical called theobromine, which is thought to increase levels of endorphins, the body's own mood-boosting hormones. To get this benefit, choose dark chocolate with over 70 percent pure cocoa solids.

● **Pay someone a compliment** The effect of negative comments can be offset by positive ones, and this is something to think about when dealing with family, friends, and colleagues. It takes about three positive comments to counteract the effect of one negative one. Boost your own mood by dishing out plenty of compliments, and try to spend time with people who accentuate the positive in life.

● **Exercise—just a little** We all know that exercise can help to lift the blues. But if even the thought of pounding away on the treadmill is enough to send your mood plummeting, here's a secret: You don't have to spend hours at it. Just 20 minutes of vigorous activity a week—anything from jogging to housework, as long as you work hard enough to build up a sweat—can send your mood sky high.

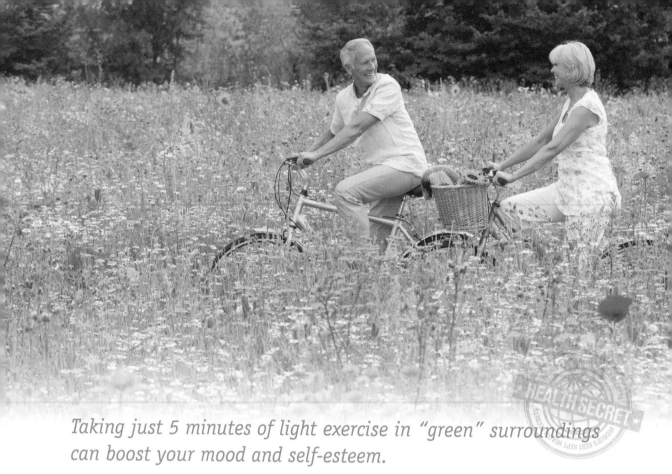

Taking just 5 minutes of light exercise in "green" surroundings can boost your mood and self-esteem.

SURPRISINGLY EASY

See the big picture

If something bad happened yesterday, everything may seem doom and gloom today. But it need not be so. Take a step back and ask yourself how your situation will look in a week, a month, a year, or five years. In most cases, you will soon realize that in that context, your worries are not so important.

● **Eat turkey—and walk** A post-dinner Thanksgiving walk will fill you with good cheer. Canadian scientists have found that exercise helps boost absorption of tryptophan, an amino acid found in turkey, which is linked with relaxed mood. Lettuce and milk are other sources. But no need to wait for November—enjoy a turkey and lettuce sandwich with a glass of milk before your next exercise session and maximize that exercise high.

● **Maintain relations** They may drive you to despair at times, but friends and family really can help you keep your emotional balance, and research has proved it. A 2002 study carried out at the University of Illinois found that one in ten students with the highest levels of happiness and fewest signs of depression were those most likely to have strong attachments to friends and family.

● **Take a "wild" swim** A gym workout is good for your body, but outdoor exercise does more for your mood and self-esteem, say researchers from the University of Essex in the UK. In their study, the benefits were felt after just 5 minutes of "green" exercise, with light activities having the biggest effect on self-esteem, and light or vigorous activity the biggest impact on mood. Walking, cycling, sailing, horseback riding, gardening, and "wild swimming" in the sea, lakes, or rivers are all good options for mood-enhancing outdoor exercise.

● **Get together** Activities carried out with friends nurture happy feelings according to psychologists. Whether you are talking, gardening, cooking, or shopping, doing it with friends should bring benefits for your mood. You could also pursue an interest or activity, such as a team sport, a club, or a class that involves meeting people and making friends.

● **Bend over backward** When researchers rated the mood-altering powers of different yoga poses, such as back bends, forward bends, and standing poses, they concluded that the best way to get a mental lift is to bend backward. Enrol at a local yoga class and look forward to raising your spirits with a back workout.

● **Relax with a cup** Next time someone suggests that you calm down with a nice cup of tea, it's worth listening—they may be on to something. Research shows that ordinary black tea with milk lowers levels of the stress hormone cortisol. Three cups a day is all you need to reap the stress-reducing benefits.

● **Get out in the sun** Sunlight is essential for you to make vitamin D, which research now shows can boost your mood. Researchers at the University of Massachusetts, studying a group of post-menopausal women, found that those with the lowest levels of vitamin D were most likely to be depressed. To reach the

recommended levels of vitamin D at 50°N latitude you need to spend about 10 minutes a day in the sun without sunscreen on cloudless days between 11am and 3 pm, when the sun is high. The more skin that is exposed, the better. You should spend less time in the sun with fair skin, but can sun yourself longer if you are dark-skinned.

● **Try some herbal help** St John's wort has been found in many studies to help combat mild-to-moderate depression. If you want to try it, it's important that you follow the instructions on the package. Be aware that it can increase sensitivity to sunlight. If you are taking any other medications, consult your doctor, because this herb can reduce the effectiveness of some drugs.

● **Learn to play** When you were five you would run to your mother to find out your next activity, but it's not only children who need distraction from boredom. Adults do, too. Relearning how to play will keep your mood flying high as long as the activity is absorbing. Try jigsaw puzzles, painting pictures, gardening, model-making, or organizing your photos.

● **Eat some sardines** Boosting your mood could be as simple as eating a plate of food that your brain appreciates, and oily

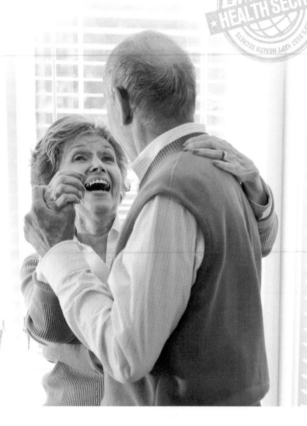

You can dance troubles away—and boost your health, too.

HEALTH SECRET

digestion leads to fluctuating blood glucose levels, which in turn lead to mood swings. The best way to avoid these highs and lows is to go for foods that release energy slowly. This approach is widely known as a low GI (glycemic index) diet. Good meal options include whole grains, such as brown rice, vegetables, and legumes that contain slow-release carbohydrates.

fish fits the bill perfectly. Finnish researchers have found that people who eat oily fish less than once a week are more likely to be depressed than those who indulge more often. Oily fish is rich in omega-3 fatty acids, which research shows to be vital for a lively, happy brain. The researchers advise that eating oily fish three times a week could help to lift your mood. Go for fresh tuna, mackerel, salmon, or maybe an old favorite—sardines.

● **Have brown rice with vegetables** Replacing foods that you digest quickly, such as potatoes or pasta with those that are broken down more slowly could have a profound effect on your mood. Rapid

● **Use the power of flowers** The Bach Flower Rescue Remedy is a natural healing system made from flower essences and used for moments of emotional crisis. A variety of products are available including drops, gum, and pastilles. Proponents of the therapy claim that some of these flower remedies can soothe troubled moods:

★ **Beech** for constantly finding fault
★ **Crab apple** for cleansing self-hatred
★ **Elm** for a sense of overwhelming responsibility
★ **Rock rose** for terror and fright
★ **Star of Bethlehem** for shock.

To learn more about this homeopathic system, visit http://www.bachflower.com.

● **Waltz away the blues** Dancing is the new antidepressant—and it's good for your health. Researchers in Britain, Germany, and the US have found that dancing lifts mood for several reasons: Exercise gives a boost to levels of the mood-enhancing hormones endorphins; learning a new skill boosts confidence; and concentrating for prolonged periods interrupts the negative thought patterns that contribute to anxiety and depression. Dance at home or join a class to raise your spirits.

● **See red** It's no coincidence that the phrase "Paint the town red" is linked to wild celebrations. Red is the most vivid, vibrant color in the spectrum and one of the best mood boosters, say color therapists. Next time you're feeling down, try wearing something red. And see if there's anywhere in your home where you could incorporate some bold red paint or accessories. You may find that it becomes your favorite place to sit and feel your spirits lift.

● **Plan a trip** Planning a vacation can be just as mood lifting as actually being on one, according to UK research. Researchers at Surrey University found that people looking forward to a vacation were much happier with life as a whole, experienced fewer negative feelings, and were more positive overall. The vacation planners also reported that they were happier with their family finances and health than those who weren't in vacation mode. So stick a pin in the map and start thinking about your next trip.

● **Splurge on a treat** Buying a new outfit or something for the home may give you a temporary buzz, but it won't last long. You'll get longer-lasting benefits to your mood if you splurge on an uplifting

experience, say US researchers. So forget that new pair of shoes and book yourself some concert tickets or a weekend escape.

● **Love yourself** The simple act of telling yourself favorable things about yourself is enough to to swing your mood in a positive direction. According to research, liking yourself is fundamental to happiness. All you need do is think up some simple phrases that encapsulate your desire to feel good. Try making positive affirmations about yourself, such as:

★ "**When I have a smile** on my face people smile back at me."

★ "**I feel happy** and I always have a good day."

Make sure your statements are set in the present, not the future, and describe the benefits of your action and the feelings that follow. Repeat these positive phrases and increase your chances of turning on your brain's happy switch.

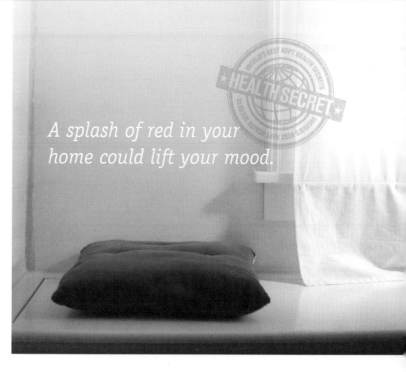

A splash of red in your home could lift your mood.

Secrets of the
POWER OF SUGGESTION

It's well known that the action of a placebo—a dummy medication or procedure—can have a genuine beneficial effect on a person's health, and thousands of scientific studies have confirmed this phenomenon. Far less studied is its sinister cousin, the nocebo effect, in which the expectation of harm creates negative health consequences.

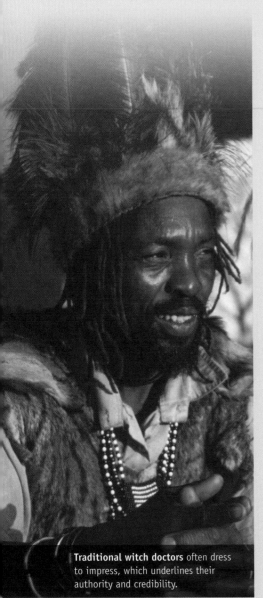

Traditional witch doctors often dress to impress, which underlines their authority and credibility.

In 1930s Alabama, Vance Vanders found himself cursed with imminent death by a witch doctor. He became very ill, did not respond to treatment and did indeed appear to be dying. His doctor eventually concocted a story—he had met with the witch doctor and extracted the secret of the curse by force: Vanders was being eaten from the inside out by a lizard. After the doctor had induced a fit of vomiting in him and produced a lizard by sleight of hand, the patient swiftly recovered. This story, reportedly corroborated by medical professionals, provides a clear illustration of the nocebo effect at work. Numerous other cases of people actually dying after being cursed have been documented over the years.

It's all in the mind

Scientists are beginning to acknowledge the power of the nocebo effect. A 2012 German review says, for instance, that it accounts for the dropout rates of people in drug trial control groups—they believe the dummy drug they are taking to be a real drug and so experience its possible adverse side effects. In an Italian study, people with and without lactose intolerance were told they would be given lactose to test its effect on their gut. Half of those with intolerance and a quarter of those without reported unpleasant symptoms—but all were taking a harmless dose of glucose. A participant in one drug trial developed dangerously low blood pressure by "overdosing" on what he thought was an antidepressant—only when he learned that it was an inert substance did his blood pressure return to normal.

Modern "witch doctors"

A patient's expectations of a treatment clearly influence the way it works. The German study's authors note that vulnerable, ill, or injured patients are highly receptive to negative suggestion, and that the subtleties of language used by medical staff when communicating with patients— for example, using words such as "hurt," "risk" or "bleed"—can have unintended adverse effects. Doctors are trained to speak with authority to their patients, and their paraphernalia—the white coat and stethoscope—

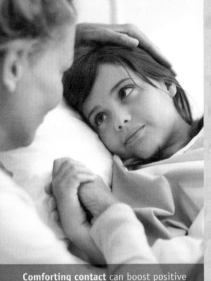

Comforting contact can boost positive feelings and aid recovery.

symbolically reinforces this impression, just as the ritual garb of shamans and witch doctors inspires awe in those who believe in their healing powers. Conversely, the power of positive suggestion may explain some of the success of complementary therapies—from herbalism to homeopathy. Most practitioners take the time to nurture patients' belief in the efficacy of their treatments, engendering optimism about the outcome. The more strongly a patient believes in the treatment, the more likely it is to be effective.

Accentuate the positive

Being aware of just how powerful suggestion can be—for good or ill—can help in every area of life. Resisting the nocebo in favor of the positive is good for health, work, and your relationships. Here are some ways you can put this knowledge into practice:

Get authoritative information Before having treatment or taking medication, get advice from a reliable source. The Internet is a vast repository of information but not all of it is reliable. If you have a tendency toward hypochondria, it can be more harmful than helpful, as the nocebo effect is known to influence those who have a pessimistic outlook more powerfully than those with a more balanced attitude.

Control your response to health experts who are treating you. Focus on encouraging phrases, such as "most people tolerate this well" or "this shouldn't hurt." Try to tune out the negative comments, such as "this may be painful," "expect a long recovery time" or "you may find that this treatment makes you feel sick."

Engage your mind Use creative imagery to stay positive while you recover from illness. If you are in pain, for example,

it may help to imagine tight muscles being massaged, visualize the muscle fibers separating and relaxing, and to concentrate on feelings of warmth. As you visualize, try to focus on your breathing and imagine that you are relaxing in the sunshine or floating in a pool.

Keep positive There is overwhelming evidence that those who heal fastest maintain a positive attitude, take responsibility for their own health, and focus on getting well. Self-awareness also helps, especially of attitudes that may hamper your health.

Use the power of touch Studies have shown that the touch of a partner, friend, or health practitioner can benefit conditions as diverse as asthma, arthritis, hypertension, and migraine. Touch therapy has also been proven to reduce pain and accelerate wound healing. Even if, as some maintain, this is a placebo effect, it is the end result that is significant.

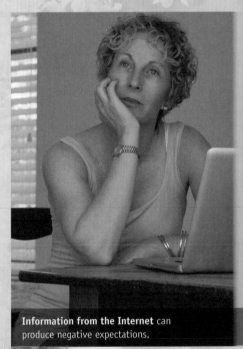

Information from the Internet can produce negative expectations.

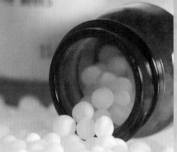

The success of homeopathic medicines may derive, at least in part, from the patient's belief in their power.

Dealing with DEPRESSION

More serious than simply a passing low mood, clinical depression is an illness described by the World Health Organization as the fourth most significant cause of disability and disease worldwide. In most cases, medical intervention is necessary, but you'll learn here about many self-help measures you can take to support prescribed treatment.

● **Stay up all night** If you're feeling down, try a sleepless night. According to worldwide studies, you could feel much better the next day. One study carried out at the University Hospital of Freiburg in Germany reported that depressed people felt better after just one night without sleep—and 75 percent of them found their improved mood stayed with them. It may be that a sleepless night resets the body's internal clock, which goes out of sync in people with depression. If you have the blues, try welcoming in the dawn and staying awake for the day. You may get your best night's sleep for some time as a result.

● **Drink coffee—in moderation** To ward off the risk of depression as you age, drink coffee each day. A study carried out at Harvard School of Public Health, found that women with an average age of 63 who consumed two to three cups of coffee a day

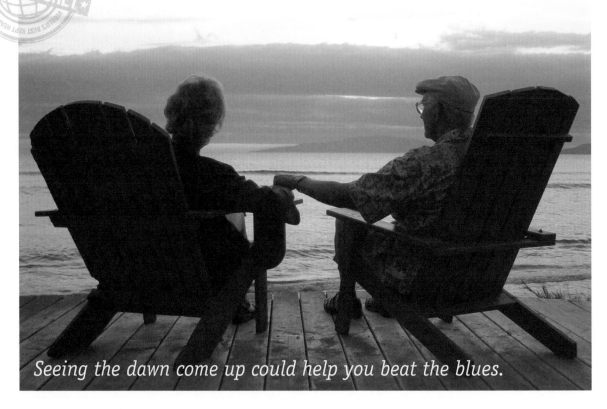

Seeing the dawn come up could help you beat the blues.

were 15 percent less likely to become depressed than those who drank no more than a cup a week. So, go ahead and drink coffee in moderation, provided your doctor does not object.

● **Dress yourself happy** Try wearing clothes that you would normally wear when you're in a good mood to pull yourself out of a low mood. A study from the University of Herefordshire in the UK found that women who were depressed were more likely to pull on a pair of jeans and a baggy top than something smarter. The researchers suggest that wearing clothes associated with feeling happy—for women, typically in bright colors and beautiful fabrics—may give your mood an upward swing.

● **Take up tai chi** If you're depressed and want to brighten your days, consider training in slow-movement tai chi. A 2011 study of people in their sixties suffering from depression found that a weekly tai chi class combined with antidepressant drugs

Instead of providing a lift, sugary snacks can dull your mood.

HEALTH SECRET

helped to improve their mood. Tai chi also improved quality of life, memory, and other aspects of mental health, as well as energy levels. Look for classes in your local health club or alternative therapy center.

● **Give yourself some TLCs** If you are depressed, you may be prescribed drugs and counseling. But a study from the University of California, shows that what researchers called therapeutic life changes, or TLCs, may be just as effective. If you want to give yourself some TLCs, spend more time outdoors, take care of others, eat well, and nurture your relationships with family and friends, advise the researchers.

● **Reduce fat and sugar** Cupcakes and croissants are starting to look a little less inviting. A study from the University of Navarra in Spain found that eating fatty, sugary foods may be linked with a 37 percent greater risk of depression. The study followed almost 9,000 people who had never been diagnosed with depression. Over six years, one in 18 of them became clinically depressed, and those with the highest intake of fast foods and bakery items were the most likely to suffer. Maybe it is time to forget comforting sweet treats and processed meals and opt for healthier foods.

SURPRISINGLY EASY

Try mood-lifting lemon balm

Lemon-scented lemon balm is known as the calming herb. Research shows that when taken as a tea or tincture, it can help ease anxiety and depression in people suffering from a range of mental health problems.

Coping with
ANXIETY

Whether a persistent feeling of worry and unease or the sudden onset of a sense of panic, we are all familiar with the symptoms of anxiety. Physical changes also often accompany the change of mood: increased heart rate and breathing, and perhaps sweating and faintness. Read on to discover ways of coping with this common problem.

● **Cry, don't laugh** You might think laughing is the best way to dispel worry, but crying is a more honest and sometimes a more helpful response, say experts. Having a good old cry helps to quite literally wash away anxiety hormones. It also signals to those around you that all is not well, enabling you to get the help you may need.

A good cry can wash away anxiety hormones.

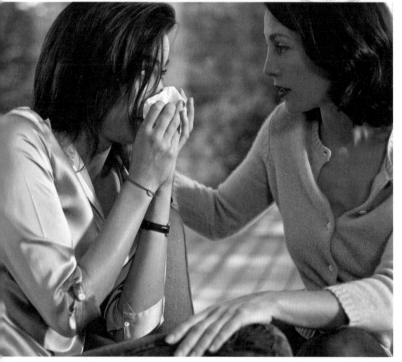

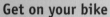

★ BODY POWER

Get on your bike
When anxiety attacks, the natural reaction is to stay rooted to the spot. Much more effective is for you to get on your bike, pull on your running shoes, or make a dash to the gym. It will get your blood moving and those happy hormones, the endorphins, pumping. So if panic strikes, get on the move.

● **Face your fears** You may imagine that avoiding things you're anxious about will help to quell them. But the opposite is true, say psychologists. It takes just 45 minutes to become familiar with an anxiety and after that it dissipates. Anxiety tends to fight back if you try to push it down. So be brave, face your fears, and watch them melt away.

● **Chew on it** When you're feeling stressed, chew some gum—the process of chewing helps to relieve stress as well as improving concentration. So say Australian researchers who put people through a variety of stress tests while chewing and not chewing gum. The results showed the gum chewers were more focused and more relaxed and were also better at complex tasks. Next time you've a problem to solve, chew it over with a piece of gum.

● **Visualize anxiety away** This effective technique, known as Autogenic Training, was developed by a German psychiatrist in the 1930s. The technique involves three daily sessions that last around 15 minutes. During each session, you repeat a set of visualizations that induce a state of relaxation. This technique can be used to alleviate many physical symptoms of anxiety. Sit or lie in a relaxed position and focus on the following throughts. Repeat the whole sequence three times:

★ My right arm is heavy.

★ My arms and legs are heavy and warm (repeat three times).

★ My heartbeat is calm and regular (repeat three times).

★ My abdomen is warm (repeat three times).

★ My forehead is cool.

★ My neck and shoulders are heavy (repeat three times).

★ I am at peace (repeat three times).

● **Focus on one thing at a time** For a busy person, multitasking may seem like an effective way of getting more done, but it can be counterproductive. For many people, trying to do several jobs at once can lead to high levels of stress, making them unable to complete any of them successfully. Reduce your anxiety levels by working on one task at a time—and make sure you make the time to relax after completing each job.

● **Try some valerian** This plant smells a bit like old rope—which might just put a damper on your mood. But if you can bear it, the pretty pink herb is an effective natural anxiety soother. Research suggests that the active ingredients in valerian attach to the same receptors in the brain that are affected by well-known anti-anxiety drugs. Take it as tea or in tablet form, sourced from your

BELIEVE IT OR NOT!

Love hormones may help overcome shyness

Oxytocin is the hormone that helps mothers bond with babies. It's also responsible for the feeling of closeness and bonding you experience during sex and when sharing a meal with family or friends. "The love hormone," as it is known, is now being used to help people overcome shyness.

local health food store. Remember to follow the instructions and, if you are on medication, check with your doctor before trying this herbal remedy.

● **Conquer social anxiety with herbal help from the North** *Rhodiola rosea* (also known as golden root) has been used for centuries to help Siberian and Arctic peoples cope with the stresses of living in a cold climate, and a 2008 study published in *The Journal of Alternative and Complementary Medicine* provided backing for its benefits in treating anxiety. Be sure to ask your doctor before using the herb if you're pregnant or taking prescribed medication.

● **Kick away your crutches** It's all too easy at times of stress to look to substances that seem to provide instant anxiety relief. Alcohol is a crutch used by many people suffering from stress, and smokers will often increase the amount they smoke when they feel under pressure. Using alcohol or nicotine as a substitute for confronting the underlying cause of the problem will only make matters worse. See your doctor if your anxiety is so severe that you feel you need such "help."

For further tips on giving up alcohol and tobacco, see Chapter 21, *Breaking Bad Habits*

17
Safeguard
YOUR BRAIN

The mechanisms that are key to healthy brain function are also vulnerable to certain disorders—perhaps most alarmingly of major degenerative diseases, Alzheimer's and Parkinson's. But science is learning much more about the causes of these conditions, and this knowledge is beginning to provide effective strategies for combating these threats.

Diet and
LIFESTYLE

The way you live has a direct effect on your brain—not only its day-to-day performance, but also how it will function as you age. You'll learn here how to make healthy choices that will benefit your brain's well-being both now and in the future.

● **Feed with fish** It's no old wives' tale that oily fish nourishes the brain. The magic ingredients are omega-3 fatty acids, which increase the blood levels of good cholesterol, known as HDL (high density lipoprotein). You can also get omega-3 fatty acids from a variety of other foods, including walnuts, monosaturated fats, such as canola oil, and omega-3 rich spreads. In a group of over-60s, those with low HDL levels were found to be 53 percent more likely to have memory problems compared to those with high levels of HDL.

● **Enjoy a yolk** In addition to omega-3 fats, the brain benefits from an essential nutrient called choline, which occurs in many high-fat foods. Egg yolk, milk, cheese, meats, and liver, as well as avocado and almonds, all contain choline. The body uses choline to produce acetylcholine, a key protective nutrient against decline in mental capabilities. Eat small amounts of all these fat-containing foods regularly to give your brain the best chance possible of staying healthy.

● **Add natural flavorings** If the recipe demands it—and your taste buds can cope—add generous amounts of ginger or rosemary to your favorite dishes. Both ingredients are powerful antioxidants and help to stimulate blood flow, and therefore the supply of oxygen to the brain.

Ginger in your cooking can boost blood flow to the brain.

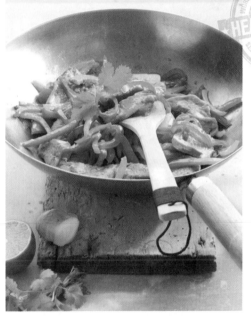

● **Avoid fried snack foods** Levels of "bad" LDL (low density lipoprotein) cholesterol are higher in people who eat a lot of fried and processed foods and baked goods. Those with high levels of LDL develop chronic inflammation in brain cells, resulting in gradual cognitive decline and memory loss. Trans fats, which are found in fast food and processed snacks such as chips, are the worst culprits for raising LDL levels. They also lead to a build up of arterial plaque that can wreak havoc with the blood supply to the brain.

● **Quit to remember** Stopping smoking could improve your memory, attention span, and ability to react quickly if you use nicotine replacement therapies (NRTs) such as patches, gum or lozenges to help.

BELIEVE IT OR NOT!

Mobile phones may boost blood flow

An international study on the long-term effects of the electromagnetic waves emitted by mobile phones found that these machines could actually be good for the brain. The research, published in the *Journal of Alzheimer's Disease*, suggests that when exposed to electromagnetic waves, the brain warms up very slightly over a period of months, boosting blood flow and energy metabolism in the brain. Despite the reassurances, many experts remain cautious, and "excessive" mobile phone use by children should be discouraged, says the UK's Health Protection Agency.

Researchers tested NRT users before and after quitting and reported significant improvements in attention and memory. But there is a risk of becoming addicted to the nicotine—the toxic chemical also present in tobacco—in NRTs. So do not use NRTs unless they are part of a plan to quit smoking.

● **Consider a daily aspirin** Clearer thinking has been noticed as a side effect in over-65-year-olds prescribed a daily low dose of aspirin. In a major study, people on aspirin tested significantly better in cognitive fluency—the ability to produce the name of words in a specific category, such as makes of cars. The researchers report in the journal *The Lancet* that aspirin-takers were 20 percent less likely to develop problems in this area, with smokers and those with high cholesterol getting the most benefit. Always seek your doctor's advice before taking daily aspirin, as even low doses can trigger dangerous internal bleeding.

● **Limit the sweet stuff** Eating too much sugar in food or sweetened drinks can increase your levels of damaging blood fats known as triglycerides. It seems that triglyceride levels could be an even more accurate predictor of stroke risk in

Mobile phones could be good for older brains.

post-menopausal women than blood cholesterol levels, according to a 15-year-long US study. Women who started out with the highest triglyceride levels were twice as likely to suffer a stroke as those who started out with low levels. Next time you have your cholesterol checked, ask your doctor to measure your triglyceride levels, too.

● **Ditch the doughnuts** If you're anxious, depressed, or under a lot of stress, avoid slipping into comfort eating and the inevitable weight gain. New research shows that it's not just the jelly doughnuts and ice cream that cause weight to pile on; high levels of the stress hormone cortisol prompt the body to store more abdominal fat—probably a primitive survival mechanism hard-wired into our brains. Stop, take stock, and try to relax. Calming the mind, say researchers, will protect the brain and prevent weight gain.

● **Check your blood pressure** Reducing blood pressure is key to protecting your brain as you get older. US scientists say that healthy blood pressure is vital for memory and an ability to think: The higher your blood pressure, the more likely you are to experience cognitive decline, including poor thinking skills and forgetfulness, particularly

in old age. High blood pressure reduces blood flow to the brain, disrupting brain function. Get your blood pressure checked and, if it's high, ask your doctor about lifestyle changes—such as regular exercise, a healthy diet, and weight loss—and whether prescription medication is appropriate.

● **Avoid noise to protect your brain** "It's so noisy, I can't think straight" is a common expression—and true. Children who attend schools near noisy airports have more learning problems than those in quiet areas, and it's been shown that in adults, loud sounds can raise blood pressure. A study near a European airport found that a 10-decibel increase in noise, caused by nighttime takeoffs, caused an average 14 percent rise in blood pressure in people 45 and over. High blood pressure is known to increase the risk of mental decline and problems with thought processes. The message is simple: Avoid frequent exposure to excessive noise and, if you have a choice, live far from major transport routes.

● **Squeeze more oranges** A UK study of 70,000 women found evidence that those who had the highest intake of flavanone, a compound found in citrus fruit had a

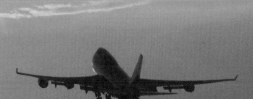

Excessive noise affects your brain and sends blood pressure soaring.

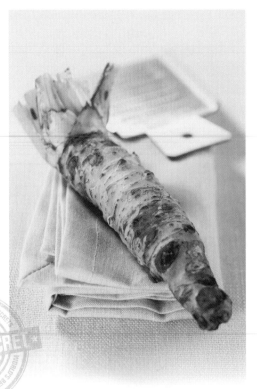

The Japanese condiment wasabi helps the growth of nerve connections.

that files memories, is interrupted and it may take a while to get back to normal. If you consistently get less sleep than you need, your memory can become unreliable.

● **Don't keep heading the ball** Studies show that repeatedly heading a soccer ball can cause lacerations to nerve fibers in the brain that affect attention, memory, sight, planning, and problem solving—damage similar to that seen in traumatic brain injury. Scientists in New York who looked at brain scans of amateur players emphasize that a single header will not cause damage. But regular heading—up to 1,000 or 1,500 times a year—"could set off a cascade of responses that can lead to degeneration of brain cells," according to a leading neurologist. There is particular concern about excessive heading of the ball by children. Although there isn't yet enough evidence to devise safe coaching guidelines, it makes sense to discourage youngsters from excessive ball-heading.

reduced stroke risk. The study did not reveal a conclusive link, but citrus fruit is a rich source of flavonoids, nutrients that improve blood vessel health in your body and brain. Whether it's squeezing juice, blending smoothies, or enjoying them as nature intended, there are plenty of ways you can increase your fruit intake and benefit the blood vessels in your brain.

● **Prioritize sleep** To avoid memory problems, you need to sleep well. The "fuzziness" that follows disrupted sleep—whether due to shift work, long-haul flights, or insomnia— won't necessarily disappear after a good night's rest. When you don't sleep properly, the work of the hippocampus, the part of the brain

For further tips on dealing with sleep problems, see Chapter 20, *A Better Night's Sleep*

● **Drink one glass of wine** A glass of wine a day staves off dementia in those over 65, according to anti-aging experts in the UK. The benefits of regular alcohol consumption based on the fact that wine is a rich source of polyphenols—natural antioxidants that provide important protection for the health of the brain. But the experts warn against excessive alcohol intake, which causes around one in ten of all cases of dementia.

● **Try spicy wasabi** This hot-tasting Japanese condiment, often served with sushi, is packed with compounds that encourage the growth of connections between nerve cells. Horseradish and broccoli are also excellent sources of these beneficial substances.

Keeping
DEMENTIA AT BAY

There's a lot you can do, even from an early age, to minimize your risk of developing dementia, often caused by Alzheimer's disease. As well as paying attention to diet and exercise, try the many simple and often surprising tips on the following pages.

● **Shrink your belly** Doctors have been telling us for years that abdominal fat can cause heart disease, diabetes, and cancer, but its effects on the brain are not so well known. But now Korean researchers have discovered that too much belly fat also puts a strain on the brain. People over 60 with a high body mass index (BMI) and a large waist are more likely to show cognitive decline and develop dementia. Fat deposits in the abdomen appear to make the hippocampus—the brain's memory center— shrink. Belly fat also damages links between brain cells. This so-called "brain rust" drains memory and thinking power in later life and increases the risk of dementia. So don't delay, ask your doctor about how to shed those extra inches around your waist.

● **Chat it up** Picking up the phone for a conversation with friends protects brain power and memory. US research shows that women with many friends who they contact every day have lower rates of dementia in later life, compared to those who mainly chat with their partner at home. Whether you phone, email, or tweet, keep in regular touch with your friends and wider family.

● **Pump up your Bs** High doses of B vitamins can halve the rate of brain shrinkage in older people showing signs of Alzheimer's disease, according to scientists at Oxford University in the UK. Certain B

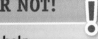

BELIEVE IT OR NOT!

A brain dye could help
Thioflavin T, a common dye that Alzheimer's researchers use in experiments to color the tangle of proteins thought to trigger the disease could turn out to be an effective anti-aging agent in its own right. US scientists have found that worms soaked in the dye live for up to 70 percent longer than undyed worms. The dye seems to preserve a healthy environment for brain proteins, preventing the tangling that occurs in people prone to Alzheimer's. It is still too early to say whether this discovery will lead to a breakthrough treatment for Alzheimer's sufferers.

vitamins—folic acid and vitamins B6 and B12—control blood levels of a substance called homocysteine, which is associated with faster brain shrinkage and Alzheimer's. The scientists found that people at risk of Alzheimer's reduced their brain shrinkage by 30 percent by taking high doses of B vitamins. But experts urge caution. Talk to your doctor before exceeding recommended daily doses of vitamins.

● **Seek early diagnosis** Hope that Alzheimer's can be diagnosed at a much earlier stage has emerged through a form of

GETTING A DIAGNOSIS

Many symptoms of Alzheimer's disease are similar to those associated with other disorders, and this means that there is no quick and easy test that provides a definite diagnosis. But it is now possible for doctors to diagnose the disease with 90 percent certainty over a period of time. Below is a three-step plan to help you obtain a diagnosis, whether for yourself or for a member of your family:

1 Take the cognitive function test
Developed at Oxford University in the UK, this online test may help you decide whether you have early problems with different components of your memory. You can find it at www.foodforthebrain.org.

2 Check your symptoms
If you (or a member of your family) have three or more of these symptoms, consult your family doctor (see Step 3).

- Memory loss that affects job skills
- Difficulty performing familiar tasks
- Poor judgement
- Tendency to misplace things
- Problems with language, such as not remembering the right word
- Disorientation about time and place
- Problems with abstract thinking
- Changes in mood, behavior or personality
- Loss of initiative

3 Talk to your doctor
Explain to your doctor why you think that you (or your relative) may need to be assessed for dementia. He or she will probably ask about your medical history, perform a physical examination, and possibly refer you to a memory clinic. Blood and urine tests and a brain scan may also be arranged to rule out conditions such as vitamin deficiency, stroke, thyroid problems, or a brain tumor.

MRI scanning—known as proton magnetic resonance spectroscopy—that can identify significant brain changes even in people who display no sign of cognitive decline. Early diagnosis is important because it allows you (or your relative) to receive treatment that can delay the progress of the disease. In some cases, such testing may eliminate Alzheimer's as a diagnosis, opening the door to treatment of the true cause of the problem. If you are concerned that your symptoms may be a sign of Alzheimer's, ask your doctor about the tests that are available.

● Reassure yourself about the risk
The risk of Alzheimer's is slightly increased in the offspring of a sufferer, but it remains a relatively low risk, since up to 100 different genes are involved. As the UK's Alzheimer's Society explains: "It is unlikely that the child of an Alzheimer's sufferer would inherit all the disease-susceptibility genes." If you have a parent with Alzheimer's, your best strategy is to live the healthiest possible lifestyle. This will ensure that you have the energy and physical strength to support your parent, and also reduce your already low chances of developing the disease.

● Try herbs to slow mental decline
Some herbs and spices seem to slow down the onset of Alzheimer's by improving circulation and alleviating the mood swings, anxiety, and sleep problems that are often a feature of the disorder. Here are a few suggestions for herbal remedies that are reputed to help:

★ **American ginseng** Take two 500mg capsules with breakfast and with lunch.

★ **Schisandra tincture** Take 20–40 drops in water three times a day.

★ **Herbal teas** Sip infusions of dried lemon balm leaves, passionflower, or California poppy to reduce anxiety.

★ **Ginkgo biloba** Take a supplement if you are an older person, especially if you have narrowed arteries. Ginkgo biloba is an antioxidant herb with blood-thinning properties. It may delay the development of Alzheimer's disease by promoting blood flow to the brain.

★ **Sage** is a traditional remedy against decline in mental function. Modern science has revealed that it may work by boosting the brain chemical acetylcholine. Add it to meat and poultry dishes or sip tea made by infusing a few leaves in boiling water.

★ **Turmeric** is thought to protect the brain from the build up of amyloid plaques, the rogue proteins that trigger Alzheimer's. This pungent yellow spice contains curcumin and is widely used in Ayurvedic medicine. Curcumin is thought to be the reason why there are so few cases of Alzheimer's in India: In people aged 65 and older in Indian villages, the incidence is only 1 in 100—the lowest rate in the world.

● **Use it or lose it** Having a mentally demanding job builds connections between brain cells that act as a "cognitive reserve" and help to ward off Alzheimer's in later life. And there is now evidence that people who have regularly engaged in mentally stimulating activities during their lives have fewer amyloid plaques in their brains, the hallmark change of Alzheimer's. In a small US study of people in their 60s, about a third developed Alzheimer's. These people were found to have had the least intellectually demanding jobs between the ages of 20 and 50. A UK study of people with early signs of dementia has shown that

BELIEVE IT OR NOT!

Coffee clears your brain

A daily cup of coffee may help prevent Alzheimer's disease—and drinking five cups appears to have an even greater preventive effect. The finding, by researchers in Finland and Sweden, may surprise coffee lovers, who are used to being told they are drinking too much of the beverage. But the study shows that three to five cups a day reduces the risk of Alzheimer's in later life by up to 65 percent. Caffeine helps to raise levels of a protein called granulocyte-colony stimulating factor (GCSF), which is thought to delay the onset of Alzheimer's. Yet caffeine on its own isn't effective. The formation of GCSF, it seems, requires the synergy of both caffeine and another, as yet unidentified, ingredient of coffee.

Sage, a traditional remedy against mental decline, boosts levels of chemical messengers in the brain.

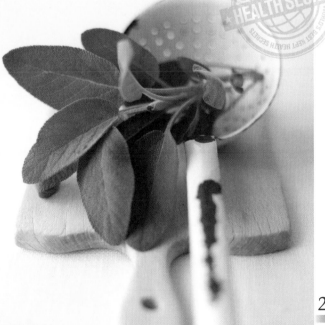

those who continued to work, despite the diagnosis, maintained sharp brain activity for the longest. If you don't have mentally demanding work, the following activities that you can do at home in your spare time could help keep your brain healthy:

★ **Play computer games**
★ **Solve puzzles**
★ **Read and write regularly**.

● **See an ophthalmologist** Regular eye tests won't just help you see better, they'll also help you think more clearly. Loss of vision in older people can often be accompanied by a decline in memory and other thinking skills. People with the "wet" type of age-related macular degeneration (AMD) who fail to get treatment and therefore suffer loss of vision, often have poorer memories than those who have been treated. And research shows that some elderly people with mild Alzheimer's disease experience an improvement in cognitive ability, sleep patterns, and mood following successful cataract surgery.

● **Take prescribed NSAIDs** People with rheumatoid arthritis who take nonsteroidal anti-inflammatory drugs (NSAIDs) to reduce the joint pain caused by inflammation are less likely to develop Alzheimer's than those who don't take NSAIDs. The reason, doctors believe, is that anti-inflammatory drugs may reduce the brain inflammation that is thought to contribute to a decline in mental functioning. Testing is now underway to discover whether the powerful anti-inflammatory drugs used to treat arthritis could have some benefit for those already diagnosed with Alzheimer's disease. However, NSAIDs can have unwanted and sometimes dangerous side effects; there are currently no grounds for taking NSAIDs as a preventive measure.

● **Go that extra mile** The more active you are between the ages of 20 and 59, the lower your risk of getting Alzheimer's, say scientists. And post-60, the benefits of exercise continue. A US study of retired men aged 71 to 93 found that those who walked less than a quarter of a mile a day were twice as likely to develop dementia compared to men who walked more than two miles daily. Another US study of women aged 70 to 81 showed that even those who walked for just 1½ hours a week did better on tests of mental function than less active females. It's particularly important to have plenty of exercise if you have a family history of Alzheimer's disease.

● **Explore "mindfulness training"** Research in Stockholm, Sweden, reveals that calm people are less likely to develop Alzheimer's than those who become easily distressed or have a negative outlook. In fact, calm people who are also outgoing and sociable are the least likely candidates for the disorder. But how can "glass half empty" people change and take a more positive view of the world? One technique that may help is "mindfulness training"—a form of meditation that aims to cultivate

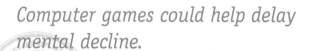

Computer games could help delay mental decline.

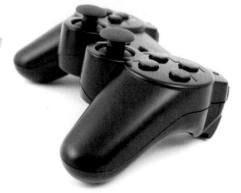

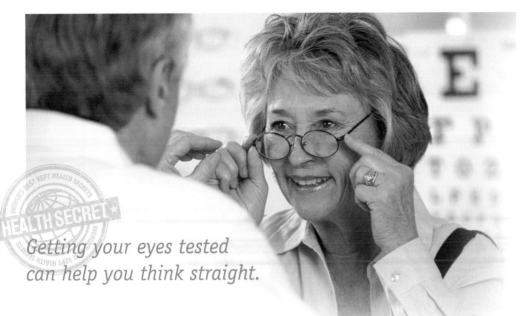

*Getting your eyes tested
can help you think straight.*

compassion, curiosity, and an awareness of the present moment. Mindfulness can reduce stress and prevent depression. Visit www.helpguide.org/harvard/benefits-of-mindfulness.htm for further information. You can achieve positive changes if you:

★ **Relax** Practice a few minutes of deep breathing once or twice a day. Try the technique described on page 305.

★ **Have a regular massage** It doesn't matter what type of massage you choose as long as you benefit from it and you can fit it into your everyday life.

★ **Try a yoga class** You are never too old to start doing yoga; opt for a class that matches your experience and suppleness.

★ **Take a break** You can get long-term gains by taking time away from your usual stresses and strains.

● **Treat sleep apnea** This condition, in which breathing pauses for several seconds or even minutes during sleep, affects six out of ten elderly people. Scientists writing in the *Journal of the American Medical Association* warn that, if not treated, the disorder leads to low levels of oxygen in the blood, which increases the risk of dementia.

The scientists found that just under half of those with sleep apnea developed cognitive impairment or dementia, compared with nearly one in three of those without the problem. Treatment, which is essential, normally involves a plastic sleep mask linked by a tube to a small bedside machine that generates sufficient air pressure to keep the airwaves open during sleep.

BELIEVE IT OR NOT!

Alzheimer's clues in the nose
The search for new ways to identify the earliest stages of Alzheimer's disease has made some surprising discoveries. One of the most promising methods is to check deposits in the mucus membranes of the nose. German researchers have shown that the tau protein—the chemical that damages brain cells in people with Alzheimer's—is deposited in the nasal passages long before there is any sign of mental decline. If further tests confirm the findings, nasal-passage testing could become a valuable tool in screening for Alzheimer's disease.

Secrets of
DEFEATING DEMENTIA

By 2012 there were more than 30 million people suffering from dementia worldwide, a figure that is expected to increase as the population continues to grow and age. Efforts are redoubling to find new treatments that can delay the onset of symptoms and reduce their severity. Here are some of the newest therapies under investigation.

In the not so distant past, it was assumed that little could be done for those suffering from the various forms of mental decline known collectively as dementia—but medical advances are at last leading to significant changes in attitudes and treatment. There are several types of dementia, and people can have more than one form—Alzheimer's disease is the most common, followed by vascular dementia.

Attacking plaques

In Alzheimer's disease, sticky plaques of amyloid proteins form in the brain and interfere with the transmission of nerve messages. Much of today's dementia research focuses on using peptides (molecules of which proteins are made) that disrupt the process of plaque formation. In 2012, researchers in Ohio were due to begin trials of the anticancer drug bexarotene, which has been associated with the breakdown of Alzheimer's plaques at "unprecedented speed." The drug appears to reduce levels of beta amyloid, a key protein in plaque production, and boost amounts of a protein that helps to remove beta amyloid from the brain and keep it functioning normally.

Other research is investigating whether drugs can be used to prompt the immune system to attack and destroy amyloid plaques. And following an intensive 20-year study, a new drug, CPHPC, has been developed that can remove serum amyloid P (SAP), a protein that accumulates in the tangles of brain cells that form as Alzheimer's progresses. More research is planned to determine whether removing SAP can prevent further deterioration.

High-protein tea

Studies at the University of South Florida have shown that a protein present in green tea may decrease production of the beta amyloid protein thought to play a crucial part in the development of Alzheimer's.

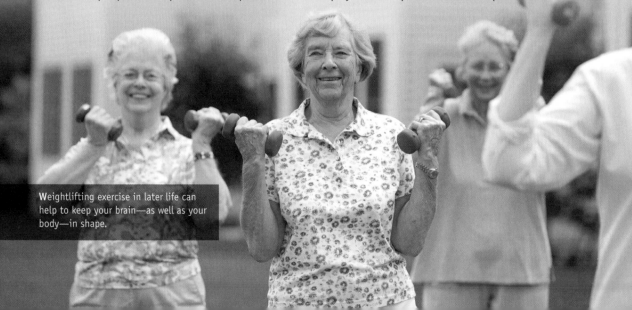

Weightlifting exercise in later life can help to keep your brain—as well as your body—in shape.

The active ingredient is an antioxidant called epigallocatechin gallate (EGCG). But the team also found that the action of EGCG is inhibited by other compounds in the tea, so the antioxidant will have to be isolated. Merely drinking the tea is unlikely to be beneficial.

Treatments today

Since Alzheimer's is as yet irreversible, treatment is based on drugs that may slow the onset of symptoms and the creation of a well-ordered, active daily routine to help those who have the disease to retain their quality of life for as long as possible.

Improving the messages

Great strides have been made with the development of drugs that inhibit the action of cholinesterase, an enzyme that breaks down acetylcholine—a key neurochemical messenger that is severely depleted in Alzheimer's. The most commonly used drug of this kind is donepezil (Aricept) but galantamine (Reminyl), the newest in this class, is more effective at boosting acetylcholine and is used to treat both severe and moderate Alzheimer's. Rivastigmine (Exelon) is also prescribed. Patients taking cholinesterase inhibitors often experience better motivation, confidence, memory, and thinking as well as reduced anxiety.

Balancing brain chemistry

In normal brains, glutamate—a type of neurotransmitter—activates neurons so that they can transmit messages around the brain. But excess glutamate is not only toxic but is implicated in the neuron degeneration found in Alzheimer's. Drugs classed as NMDA antagonists, including memantine (Ebixa), block glutamate activity, slowing the progression of symptoms and helping calm aggression. They are effective in people with severe Alzheimer's and those who are unable to take cholinesterase inhibitors.

Varied daily activities

A year-long study in Bavaria compared two groups of people with different degrees of dementia. Both groups continued taking their regular antidementia drugs, and one group also took part in 2 hours a day of varied activities, including doing puzzles, gardening, bowling, exercising, and singing. In this group, symptoms got no worse; in the "drugs only" group, they continued to deteriorate. The team concluded that the effect of such activities on the ability to perform everyday tasks was twice as high as that achieved by medication alone.

Exercise benefits

In a study at the University of British Columbia a group of 86 women, all between the ages of 70 and 80 and with mild memory problems, were divided into three different exercise groups: weightlifting, walking, or balance-and-tone exercises. Each group did the exercises twice a week for 6 months. When their brain activity was examined using MRI scans, and participants were tested for cognitive functions including memory, attention, and planning, those in the weightlifting group showed most improvement, but all benefited to some extent, confirming how vital it is that people with dementia get some exercise every day.

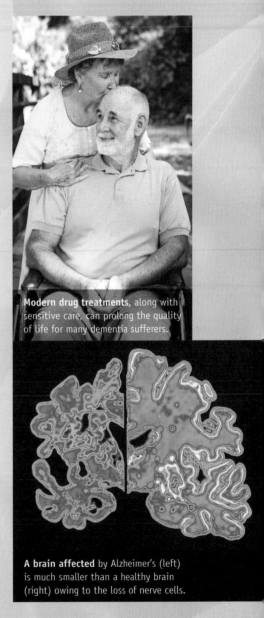

Modern drug treatments, along with sensitive care, can prolong the quality of life for many dementia sufferers.

A brain affected by Alzheimer's (left) is much smaller than a healthy brain (right) owing to the loss of nerve cells.

Parkinson's disease:
SLOWING THE SYMPTOMS

The degenerative condition, Parkinson's, affects 7 to 10 million people worldwide. As yet there is no cure, but there are many ways to help protect yourself against the disease and also to relieve symptoms if you already have Parkinson's.

● **Drink polyphenol-rich green tea** Green tea contains plant chemicals called polyphenols—antioxidants that may protect against Parkinson's disease—according to research published in the US journal *Biological Psychiatry*. Polyphenols help to prevent the breakdown of the nerve cells in the brain responsible for producing dopamine, a brain chemical essential for transmitting signals that coordinate movement. The reduction in the number of these cells makes it difficult for people with Parkinson's to move normally and maintain balance. Try to make green tea a daily habit, whether or not you are at risk of Parkinson's.

Giving newly painted rooms a thorough airing will reduce your exposure to dangerous fumes.

● **Beware of solvents** Researchers have discovered that exposure to the dry-cleaning solvent perchloroethylene (PERC, also known as tetrachloroethylene) increases the risk of developing Parkinson's disease ten-fold. Exposure to other industrial solvents was found to hold similar risks. Chemicals of this type are also used in some glues, paints, and carpet cleaners. To protect yourself, try to avoid spending time in places where these chemicals are used and give rooms that have been newly painted or recarpeted a thorough airing before you use them again.

● **Have lots of berries** Eat raspberries, strawberries, and chocolate as often as you can (though not necessarily together) say nutritionists. Summer berries are a good source of anthocyanins—plant chemicals that may help protect brain cells and reduce the risk of Parkinson's disease. Both chocolate and berries are rich in flavonoids, which have also been shown to protect against this neurological disorder.

● **Be alert for deep-brain therapy**
Researchers in the UK discovered that they could make healthy people move in slow motion by applying an electric current to the scalp to boost their brain waves. Deep-brain stimulation, involving an implantable chip powered by a battery, could be used to regulate brain waves, thereby reducing the impact of Parkinson's symptoms. In the USA, scientists have created a computer model of the brain's neural networks to improve understanding of Parkinson's. If they can find the precise area to stimulate, deep-brain stimulation could become a standard treatment.

● **Calm with a herbal tea** Have a regular cup of herbal tea or a dose of a preparation with calming and muscle-relaxant qualities to help combat the symptoms of Parkinson's disease. Here are some suggestions:
★ **Try a teaspoonful** of dried St John's wort or lavender in a cup of boiling water.
★ **Add 25 drops** of tincture of passion flower to a glass of water.
★ **Take a couple** of valerian capsules.

● **Be a proactive patient** Don't assume that because your doctor has prescribed medicine for your condition that there's no more that can be done, even if your condition worsens. The brain's response to levodopa, the drug most commonly used for Parkinson's, changes over time. Always tell your doctor about any increase in symptoms; he or she may decide to adjust the dose or type of drug prescribed.

● **Don't mix protein and medication**
Protein, found in meat, fish, eggs, and dairy products, can interfere with the absorption of levodopa, the drug often used to treat Parkinson's. The UK's Parkinson's Disease

Gou teng, a traditional Chinese remedy, contains a chemical that normalizes vital brain cell functions.

HEALTH SECRET

Society advises taking this medication 45 minutes before a meal but not with a milk-containing drink.

● **Try Chinese gou teng** Used for centuries in China, the herb gou teng has produced positive results as a treatment for Parkinson's in Western drug company trials. Sufferers reported better sleep and more fluent speech after just 13 weeks on gou teng, according to the journal *Parkinson's Disease*. Researchers found that the herb contains an alkaloid called isorhy, which appears to normalize the brain-cell death process that often becomes disrupted by Parkinson's. A synthesized version of the herb is being developed that may eventually lead to a new treatment for Parkinson's. If you are considering using this remedy, or especially if you are already on medication, discuss it first with your doctor.

● **Seek expert physiotherapy**
Increasing stiffness is common in Parkinson's sufferers. But there's much that can be done by following an exercise program under the guidance of a physiotherapist. Similarly, you may notice problems with speech for which specialized speech therapy can be helpful. Ask your doctor if you think you could benefit from either or both therapies.

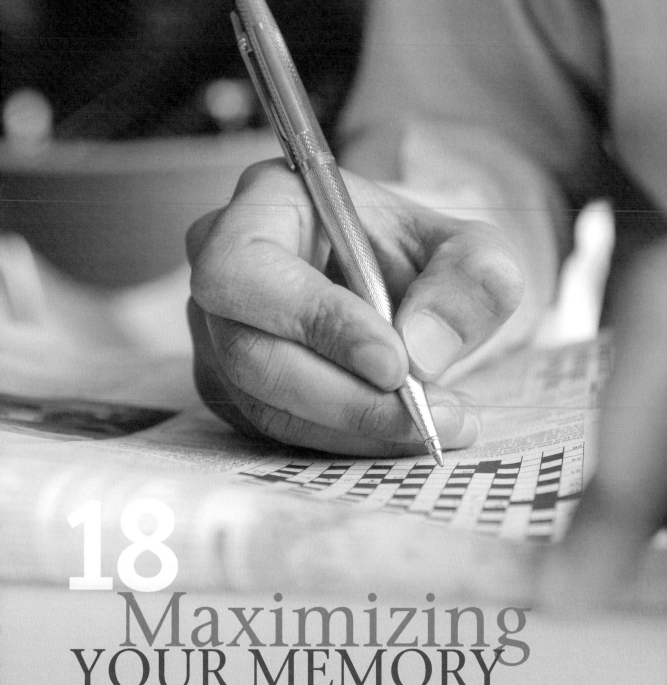

18
Maximizing
YOUR MEMORY

The human brain's capacity for recall is truly mind-boggling, but memory is more than a mental filing cabinet. From childhood memories to knowing where you've left your keys, it plays a vital role in your life. Nobody wants to become forgetful and, fortunately, research now shows that serious lapses are not inevitable as we go through life. Read on for tips to help you retain your precious memories.

Fuel your POWERS OF RECALL

As with your physical health, your memory can be affected by how you look after it, and specifically by what you eat and drink. To keep it functioning well into old age, nourish your brain with a healthy, varied diet that includes as many as possible of the brain-boosting foods suggested on the following pages.

● **Drink blueberries** Consuming the equivalent of 2 to 2½ cups (500–600ml) of blueberry juice a day can boost your memory, according to a study at the University of Cincinnati. When a group of volunteers in their 70s with early memory decline did this for two months they performed significantly better in learning and memory tests. A second group given a placebo did not appear to benefit. So try blueberry juice instead of your usual drink and see the difference. For extra benefit, include blueberries in your regular diet.

● **Dine on greens** Green leafy vegetables contain an abundance of folates, a type of B vitamin that can help to improve memory and information-processing skills. In a study carried out in the Netherlands, researchers gave a group of volunteers either a low-dose folic acid supplement (a synthetic form of folate) or a placebo for three years. At the end of the study, tests showed the folic acid group had significantly better memory than the placebo group. Leafy greens, broccoli, and green beans are all excellent sources of folate, so eat these delicious vegetables as often as possible.

● **Eat oily fish twice a week** Among the many studies confirming the benefits of fish oils for the brain, a review by researchers at the London School of Hygiene and Tropical Medicine revealed that higher levels of an omega-3 fatty acid called docosahexaenoic acid (DHA)—found in oily fish, such as salmon, sardines, and mackerel—improves cognitive function, including memory, and reduces the risk of dementia in older people. A separate study at the University of California found that omega-3 fatty acids help to strengthen synapses, the connections between brain cells. Two to three portions of oily fish a week will provide sufficient omega-3s to

BELIEVE IT OR NOT!

Breathe insulin

Inhaling insulin helps improve memory in people with memory impairment, according to scientists from Brazil and the USA. In a study, people who breathed in insulin twice daily had improved memory and ability to carry out everyday tasks. Insulin has a positive effect on the memory by feeding the brain extra glucose, which it needs to function efficiently. Insulin also helps to cancel out the effects of cortisol, a stress hormone that interferes with retrieving memories. But breathing insulin is not practical for most people; instead make sure your brain gets the glucose it needs by taking daily exercise and eating less fat and refined sugar.

keep your memory in good shape. If you're not keen on eating fish, try a daily fish oil supplement in capsule form.

● **Eat a starchy breakfast** Always eat breakfast, say researchers at Canada's University of Toronto. Their study of a group of healthy men and women aged 61 to 79 found that they performed better in memory tests after a morning meal. It did not matter whether the food source was protein, starch, or fat. Another study from the same institute compared the memory-improving effects of different breakfasts eaten after an overnight fast. A starchy meal of potatoes or barley produced better results in short- and long-term memory tests than a glucose-laden lemon drink. The sugars in starchy foods increase the blood levels of the brain's essential fuel—glucose. Here are some ideas for a memory-boosting breakfast:

★ **A bowl of oatmeal** or cereal topped with dried cranberries and sliced almonds

★ **An omelet** filled with chopped vegetables

★ **A whole-grain bagel** topped with sliced tomatoes and cucumber, followed by a handful of berries

★ **A slice of whole-wheat toast** spread with peanut butter, followed by a sliced banana or low-fat yogurt sprinkled with granola and fruit.

● **Try memory-boosting guarana** This Amazon rainforest fruit has long been used by the indigenous people as a natural stimulant. Its reputation has now been confirmed by research at Northumbria University in the UK. The study showed that guarana can reduce mental fatigue and make you feel more alert. Other research has also found that it can help boost memory, alertness, and mood. Guarana contains a compound called guarine, which is thought to stimulate the brain gradually over several hours rather than producing the "peaks and

---

CATEGORIES OF MEMORY

Memories are of different types and the brain handles them in different ways. There are three main categories of memory identified by doctors and used to define and diagnose the different conditions that can affect the memory.

● **Sensory memory** retains the transitory impression of a sight, sound, taste, or smell as soon as you experience it. This form of memory tends to be lost soon after the stimulus ends. But the memory of particular smells is longer lasting and is often linked to the emotions that you felt at the same time.

● **Short-term memory** is a temporary bank where information is stored for a few seconds or minutes. For example, a telephone number you're about to call or the name of someone you've just met. As you age, your short-term memory becomes progressively less effective.

● **Long-term memory** is a more permanent archive, in which information is stored over hours, days, or years. This includes declarative memories (simple facts or recollections of specific periods in your life) or procedural memories (relating to the retention of skills such as swimming or riding a bike). Our procedural memories are often preserved even when short-term memory is impaired.

troughs" so often associated with caffeine-laden drinks. Look out for guarana drinks, gums, and other guarana products in health food stores.

● **Say "no" to pudding** Carrying extra pounds can dim your memory. One easy way to control your weight is by saving desserts for special occasions only. When French researchers checked the body mass index (BMI) and thinking skills of 2,223 women and men aged between 32 and 62 on two occasions over five years, they found that those with high BMIs scored lower in memory tests and had a steeper mental decline. Substitute fresh fruit or low-fat yogurt for creamy puddings.

● **Fill up on legumes** Lentils, peas, and beans are rich in B vitamins, which can help protect your memory and nervous system. Vitamin B12 (cobalamin) and vitamin B9 (folate) are especially good for memory. This family of vitamins helps break down homocysteine, an amino acid that can trigger inflammation in blood vessels, which in turn can lead to clogged arteries and poor memory. Good food sources include leafy green vegetables, broccoli, and other vegetables from the cabbage family, yeast extract, cottage cheese, peanut butter, and eggs. If you think your diet could be lacking in B vitamins, ask your doctor if you should take a B-complex supplement.

● **Go veggie** Changing to a mainly vegetarian diet is just one way to reduce your cholesterol levels. Red meat is high in saturated fats, which boost levels of "bad" LDL cholesterol. High LDL levels have been shown to damage blood vessels, which in the long term may affect memory. In a study of more than 3,600 British civil servants, those with the lowest levels of "good" HDL

Extracts of the guarana fruit from the Amazon can stimulate the brain.

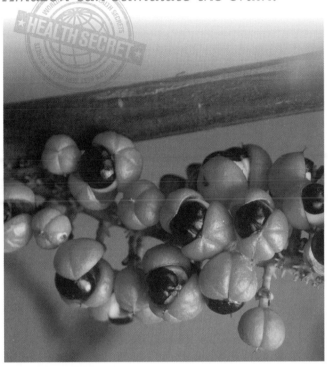

cholesterol were 60 percent more likely to have poor memories than those with high HDL levels. When researchers revisited the men five years later they found that those whose HDL levels had continued to decline were two-thirds more likely to have memory problems. Vegetarians tend to have lower cholesterol levels than those who include meat in their diet. And vegans, who eat no animal products, have even lower levels. It makes sense to cut out meat and fill up your plate with vegetables instead—even if you do this only a few times a week.

For further tips on reducing your cholesterol levels, see Chapter 2, *Blood and Circulation*

● **Savor more sage** To boost your powers of recall try to include more sage in your meals. A group of British scientists invited young adults to take part in a word recall test. Some were given capsules containing sage oil and others a placebo. Both groups were tested at intervals to see how many words they could remember. The sage oil group performed consistently better than the placebo group. To harness the herb's benefits, drink a tea made with a few fresh leaves, include sage leaves in salad dressings, or use them to flavor pork, poultry, or fish. It is thought that the anti-inflammatory effects of sage can boost the memory for several hours.

● **Give ginkgo a try** An extract from leaves of the ginkgo, or maidenhair tree contains antioxidant compounds that help to dilate blood vessels, increase blood circulation, inhibit blood vessel blockages, and encourage blood flow to the brain. These effects can help protect against memory loss caused by lack of oxygen reaching the brain.

● **Snack on grapes** Retrain your palate so that you choose healthy snacks, such as fruit, between meals. Grapes, in particular, are rich in phytochemicals and antioxidants, which help improve blood circulation to the brain and so improve cognitive function, including memory. Studies have shown that people with a high intake of trans fats, which are found in baked foods such as cookies, are at a higher risk of memory problems than those who snack on healthy foods. Portable and easy to eat, grapes are the perfect nibble.

● **Recall more with rosemary** This common herb has long been associated with remembrance. Now scientists from the UK's Northumbria University have discovered a scientific basis for this. When a group of people inhaled the aroma from essential oil of rosemary, their powers of memory and concentration showed a significant

SURPRISINGLY EASY

Drink plenty of fluids

Our brains consist of up to 85 percent water, so it's no surprise that lack of fluid has an immediate effect on memory—dehydration can lead to confusion and other problems related to brain function. A mere 2 percent drop in body water can trigger fuzzy brain syndrome. If you don't like plain water, add some interest with a sliver of orange, lemon, or lime. Alternatively, drink fruit and herbal teas, which count toward your daily fluid intake.

improvement. Pop a few drops of rosemary essential oil in an aromatherapy burner. Not only will the sweet aroma pervade your home, it will also boost your mental focus and powers of recall.

● **Drink decaffeinated coffee** A cup or two of decaffeinated coffee may help protect the memory of people suffering from age-related forgetfulness and may even prevent it—so say scientists at the Mount Sinai School of Medicine in the USA. Their research showed that consumption of decaffeinated coffee could increase the brain's ability to utilize (metabolize) glucose in the blood over a period of months. People with type 2 diabetes are particularly susceptible to memory problems caused by impaired glucose metabolism in the brain. The scientists say that drinking decaffeinated coffee may provide special benefits for those suffering from this condition.

● **Eat kale and lentils** These foods are rich in iron, which can help preserve memory. This mineral is an essential component of hemoglobin, the oxygen-carrying substance in red blood cells. And all brain functions, including memory, depend on a healthy blood supply. Iron is found in legumes, green leafy vegetables, and seeds. However, the most easily absorbed type—known as "heme" iron—is found in red meat. By treating yourself to the occasional steak, you'll be doing your memory a huge favor. Vegans, vegetarians, and people who don't eat red meat for other reasons should consider a supplement.

● **Get enough calcium** Ensure your diet contains plenty of calcium-rich foods to help keep your memory fine-tuned. Too little of this vital mineral can encourage protein build-up in the synapses—the connections between brain cells—and disrupt their functioning. Just three slices of Cheddar cheese and two glasses of milk will give you enough calcium to meet your daily quota. Leafy green vegetables such as kale and cabbage are also good calcium sources. It's worth bearing in mind that caffeine can increase the excretion of calcium and it may therefore be wise to limit your intake of coffee, tea, and cola drinks.

● **Cut your calories** Research from the Mayo Clinic in the USA suggests that eating between 2,100 and 6,000 calories a day can double your risk of memory loss or mild cognitive impairment (MCI). In a study of 1,233 people between 70 and 89 who ate different amounts of calories, the odds of developing MCI more than doubled for those eating the most. Cut calories and follow a healthy well-balanced diet to help preserve your memory as you age.

● **Don't ditch carbohydrates**
If you're trying to lose weight, don't follow a low-carbohydrate diet because it could affect your mental acuity. Your memory needs a continuous supply of glucose to function properly. By restricting your intake of carbohydrates, you are reducing the amount of glucose reaching your brain. Researchers from Tufts University found that women on a low or zero carbohydrate diet performed worse on thinking and memory tests than when they reduced calories without cutting back the carbohydrates. If you need to lose weight but want to stay at your peak mentally, don't ban carbohydrates completely.

The aroma of essential oil of rosemary could enhance your mental powers.

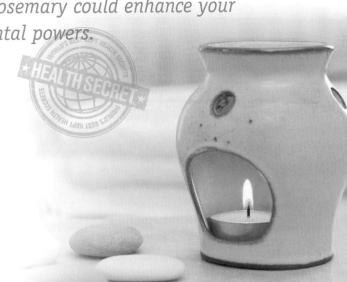

BELIEVE IT OR NOT!

Chewing gum helps your memory
When researchers put a group of 75 adults through a battery of memory and attention tests, those who were chewing gum scored higher in tests of word recall than those who merely mimicked chewing movements and another group who did not chew at all. The gum-chewing group was also more accurate in spatial working memory tests—involving items such as finding your way around a new area. Chewing is thought to boost oxygen delivery to the brain and may trigger the release of insulin, also believed to stimulate memory.

Secrets of
BOOSTING MEMORY

Before most people were literate, societies developed other ways of passing on and retaining knowledge. In the 21st century, when many of us are bombarded with information 24 hours a day, there is much we can do to improve our memories by taking our cues from cultures less sophisticated than our own. Learn their secrets here.

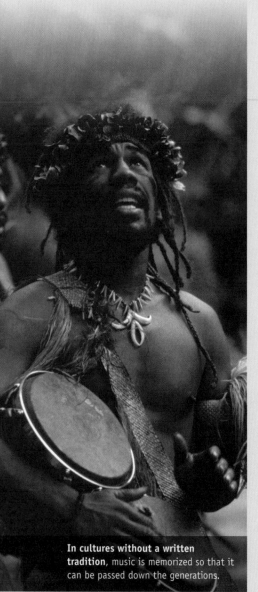

In cultures without a written tradition, music is memorized so that it can be passed down the generations.

Humans first spoke some 50,000 years ago and as societies and language evolved, experience began to be passed from generation to generation. Histories, myths, and folk tales were also communicated by word of mouth. In ancient societies such as the Yoruba of West Africa, keepers of oral lore were revered as "official" historians. Reciting information helped people to remember it. The Luba of Central Africa, for example, still recite lists of kings. They also use necklaces as memory triggers and create *lukasas*—memory boards covered with colored pins and beads to represent specific names or places.

Remembered with music and landscape

In every part of the world, music, song, and dance are central to oral tradition. Written and sung as ballads, events key to a people's history have been preserved. The Aboriginal Australians, whose ancestors are said to have sung the world into existence, identify every feature in their landscape with a different song and remember them in this way.

In cultures such as those of the Amazon rainforest, people remember how to get from one place to another by making a mental note of the subtle differences in vegetation in each small "chunk" of the landscape. By creating visual and spatial memories of each route, using the sun and stars to orientate themselves as they travel, they can journey on foot for long distances without getting lost.

Memory practice

The 2010 and 2011 World Memory Champion, 21-year-old Wang Feng, was able to recall 300 of 400 numbers spoken at a rate of one per second and remember the sequence of a shuffled pack of cards in a mere 24.21 seconds. His ability is honed by 5–6 hours of daily practice using various methods, including visualization. The "practice and performance" method dates back to ancient Greece and Rome, when—although much important information was written down—orators with exceptional powers of memory were held in great respect.

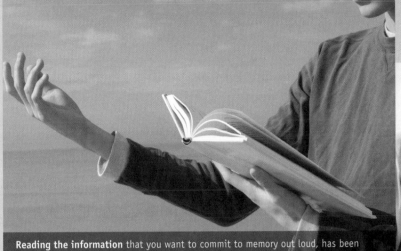

Reading the information that you want to commit to memory out loud, has been shown to fix it more firmly in your mind.

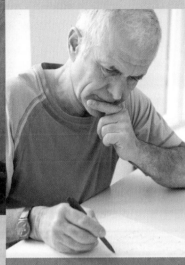

Memory tools for you to use

The memory "systems" of other cultures include a number of techniques that most of us would be able to use. Try employing some of them and you will soon see an improvement.

Memorizing in chunks Split information such as telephone numbers into manageable chunks—they will be far easier to recall.

Tell yourself a story Weave information into a story in which people and events represent things to be memorized. Studies show that this technique, akin to the oral tradition of relating myths and folk tales, makes information easier to remember and retrieve.

Say it out loud Reading information aloud makes it easier to recall. You can do this either by yourself or with someone else. Relating something to another person has been proved to help embed facts in your own memory.

Memorize to music The brain is more adept at storing and recalling information that is associated with music and rhyme, studies show. It seems that familiar music acts as a soundtrack for a "mental movie" playing in the brain. So try setting information to a well-known tune, making up your own rhymes.

Create colorful visual images in your head and associate them with the names of people and places you want to recall. To link pieces of information, draw "memory maps" made up of strong images. You could also use smells and textures in your memory maps.

Daily practice Take a leaf out of the champion's book and practice memory tasks—even simple ones like shopping lists. Rehearse over and over again until you have perfect recall. If you concentrate hard you'll find that these challenges get progressively easier.

File your memories Use the example of American Jill Price, who remembers 99.9 percent of everything that has ever happened to her, by creating your own mental filing system. By storing information in separate "compartments" in your mind, you'll greatly increase your powers of recall.

Recalling by route Imagine a familiar journey or route and place things you want to remember along it at specific locations to create spatial memories.

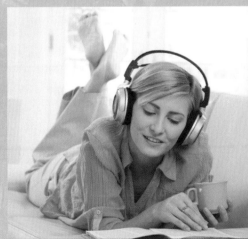

Associating information with music can make it more memorable.

Remember
YOUR LIFESTYLE

As well as watching what you eat, your memory will be helped by other lifestyle changes and tips. Most of these dos and don'ts are easy to incorporate into even the busiest life and the more of them you try and stick to, the better for your memory.

● **Forget which bus you took** By forgetting things you don't need to know—such as which bus you took last week—you are freeing up space in your memory. Research carried out at the University of Illinois showed that people who were good at discarding unnecessary information were also good at problem solving. They were also better at hanging on to memories when they were in distracting situations. Trying to remember too much can cause loss of mental acuity. So don't fret if you can't remember things of no great consequence, it just means your brain is doing its job of prioritizing information.

● **Learn a poem a day** Learning verses by heart gives those memory muscles a helpful workout. According to research carried out in the USA, a septuagenarian who started training his memory at the age of 58 can now recite all 60,000 words of John Milton's *Paradise Lost* with amazing accuracy. With enough time and effort

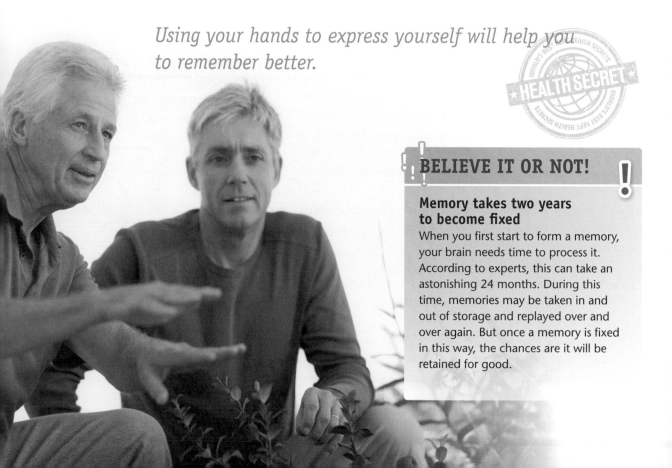

Using your hands to express yourself will help you to remember better.

HEALTH SECRET

BELIEVE IT OR NOT!

Memory takes two years to become fixed

When you first start to form a memory, your brain needs time to process it. According to experts, this can take an astonishing 24 months. During this time, memories may be taken in and out of storage and replayed over and over again. But once a memory is fixed in this way, the chances are it will be retained for good.

anyone can do it. If you don't fancy poetry, try memorizing some useful telephone numbers or zip codes.

● Let your hands do the talking

Using your hands to express what you are saying can help you to remember better. A study conducted by the University of Chicago revealed that people who gesticulated most had a more retentive memory than those who kept their hands to themselves. The researchers think using gestures may free up thinking space and therefore leave more room for memory.

● Work up a sweat
Try to do some type of regular activity that gets you slightly sweaty and breathless. You know this is good for your general health but, in addition, aerobic exercise boosts blood flow to the brain helping the hippocampus, the area associated with memory, to flourish. A small study of adults in their 60s found that going on the treadmill just three times a week for a year reversed age-linked loss of brain volume by one or two years and improved spatial memory. Choose exercise that is not so intense that you can't chat to a companion—brisk walking, jogging, or running, swimming, dancing—anything that works up a sweat.

● Be a chatterbox
Chatting could help you remember. A team of psychologists from the University of Michigan Institute for Social Research found that talking to someone for at least 10 minutes a day was good intellectual exercise—in fact, they discovered that chatting was as effective as more traditional kinds of mental exercise, such as puzzles and games, for boosting memory. So cement your memories by having a regular gab fest with your friends and family.

SECRETS OF SUCCESS

Protective headgear
Wearing a helmet when engaging in potentially risky sporting activities could save your brain. While a mild bump may have little or no effect, medical science has shown that moderate and severe head injuries can cause changes to blood flow patterns in the brain and affect connections between brain cells, contributing to memory loss. Manufacturers design helmets to withstand the impact of a fall or blow, so it's vital to wear one appropriate for your sport. Whether you're biking, motorcycling, skateboarding, horseback riding, skiing, or rock climbing, protect your memory with a helmet.

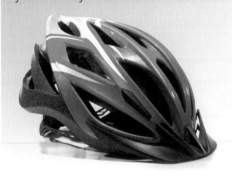

● Get 8 hours sleep
While you're asleep your memories are fixed in the brain, making later retrieval possible. A study carried out by American researchers in 2010 showed that as well as consolidating information, the brain is also organizing memories and picking out the most salient information during those nighttime hours. Scientists think sleep may not only make memories stick but could also help you to come up with creative new ideas. Numerous experiments have found that going to sleep shortly after learning new facts or skills helps your brain reinforce its memory traces. It doesn't matter if it's a good night's sleep or a quick afternoon nap, as long as you go

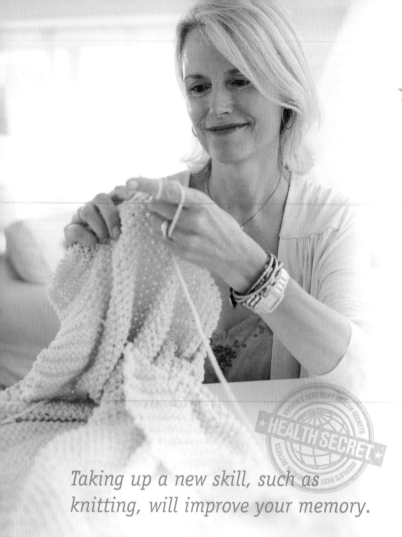

Taking up a new skill, such as knitting, will improve your memory.

BODY POWER

To learn it, do it

When it comes to remembering, physical actions are as important as thoughts. You will learn and remember something faster if you involve your body as well as your mind. For example, it is easier to remember the layout of a town if you walk the streets rather than trying to learn it from a map alone.

into a deep sleep. And to maximize the benefit to your memory, try to get about 8 hours sleep most nights.

● Build memory with "me" time

Keep your stress levels down by taking time out to do something relaxing and enjoyable every day. Studies show that high levels of cortisol, one of the main stress hormones, can damage the hippocampus, the part of the brain most closely involved with memory.

● Don't concentrate too hard

The secret to better recall could lie in timing. Give yourself time to ruminate but move on from those "tip-of-the-tongue" moments. Humans move between "areas" in their memories much as bees flit between flowers for pollen. A US study in which college students were asked to name as many animals as they could in 3 minutes found that those who stayed too long or not long enough on one task recalled fewer animals than those who were adept at switching between areas. Chances are that the information you want to retrieve will come to you if you don't dwell too long on one illusive challenge.

● Focus to fix it

Your brain needs at least 8 seconds of focused concentration to process information and send it successfully into long-term storage. To ensure efficient recall, give up multitasking and apply your mind to one thing at a time.

● Test yourself

To be sure of recalling something, repeatedly bring it to mind. Cognitive scientists are starting to appreciate this retrieval practice. In a key US study, a small group of students were asked to learn the meaning of 40 Swahili words; those who were repeatedly asked to recall the words during the learning session scored an average of 80 percent in a test a week later. But those who simply studied the words without actively testing themselves scored an average of just 36 percent. If you want to remember something, self-testing can help to make it stick.

● **Learn to draw** or take up any new skill and you'll be surprised how it can improve your memory. Anything that stretches your brain or pushes you mentally just a little bit further or in a different direction helps strengthen synapses—the connections between brain cells that enable us to learn, adapt, and form memories. If you work in an office, learn to dance; if you are a dancer, learn how to use a computer; if you are a programmer, learn how to draw. Skills such as knitting that involve brain, eye, and hand coordination are as beneficial as mentally challenging games such as bridge or chess. Whatever activity you choose, it should provide a challenge to yield the full benefit.

● **Stroll down memory lane** Walking is good for your physical health and now there is evidence that it's good for your memory, too. Research indicates that walking can prevent brain shrinkage and memory loss. In a US study, older adults who walked between 6 and 9 miles a week had more gray matter—a type of brain tissue—after nine years than people who didn't walk as far. Those who walked the most also cut their risk of memory loss in half. Make a daily walk part of your memory boosting strategy.

● **Find a quiet place** Shut yourself away in a quiet room or go to the library if you want to learn something. Studies reveal that exposure to noise can slow your ability to rehearse things in your mind—one of the ways in which you build memory links. Whether you are trying to study for exams or learning for some other reason, make sure you are not within earshot of the television, radio, or computer.

● **Clear your mind** Our ability both to recall and process information at the same time dwindles as we grow older. According

SECRETS OF SUCCESS

Expanding your brain power

Scientists have made the exciting discovery that brain cells continue to forge new connections throughout life. You are therefore capable of learning and forming new memories whatever your age. Even more amazing is that some parts of the brain—notably the hippocampus, the center of memory and emotion—can actually form new cells. This regrowth and rewiring is something you can influence, as a study of London taxi drivers proves. Magnetic resonance imaging (MRI) of the drivers' brains revealed enlargement of the area of the hippocampus used for navigating in three-dimensional space. The drivers' experience of negotiating complex London streets had exercised a part of their brains, which had grown as a result. The scientists concluded that stimulating the brain by giving it complex tasks can actually help it to grow.

to a 2011 study from a Canadian university, a cluttered mind may be to blame. The researchers suggest relaxation exercises, yoga, or meditation to give your mind a clean start. Ask at your local community center about classes in your area.

● **Get rid of the smoke** from your lungs and you will be doing your memory a favor. Smokers have poorer recall because less oxygen reaches the brain. But the encouraging news is that research reveals that once you quit, your ability to remember everyday things can improve. In a recent UK study, a group of smokers, previous smokers, and people who had never smoked were asked to do certain tasks at specific places on a tour of the campus. Smokers remembered 59 percent of the tasks, those who had given up smoking remembered 74 percent, and the nonsmokers, 81 percent. If you want to keep your memory strong, give up smoking without delay. Ask your doctor for the help you need to do this.

● **Work out to remember** Abdominal fat, the source of so many risks to bodily health, can also affect mental performance. French researchers gave word recall tests to a large group of middle-aged men and women and they found that the more svelte participants performed 35 percent better than those with the largest waist sizes. Reduce the excess fat that tends to accumulate around your middle by combining regular exercise with a calorie-controlled diet to improve your memory and other mental functions.

BODY POWER

Clear your head

Try this quick and easy relaxation exercise to clear your mind of unnecessary information. Choose a quiet time of day and a place where you won't be disturbed:

● Lie on your back on a firm bed or mat on the floor.

● Let your feet flop outward and your hands rest, palms up, by your sides.

● Close your eyes and sigh to release tension. Breathe slowly, pausing after each exhalation.

● Release tension in your toes, feet, and legs. Then do the same with your fingertips, arms, and neck. Ease tension in your shoulders by lowering them away from your ears.

● Visualize the muscles of your face becoming smooth and relaxed.

● Be aware of the relaxation in the muscles throughout your body.

● When you're ready, slowly open your eyes and stretch.

● Bend your knees and roll onto your side before slowly getting up.

● **Surf the web** Spending time searching the Internet may help to stimulate your memory. It requires you to make multiple decisions, which in turn engages the circuits associated with attention, memory, and reasoning. It could be time to stop feeling guilty about spending all those hours online. But bear in mind that meeting people in person, socializing, going for walks, and doing puzzles can be just as stimulating for your brain's memory centers.

● **Rehearse that name** When being introduced to someone new it's easy to forget their name as it goes in one ear and out the other. Try these tips to help you remember new names:

★ **Stop and listen** carefully and repeat the name in your head or out loud by saying, for example, "It's nice to meet you, Jane."

★ **Practice the names** of the people you are introduced to in the evening and the morning after the encounter.

Brain scientists call this "spaced rehearsal" and believe it to be more effective than trying to recall the names 5 minutes before the next meeting or social occasion. This technique can also help you to remember other kinds of information such as where you parked your car. Repeat to yourself the name of the road or a nearby landmark, and you'll be less likely to find yourself wandering the streets later on looking for it.

● **Brush and floss twice a day** It may surprise you to know that taking care of your teeth can help to keep your brain sharp. Numerous studies have shown that gum disease caused by poor oral hygiene may trigger inflammatory chemicals, which could affect areas of the brain involved in memory loss. Brush and floss twice daily and see your dental hygienist regularly.

● **Become a sightseer** Pick a town or city that you have always wanted to visit and spend a day exploring it. Map reading will challenge your mind, while new sights, smells and sounds will stimulate it. This in turn can help to create new synapses—those vital connections between brain cells that memories are made from. If you live in a big enough town or city, you can pick an area you don't really know, and spend some time scouting around.

● **Get dressed with your eyes closed**
Trying out new activities or performing familiar ones in a new way may help to stimulate underused nerve cells in parts of the brain linked to memory and abstract thought, according to research from the Duke University Medical Center. Nerve cells in these areas tend to shrink with age, which can reduce the brain's ability to process new experiences and retrieve old memories. To keep your brain alert and improve its processing power, give it an occasional surprise—for example, try getting dressed with your eyes closed, or try brushing your teeth, holding your fork, or using your computer mouse with your nondominant hand.

● **Take a break** A rest may be as effective as sleeping in terms of refreshing your brain. US researchers asked a group of people to do a mental task before instructing them to rest and let their minds float free. Using a brain-scanning technique that shows the brain at work, they found that during rest periods the areas of the brain concerned with memory were as active as when the participants were engaged in the task. It would seem that your brain is working for you even when you're resting. So take that coffee break even if you're busy; it may help you to remember.

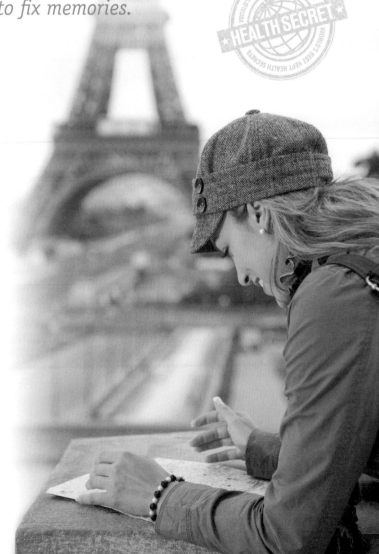

Using a map to explore new places stimulates your mind and helps to fix memories.

HEALTH SECRET

What the
EXPERTS KNOW

If you are experiencing memory problems, there could be a variety of causes—many of which are unrelated to age. Some drugs can interfere with the brain, as can fluctuations in hormone levels and certain illnesses. Read on to find out more about what the professionals know and what they can do to help.

● **Select your statin** Cholesterol-lowering statins offer excellent protection against heart disease and stroke, but several drugs in this group can affect memory. A recent overview of many thousands of people taking statins found that some statins could impair recollection of recent events. If you feel that the statin you're taking is having this effect, speak to your doctor about changing to a different variety, but don't stop your medication without medical advice.

● **Get help for depression** Consult your doctor if you're feeling depressed. Depression slows your brain's ability to process information, hinders concentration, and can deplete memory. It has also been linked with physical changes in the brain itself. When researchers from King's College London scanned the brains of a group of depressed people, they found a reduced volume in the hippocampus—the area of the brain related to memory—compared with a group of happier people. Depression appears to interfere with neural connections, making memories difficult to form and retrieve. If you are feeling low as well as having problems of recall, don't delay in consulting your doctor.

● **Combat baby drain** Maternal amnesia or "baby drain" may be more than just a popular myth. When Australian researchers compared the memory performance of pregnant and nonpregnant women, the pregnant group fared worse, especially when it came to remembering new phone numbers or people's names. As well as hormonal changes, it's thought that changes in lifestyle together with the disruption and loss of routine that pregnancy brings may be to blame. You can't do anything about the hormones, but you can try to get as much sleep as possible and eat a nutrient-rich diet to help keep your memory sharp.

● **Replace estrogen** If you're menopausal and becoming forgetful, it may be the result of low estrogen. A study from the University of California has found that dwindling levels of the female hormone estrogen affect the neurotransmitters—the

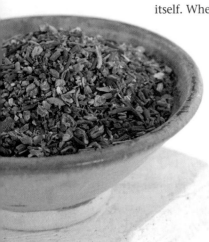

Black cohosh may help post-menopausal memory problems by boosting estrogen levels.

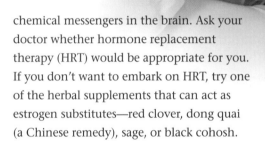

A nutrient-filled diet can help keep your memory sharp while you're pregnant.

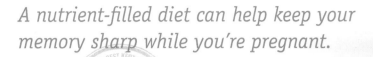

chemical messengers in the brain. Ask your doctor whether hormone replacement therapy (HRT) would be appropriate for you. If you don't want to embark on HRT, try one of the herbal supplements that can act as estrogen substitutes—red clover, dong quai (a Chinese remedy), sage, or black cohosh.

● **Get your thyroid checked** If you're forgetful and also feeling tired, putting on weight and feeling down in the dumps, you may be suffering from low thyroid levels (hypothyroidism), a condition that affects 15 in every 1,000 women—it's less common in men. If the thyroid gland is underactive, many functions, including mental acuity and memory, can be affected. The condition is easily diagnosed and treated. If you're concerned, ask your doctor to arrange for you to have a thyroid check.

● **Reconsider your sleeping pills**
Sleeping pills can damage memory and performance both immediately and on the following day. If they affect you in this way, consider lifestyle changes as an alternative to pills. Are you drinking too many caffeinated drinks or eating too late? Are you getting enough exercise? Are you exercising too late in the evening, which makes it harder to wind down? Good sleep hygiene—going to bed and getting up at the same time each day and keeping your bedroom for sleep and sex—is also important. If all else fails you might consider a natural herbal supplement such as valerian. Discuss your options with your doctor.

BELIEVE IT OR NOT!

A memory-boosting pill
A drug that boosts memory could be on the horizon, according to researchers from the Baylor College of Medicine in the USA. They found that blocking the action of a molecule called PKR increased the excitability of brain cells and significantly enhanced their powers of learning and memory. The next step could be to develop a memory-enhancing drug that specifically targets PKR, which could hold the key to how we can keep our memories longer as well as how we create new ones.

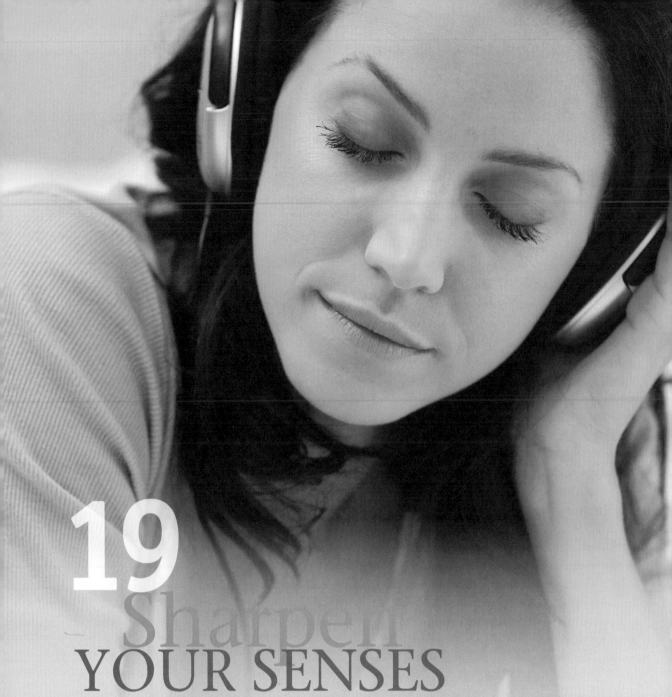

19
Sharpen
YOUR SENSES

The acuity of your five senses inevitably declines with age—
and in some cases because of mistreatment—but scientists are
developing new solutions and there is also much you can do to
protect and preserve them. And in some cases, there are
strategies to help you increase their sensitivity—which will
also enhance your enjoyment of their powers.

Protecting
YOUR EYESIGHT

Your brain receives more input from your eyes than all your other senses combined: They supply half the total information in your conscious mind. You can help protect these vital organs from damage and disease by acting now on these effective and intriguing tips and hints.

● **Smell your eye makeup** You have probably never thought about bacteria lurking in your mascara and other eye cosmetics—but they love it and can end up causing eye infections. Health experts suggest that you should discard your makeup every three months. If you balk at throwing away unfinished (and often pricey) cosmetics four times a year, an alternative way to stay safe— according to the authoritative Mayo Clinic —is to treat your cosmetics in the same way as food and smell them before use. If it has gone bad, mascara will smell just as bad as fish does when it's not fresh.

● **Eat sunshine-colored foods** Make sure your dinner plate contains a splash of yellow or orange. Egg yolks and a wide range of orange or yellow vegetables, including carrots and squash, are good sources of zeaxanthin and lutein. These vital nutrients help protect against age-related macular degeneration (AMD), which is the most common cause of blindness in older people. Researchers at the University of Wisconsin, have reported that people in their 50s who regularly eat food containing the yellow pigment that gives egg yolks their bright color are less likely to develop AMD. Dark green vegetables including kale, cabbage, red lettuce, arugula, spinach, romaine, broccoli, and zucchini have the same beneficial effect.

BELIEVE IT OR NOT!

Fish provides insight for eyes

A tiny striped tropical fish is helping doctors develop new strategies to slow or reverse eye conditions such as glaucoma, cataracts, retinopathy, and age-related macular degeneration (AMD). The similarities between human eyes and those of the zebra fish—a striped freshwater fish of the minnow family native to the southeast Himalayas—have thrown light on how these potentially devastating eye diseases develop as we age. Research into the mechanisms by which zebra fish regenerate their retinas after injury may lead to new eye treatments.

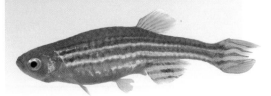

● **Send your children outside**
The indoor lifestyle led by many families in the West could have a surprisingly negative effect on children's eyesight, leading to an increased risk of myopia (short-sightedness). Scientists at Cambridge University in the UK, who carried out a review of research in this area, found that children today are spending too little time outside, where the

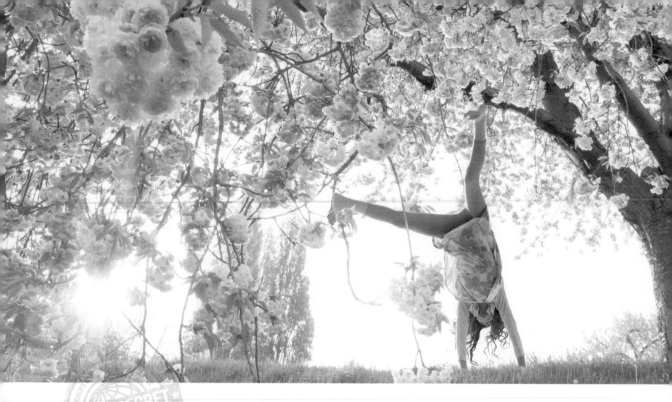

Every hour that children regularly spend outside reduces their risk of short-sightedness by 2 percent.

BELIEVE IT OR NOT!

A source of new eye cells

Stem cells from human embryos could soon produce an unlimited supply of retinal pigment cells that can halt, and even reverse, blindness caused by degenerative disorders such as age-related macular degeneration (AMD). These disorders damage specialized neurons or brain cells, known as photoreceptors, in the retina. Now doctors are testing therapies to repair this damage. One approach, by a leading California biotechnology company, involves injecting retinal pigment cells directly into the eye.

light is natural and the horizons are further away. Making more use of distance vision and increased exposure to ultraviolet light are the principal health gains of having

regular time playing outside, the scientists report in the journal *Ophthalmology*. Studies show that every hour children regularly spend outside reduces their risk of short-sightedness by 2 percent.

● **Get tested for glaucoma** Ask your ophthalmologist about having a test for this serious eye condition. The disease, a leading cause of blindness, is caused by a rise in pressure inside the eye. Early diagnosis can save your vision because prescription eye drops can prevent the otherwise inevitable damage to the optic nerve. The International Glaucoma Association recommends testing at least every two years if you are:

★ **Over 40**
★ **Closely related to someone with glaucoma**
★ **Short sighted**
★ **Diabetic**
★ **Of African-Caribbean origin.**

● **Take a break** If you work long hours in front of a screen in artificial light, you are increasing your chances of becoming short sighted, according to California eye specialists. Take regular short breaks away from the screen and walk around the office to exercise your eyes as well as your legs. If possible, alternate your work duties so you reduce the length of periods spent in front of a screen. And make a determined effort to get out of the office at lunchtime.

● **Don't tell the children** You may constantly warn your children of the dire consequences of sitting too close to the TV, but this causes no long-term damage to eyes. The worst it can do is tire your eyes or stress them temporarily, which may cause problems in focusing until they have rested. All the same, it's better for your child's eye health to play outside than to sit in front of a screen—at whatever distance.

● **Wear eye protection** You may wear goggles to protect your eyes from chlorine in the swimming pool—but what about other occasions when your eyes may be at risk? If splinters, dust, and other small particles get into your eye, there is a risk of corneal abrasions that could threaten your vision. The American Academy of Ophthalmology estimates that 90 percent of eye injuries could be avoided by wearing protective eyewear. Be sure to safeguard your eyes while cycling, doing DIY jobs (particularly sanding and sawing), and even gardening— bamboo canes, twigs, and thorns can pose a serious hazard to your eyes.

● **Walk for 40 minutes** If you have glaucoma or are in a high-risk group—for example, if a close member of your family has the disease—being physically fit can reduce symptoms. Research over 20 years has shown that people with glaucoma who walked briskly for 40 minutes four times a week reduced their intraocular pressure enough for them to stop taking medication for the condition.

Protective eyewear could prevent 90 percent of accidental eye injuries.

HEALTH SECRET

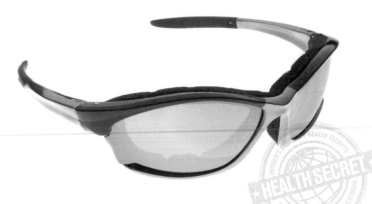

Wraparound sunglasses reduce the risk of eye damage, even on a cloudy day.

irritating condition, which is common in older people, occurs when the eyes do not produce enough tears or when the tears evaporate too quickly. The result is itchy, red eyes that can be slightly painful. Harvard University researchers, who studied the diets of thousands of women, found that those who ate the least amount of oily fish—and therefore had the lowest intake of omega-3 fatty acids—had the highest risk of dry eye syndrome. If you're not keen on eating oily fish, you could choose supplements, which work as well as having fresh fish, according to the researchers.

● **Keep clear of smoke** Smoking is as bad for your eyesight as it is for the rest of your body. Research showing a link between age-related macular degeneration (AMD) and smoking is now as robust as that between smoking and lung cancer—with evidence that cigarette smokers are up to four times more likely to be blinded by AMD compared to nonsmokers. What's more, this risk continues for up to ten years after smoking cessation.

For tips on how to give up smoking, see *Chapter 21, Breaking Bad Habits*

● **Cool your feet** Make sure that the vents that deliver cool air into your car are aimed at your feet rather than at eye level. Specialists warn that the dry air from car air conditioning systems sucks moisture out of your eyes, which can cause discomfort and put you at greater risk of eye infections and even ulcers. The same goes for the air conditioning in planes, trains, coaches—and even in offices. Check where you are sitting and adjust the vents if you can.

● **Eat fish for moist eyes** Scientific research has found that eating oily fish helps to prevent dry eye syndrome. This

● **Get wraparound protection** You may already know that wraparound sunglasses offer the best protection for the eyes against the damage of ultraviolet rays during sunny weather. Researchers now suggest that wearing sunglasses of this type on a cloudy day is also beneficial for your eye health. Exactly why this is so is not fully understood, but one theory is that the glasses also protect against the drying effects of wind and against pollution. The Mayo Clinic offers the following tips when choosing sunglasses:

★ **UV protection** Choose glasses that offer 99–100 percent UV protection.

★ **Polarized lenses** While these are useful for reducing glare, make sure that they also offer the eyes UV protection.

★ **Lens size** Opt for large lenses, which exclude the most light. Wraparound styles are the best.

● **Lower the screen** You can reduce your risk of suffering from dry eyes while working at a computer simply by positioning the screen just below eye level. This will mean that your eyes will naturally close slightly when you're viewing the screen, which minimizes fluid evaporation.

Hearing
AND BALANCE

You know that your ears enable you to hear a beautiful symphony, a bird singing, or your alarm clock, but you may not be aware that they have another function—they help you keep your balance. The ear's delicate structures can be damaged by excess noise and disease. Read on to discover ways to care for your hearing.

● **Sip red wine** Good news—a moderate intake of red wine can help preserve your hearing. Scientific evidence shows that regular consumption will improve your hearing over time. The protection comes from a powerful antioxidant—resveratrol—which is known to protect against damage caused by free radicals in many parts of the body, including the inner ear. Red wine is one of the best sources of resveratrol, but follow healthy guidelines and stick to one or two glasses. If you don't drink alcohol, try purple grape juice or eating red grapes, which are also rich in resveratrol.

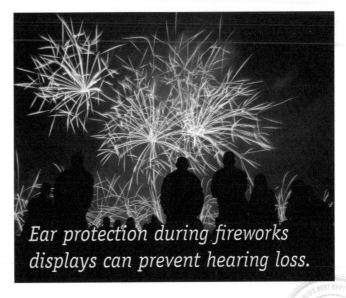

Ear protection during fireworks displays can prevent hearing loss.

SECRETS OF SUCCESS

Stopping the buzz
A drug that is given to alcoholics to reduce cravings for alcohol has been found to have the side effect of reducing tinnitus symptoms. Volunteers with the disorder have found the prescription drug, acamprosate (Campral), gives some relief, according to a Brazilian study. Although more research is needed, the researchers say the drug appears to reduce the excess nerve cell activity underlying the sensations produced by the disorder, offering the possibility of new treatment approaches for this often distressing common condition.

● **Beware of fireworks** Modern fireworks are much louder than older ones and can pose a risk to hearing—especially in babies and young children. At a major fireworks display, young children should wear ear protectors or ear plugs. Avoid displays in enclosed spaces, such as small gardens, particularly if there are likely to be large, explosive fireworks. Protect yourself in similar ways against other types of loud noise, such as that caused by:
★ **Rock concerts** (try special noise-reducing earplugs)
★ **Road work**
★ **Motorized lawn mowers**
★ **Power tools**
★ **Industrial machinery.**

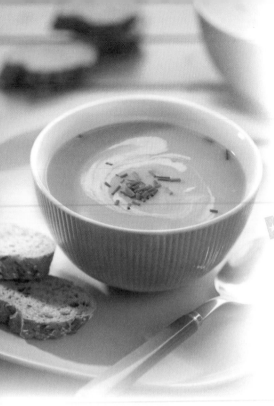

Whole-grain bread and pea soup are packed with B vitamins, which help you to hear better.

BELIEVE IT OR NOT!

Implants can combat deafness in one ear

Being deaf in one ear is a common problem that makes it difficult to pinpoint the exact source of sounds, making crossing roads hazardous, and conversations in noisy rooms difficult to pick up. The condition is considered problematic to treat, but several new solutions coming on the market include a device that picks up sound from the hearing ear through a small titanium implant and creates the impression of stereo sound. Another high-tech solution is a device, which is wrapped around the teeth, that "tunes" the deaf ear. Noises that are picked up in a tiny microphone in the deaf ear are turned into vibrations and then transmitted to the brain through a process of bone conduction, in the same way that we hear our own voices.

● **Hum to protect your ears** It may seem slightly eccentric, but getting into the habit of humming whenever you approach a loud noise without ear protection will help you hear better in later life. The inner ear has a mechanism to protect itself from noise damage by tensing muscles around the eardrum and to reduce the volume of the sound that reaches the inner ear. You can boost this automatic reflex by the simple measure of pressing your lips together and starting to hum—a process that helps to tighten these muscles, protecting your eardrums even further.

● **Choose headphones wisely** The small headphones that fit neatly inside your ears are, contrary to expectations, not good for your hearing—sound leaks so badly that you are likely to turn up the volume to a dangerous level, risking hearing damage. According to Deafness Research UK, larger headphones that fit over your ears have been shown to be much more protective of hearing—simply because it's possible to get lost in the music at a lower volume.

● **Have some sweet potatoes** Getting the right nutrients into your diet is a vital strategy for safeguarding your hearing. Sweet potatoes are rich in vitamin A, which increases the inner ear's sensitivity to noise. B vitamins are also vital for hearing; they protect the neurons and blood vessels connected to the cochlea in your inner ear. Whole-grain bread with pea soup provides a vitamin B-rich light meal.

● **Check your medications** If you've noticed that you've become hard of hearing, consider the possibility that your medications may be to blame. Ask your pharmacist or doctor whether any drugs you're taking are "ototoxic" (dangerous for the ears). Many drugs can cause hearing loss or noises in the ear (tinnitus) as a side effect, especially at high doses, including aspirin, other nonsteroidal anti-inflammatory drugs (NSAIDs), some antibiotics, diuretics, blood-pressure lowering drugs, oral contraceptives, and antimalarial pills. If you think a drug might be causing your hearing problem, speak to your doctor.

● **Focus on birdsong** Isolate specific sounds, whenever the opportunity arises. This helps you become a more perceptive listener, able to distinguish speech from background hubbub. The key is to practice extracting particular sounds from the mixture of noises that surround you—for example, listening to a bird singing against the drone of traffic or picking out the sound of a specific instrument in an orchestral recording. Scientists at Northwestern University in the USA report in the *Journal of Neuroscience* that making this a habit will improve your hearing. Their research has revealed that musicians who play in an orchestra are better at picking out speech from background noise than nonmusicians.

● **Keep on the move** to slow age-related hearing loss. Regular aerobic exercise improves blood flow to the ears—and the fitter you are generally, the better your hearing will be.

● **Reduce your smoke risk** As well as stopping smoking yourself, it's important to stay away from other smokers for the sake of your long-term hearing. The more you're

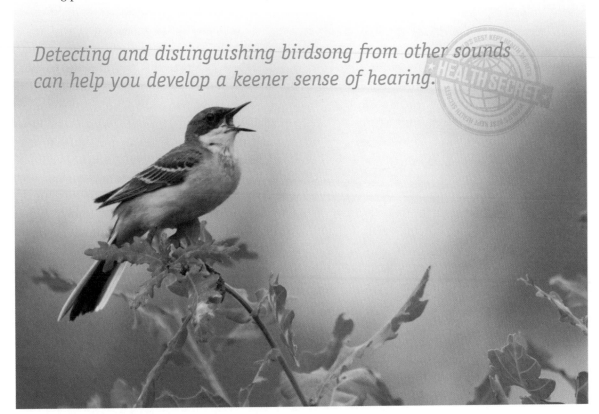

Detecting and distinguishing birdsong from other sounds can help you develop a keener sense of hearing.

exposed to cigarette smoke, the more likely you are to experience age-related hearing loss, according to a research paper published in the *Journal of the American Medical Association*.

● **Ditch the remote** It's well known that TV ads are often louder than the programs you're watching. The natural response is repeatedly to adjust the sound at the beginning and end of the commercial breaks. Surprisingly, the experts advise that you keep the sound at a comfortable level for the ads and, when your program resumes, you neither turn up the sound nor move closer to the TV to compensate. Listening more carefully seems to be the best strategy. The effort you make to detect quieter sounds actually helps to prevent hearing loss.

Keeping the TV volume low could help keep your hearing sharp.

● **Drink with restraint** The occasional glass of wine or beer will help to protect your hearing. But bear in mind that over the years, excessive drinking will eventually contribute to hearing loss.

● **Try yoga** If you have Ménière's disease—a condition in which sudden attacks of vertigo occur along with tinnitus and hearing loss as a result of a build-up of fluid in the inner ear—you may feel despondent at being told there is no real treatment because of its inaccessible location. But help is at hand. Therapies such as mainstream physiotherapy and yoga have been found to help to reduce the symptoms. If your doctor thinks yoga might help you, ask him or her for a recommendation, or try yogafinder.com for a yoga class in your area.

● **Have less salt** Some people affected by Ménière's disease have found that cutting back on salt can improve their symptoms. Since reducing salt intake is beneficial for health in other ways—notably for lowering blood pressure—this strategy is well worth a try. To start, cut back on salty snacks.

● **Retune your radio** If you're a tinnitus sufferer, try leaving your radio tuned to a space between stations. The static that is picked up may help cancel out the buzzing

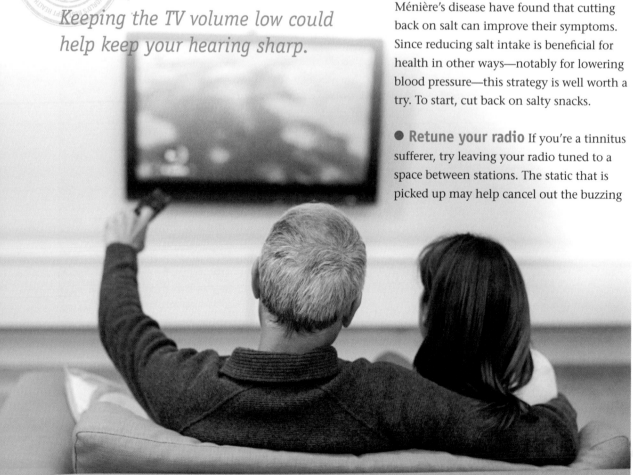

in your ears. According to the National Foundation for the Deaf in New Zealand, the problem can be held in check by listening to the "white" noise from a mistuned radio; it says the noise effectively masks the irritating sounds of tinnitus.

● **Try ginkgo** A herbal remedy extracted from the leaf of the maidenhair tree—*Ginkgo biloba*—may help to reduce tinnitus and ringing in the ears. It is also thought to reduce hearing loss by boosting blood flow to the ears. A word of caution though—it won't work immediately and you will need to take the herb for several weeks before noticing any changes. Products vary in their strength, so follow the dosage instructions on the label.

● **Get a hearing aid** Getting fitted for a hearing aid will not only enable you to hear better, but will also slow down any further decline into deafness. The longer your brain is deprived of auditory stimuli, the less it responds to sound, making it more difficult for your brain to adapt when you finally get a hearing aid. If you have an inkling that your hearing is not as good as it used to be, don't delay getting a hearing test and being fitted for a hearing aid.

● **Look away to listen** It may seem rude, but if you turn your head 45 degrees away from the person you want to listen to, you may hear them much better. Sound waves travel around the head—and your skull can sometimes get in the way of hearing properly, especially if you are looking straight at someone in an environment where there is background noise. The tip comes from Deafness Research UK as part of a campaign to educate people with hearing loss about ways to make the most of their hearing.

BELIEVE IT OR NOT!

An invisible hearing aid

You'll soon be able to wear an aid that is not just small but invisible. At present only part of the electronic device can be surgically implanted inside the cochlea—the part of the inner ear that conducts sound to the auditory nerve. The tiny microphone that amplifies external sound has to be hooked onto the outside of the ear because of the need to exclude internal body noises, such as eating and the heart beating. Scientists say they are finally getting close to providing a way around this problem, with the first fully implantable hearing aids now being tested on humans. The only down side to this amazing development is that every ten years surgery will be required to replace the battery—perhaps a small price to pay for an invisible device.

● **Consider the possibility of wax** Older people often think their increasing deafness is simply caused by age. In fact, wax accumulation, which can be easily remedied, is often the cause. Always see your doctor to check out the underlying cause of any hearing loss.

● **Don't clean your ears** by inserting cotton swabs into the outer ear canal. These cotton-tipped sticks are likely to poke bacteria and bits of debris further into your ear canal. And there is a real risk of ear drum damage. If your ear feels blocked by excess wax, loosen it by inserting a few drops of olive oil into your ear or you can buy wax-softening eardrops from a pharmacy. If self-help methods don't help, see a nurse or your doctor, who will be able to relieve the blockage safely.

Secrets of
SUPER SENSES

Humans cannot compete with the extraordinary sensory powers of many animals, which can see and smell things miles away. Yet there are examples of people developing their senses to a remarkable extent. With the right focus and technique, it's possible for most of us to make greater use of our senses that we ever thought possible.

Our environments attune our senses to help us survive. Just as jungle dwellers are highly sensitive to the sights, sounds, and smells of their ecosystem, always on the lookout for danger or opportunities for food, new mothers the world over sleep on survival alert for the sound of their baby crying. We all learn to use our senses effectively but a small proportion of people are endowed with "super-senses" that give them a special edge.

A matter of taste

One in four of us is born with up to twice as many taste buds as everyone else. These supertasters can distinguish subtle nuances of flavors with great confidence, a particular advantage for chefs and wine tasters. Supertasters are sensitive to 6-n-propylthiouracil (PROP), a bitter chemical found in foods such as coffee, beer, grapefruit, cabbage, sprouts, and spinach, which they often dislike, along with hot, spicy, or sugary foods. Children are also more sensitive to PROP than adults, which may explain why many dislike PROP-rich foods. Women are more likely to be supertasters, as are people from Asia, Africa, and South America.

A person with a super-developed sense of smell will also have a powerful sense of taste, since these senses work together to create our perception of flavor. People who make perfumes (known as "noses") have a highly developed sense of smell—they aim to be able to identify and name as many as possible of the 3,000 raw materials that can be used in perfume-making, describing them with terms such as "fruity," "flat," "rounded," "grassy," or "juicy."

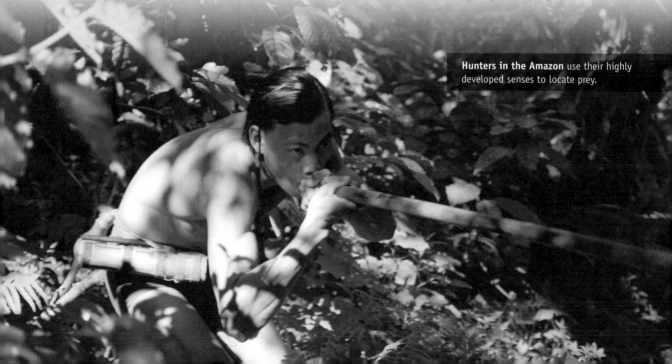

Hunters in the Amazon use their highly developed senses to locate prey.

Do I see what you see?

Do super-sighted people exist? Some scientists think so. Most humans are trichromates—they have three types of cone cells in their eyes that detect light in the blue, green, and yellow wavelength ranges. Each cone type can distinguish about 100 shades, so the total number of shades we can see is 100^3 or a million. Some people—tetrachromates—have a fourth type of cone that may allow them to see up to 100 million shades. The most likely candidates for super-sight are the mothers and daughters of colorblind men, who possess a fourth, mutated type of cone. However hard they try, trichromates will never be able to see the world as tetrachromates do.

Supertasters, such as many wine tasters, may have more taste buds.

Daniel Kish is blind but has developed his use of echolocation to guide him—even when cycling.

Bouncing off the walls

As for hearing, the best-known supersensers today are the growing number of visually impaired people who can learn to understand and navigate the world using senses other than sight. The lack of one sense means that they rely on others, allowing them to become adept at using them in ways that sighted people do not. They not only have a highly refined sense of touch but can also develop an aspect of hearing better known in the animal kingdom: echolocation—a system of navigation that is used by bats and dolphins. It involves interpreting echoes of clicks made with the tongue—and working out an object's location by timing the echo and noting which ear it reaches first. MRI scans show that echolocation actually triggers the visual rather than the hearing cortex of the brain, helping its practitioners build up a mental image of the world. Some totally blind people are even using the system to gain an unprecedented level of personal freedom, from mountain biking and jogging to playing ball games and even rockclimbing.

Some bats use echolocation to locate their insect prey in the dark.

Hone your senses

With a little concentration and practice, most of us could improve our perception of our surroundings.

Language Devise a vocabulary to describe different smells and tastes. This will allow you to become more adept at perceiving, recognizing, and identifying nuances of flavor and aroma.

Focus The familiarity of many smells and tastes means that we don't really notice them. Help yourself to focus on these senses by recording both notable and everyday aromas and flavors in a diary, in which you can describe the sensory experiences of meals and aromas you encounter on your way to work, in the park, or at home. This will help you build up a fragrance vocabulary.

Practice Find time to practice using a particular sense and identify the best opportunities for this. For example, you can use a walk in the park to give any of your senses a workout. Try to pick out particular sounds—birdsong is a good one—and sights, such as certain colors or the aromas of plants and flowers.

Protection Keep your sense organs healthy to ensure you enjoy their powers to the full—find out more in the rest of this chapter.

Making the most
OF THE SENSE OF TOUCH

Your skin has a plentiful supply of touch receptors, some at the surface and others deeper down, that are responsible for passing messages to the brain. Gentle touch can be a source of pleasure and comfort, and this sense also helps to protect us from danger. Here are some tips to help maintain touch sensitivity.

● **Walk barefoot** to increase your awareness of the textures underfoot. This exercise is particularly helpful for those with impaired vision, who need to boost the sensitivity of their sense of touch. But people with normal vision can also benefit— do it with your eyes closed.

★ **Take off** your shoes and socks and ask a companion to guide you.

★ **Walk** over different floor surfaces in your home, and if it's safe, the garden.

★ **Focus** on the different textures and temperatures of carpets, tiles, wood flooring, and perhaps concrete and grass.

You can also try these simple exercises to enhance the sense of touch in your hands and fingers.

★ **Use** your hands and fingertips to feel a variety of surfaces from counters to tabletops and soft furnishings, noticing the different sensations they create.

★ **Handle** small household objects, feeling their features such as grooves, buttons, and handles. Try to work out what materials they are made from and identify what the objects are.

● **Cuddle your baby** Most parents don't need to be prompted to hold their baby—it's the most natural thing in the world. But you may be surprised to learn that this loving physical contact is essential to your baby's health and development. The sense of touch is perhaps the most primitive of our senses and the stimulation of touch sensors in infancy seems to activate essential nerve connections in the brain.

Babies who don't receive sufficient physical affection can grow up more prone to violent behavior and are at increased risk of psychological problems such as depression. It can also have a serious impact on their physical health, such as failure to gain weight and increased susceptibility to infection. Give your baby and young children all the cuddles they want and boost their chances of future well-being.

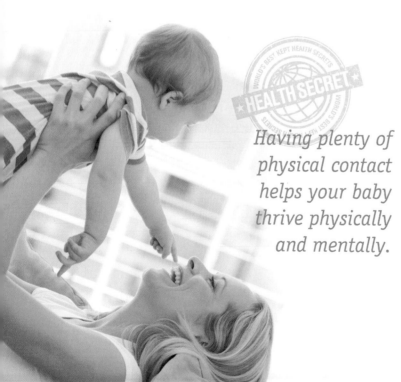

Having plenty of physical contact helps your baby thrive physically and mentally.

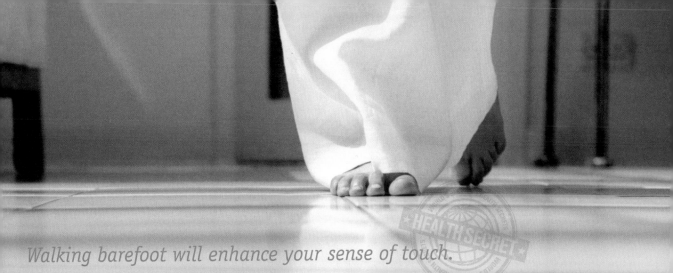

Walking barefoot will enhance your sense of touch.

● Look out for loss of sensation

Watch out for a loss of touch sensitivity—whether in yourself or in an older relative. You start losing sensation and elasticity in skin cells from your fifties, which means you are slightly less likely to notice a cut, burn, or bruise—you may not respond to pain until after your skin has been damaged. First signs of the problem are the coins in your purse or pocket suddenly feeling identical or small objects becoming difficult to pick up. People with diabetes need to be particularly alert to this risk as the condition can be a warning sign of damage to the peripheral nerves, notably in the feet. If you think that your sense of touch has deteriorated, seek your doctor's advice. Medical treatment may be needed.

● Sit in the sun

Get sufficient sun on your skin to keep up your vitamin D levels. This vital vitamin has been found to protect against loss of sensation caused by peripheral neuropathy, a problem that is particularly likely to affect people with diabetes. You can boost your vitamin D levels by exposing your skin to sunshine for just 10 minutes a day. Protect yourself from sunburn if you expose your skin for longer. And when the skies are gray, include plenty of vitamin D-rich foods such as oily fish in your diet.

● Take a break—from repetitive actions

It's always a good idea to avoid making the same limited movements for long periods of time, whether at work or when engaging in sports activities. Repeated movements can lead to RSI (repetitive strain injury) and one of the main symptoms of this often disabling condition is numbness in the affected part of the body—the hands and arms are the most commonly affected. Take breaks from repetitive activities and vary your tasks whenever possible.

● Enjoy the pleasure of stroking

It's not just for cats and dogs: Being stroked is good for humans, too. Researchers at the University of North Carolina, measured hormone levels in women before and after their hands, necks, and backs were stroked by their partners for 10 minutes. The "after stroking" tests showed a dramatic increase in levels of the hormone oxytocin, often dubbed the "love hormone," which promotes feelings of attachment. The health benefits of increased levels of oxytocin include slowing of the heart rate and a reduction in blood pressure. Stroking raised oxytocin levels in women by an average of 20 percent. Research suggests that stroking works anywhere on the body and benefits both genders, although women seem to be particularly responsive.

Boosting
SMELL AND TASTE

Your senses of smell and taste are inextricably linked. You only have to think about the last time you had a cold to realize that when you can't smell, you can't taste. While these senses can give you enormous pleasure, their primary function is to protect you from dangerous substances. Read on to discover what you can do to improve the acuity of these vital senses.

● **Savor your meals** Here are some taste-boosting tips to help you enjoy the flavors in your food:

★ **Stir your food** before you eat to aerate the molecules and release more of the aroma, which will enhance the flavor of your meal.

★ **Eat slowly** Chewing your food thoroughly releases more flavor and keeps the food in contact with your taste buds longer, enhancing the taste experience.

★ **Take separate mouthfuls** If your sense of smell is getting jaded, eat the different foods on your plate separately—for example, have a piece of steak, then a bit of potato, and then some salad, and then go back to the steak.

BELIEVE IT OR NOT!

Unblocked by a balloon

A new minimally invasive procedure called balloon sinuplasty involves inserting a small, flexible balloon catheter into your nose. This is then gently inflated to open up and widen the blocked passageways to restore normal sinus drainage without damaging the delicate nasal lining. The treatment can bring about an almost immediate restoration of the sense of smell.

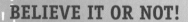

Chewing for longer will maximize the taste experience.

● **Wake up to the essentials** Dab a few drops of essential oil—jasmine, peppermint, or vanilla are good choices—on your arm and sniff them from time to time to wake you up and make your senses more alert. According to the US Smell and Taste Treatment Research Foundation, these scents boost the activity of the beta waves in the frontal lobes of your brain, which can help improve awareness and alertness.

● **Pare back the presentation** An over-fussy dinner offering can ruin the taste of that special meal you've slaved over. Your sense of taste is stronger if the brain can connect what you're eating with how it looks, according to research. For example, say scientists, if you're serving fish, it'll taste more intense if you present it with its fishy form intact rather than cut into pieces.

● **Name it** Developing a terminology to describe different smells can enhance your ability to recognize and recall specific scents. Professor Tim Jacob from the School of Biosciences at Cardiff University in Wales explains that creating two different information stores—in the olfactory part of the brain and in the language center—helps to reinforce the memory of the smells you have encountered. So when you want to be able to remember a scent, make an effort to describe it in words.

● **Detect it** As you get older you can't rely on your sense of smell to warn you of leaking gas, smoke, or food that has gone bad. A report in the journal *Neurobiology of Aging* suggests that people 60 and over are less adept than a group of 45-year-olds at distinguishing between different smells. The younger group could easily differentiate between two odors that had been blended together while the older group could not. To

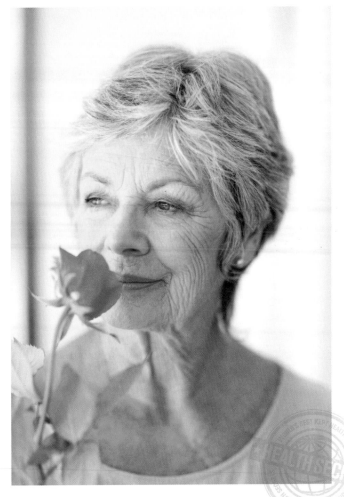

Finding words to describe a scent can help you recognize it when you next encounter it.

reduce your risk of failing to smell smoke or gas, install smoke and gas detectors and test them regularly. Observe "use-by" dates for food and if in doubt, throw it out.

● **Exercise your nose** Our sense of smell can become dulled by lack of challenge. Give the receptors in your nose a regular workout by exposing them to new smells. You might even try keeping a scent diary of different smells you have noticed or try to identify a variety of different smells with your eyes closed or while blindfolded.

● **Add zinc-rich foods** Many experts believe that an impaired sense of smell, known as hyposmia, can sometimes be caused by a deficiency of zinc in the diet. If you've noticed a reduction in your sense of smell, perhaps following a cold, give your zinc reserves a boost by including more shellfish, lentils, and sunflower seeds in your diet. Alternatively, try taking a supplement of this mineral.

● **Whip up an appetite** Taking a brisk walk or run before mealtimes will make your food smell and taste stronger. The sense of smell is heightened by exercise, probably because the activity creates additional moisture in the nose, say researchers. The extra moisture in the air also increases the sensitivity of our sense of smell in spring and summer.

● **Steam cleaning** Blocked sinuses are a common cause of loss of the sense of smell. They are also painful and uncomfortable, triggering headaches, sore throats, coughing and tiredness (as a result of disturbed sleep). An effective and easy way of relieving this condition is to inhale steam—either by the time-honored method of breathing the vapors from a bowl of hot water with a towel over your head, or by investing in a vaporizer. If steam fails to clear the congestion, see your doctor, who may recommend a decongestant nasal spray, drops, or medication.

● **Cool that hot chile burn** To dampen down the burning sensation from eating chiles, a drink of full-fat milk or a spoonful of yogurt is the best solution. Capsaicin, the chemical that makes chile pepper hot, is fat

Using spices in cooking instead of salt and sugar provides plenty of flavor without compromising your health.

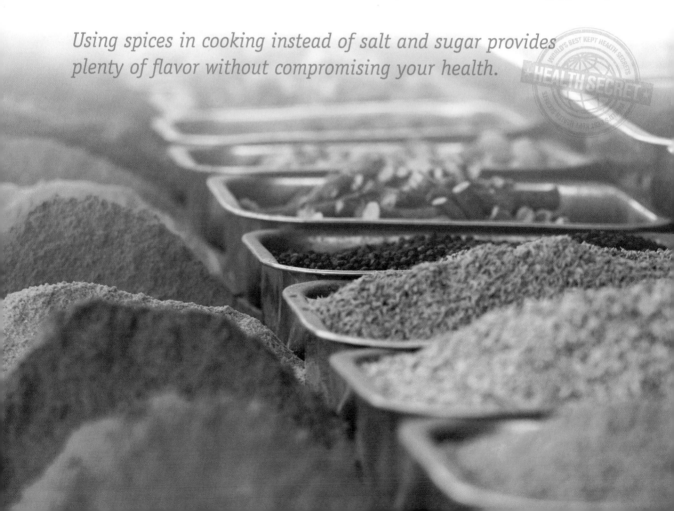

soluble so any fat-containing beverage, such as a yogurt-based smoothie, helps to counteract the heat of the chile. This is why yogurt-based lassi and raita are often served alongside curries. Water and soft drinks have no effect on chile's heat.

● **Fight blandness with spices** As you get older, you may find yourself adding more salt and sugar to your food. The number of taste buds declines by as much as 60 percent by the age of 60, and it is your sweet and salty receptors that are first to be affected. You can counteract the reduction in your taste without increasing your health risks by using more herbs and spices and by adding more acid notes with lemon and vinegar. Varying food textures can also help to make your meals more interesting.

● **Avoid salt in the air** Airline chefs face many challenges in providing healthy, tasty meals, not least of which is the dry air in the plane that affects your sense of smell and taste, making food seem blander than on the ground. As a result, airline food is often laced with large amounts of sugar and salt to make it appealing. But provided you order it in advance, you can eat well in the air by requesting a healthy option meal designed for people with special dietary requirements, such as diabetics and those with high blood pressure or high cholesterol.

● **Miss a meal** Go hungry and you'll find you become more sensitive to sweet and salty tastes. Researchers at the University of Malawi persuaded male undergraduates to forgo breakfast, having eaten dinner the previous evening. Students were then asked to sip sugar, salt, or bitter solutions of different concentrations and to say what flavors they were tasting. The volunteers repeated the taste tests 1 hour after lunch.

With empty stomachs, the students were more sensitive to the presence of sugar and salt but not to bitter tastes. This explains why food seems to taste better when you're hungry. Knowing this could also help you reduce the amount of salt and sugar in your diet—and cut your heart attack and stroke risk. Wait until you're hungry before you eat and you'll be less inclined to supplement natural flavors with unhealthy extras.

● **Stick to "natural MSG"** Research has revealed that the fifth taste known as umami is produced by an amino acid named L-glutamate, which is found naturally in foods such as mushrooms, ripe tomatoes, and ginger. In much Asian cookery and increasingly in many western packaged foods, this flavor is added artificially by the use of monosodium glutamate (MSG). Many people report suffering symptoms such as headaches after eating foods containing MSG. Although the Mayo Clinic has found no clear link between the symptoms and this ingredient, it's probably worth limiting your intake of MSG, if only because its compelling flavor may draw you to consume foods that you know to be unhealthy when you're not even hungry.

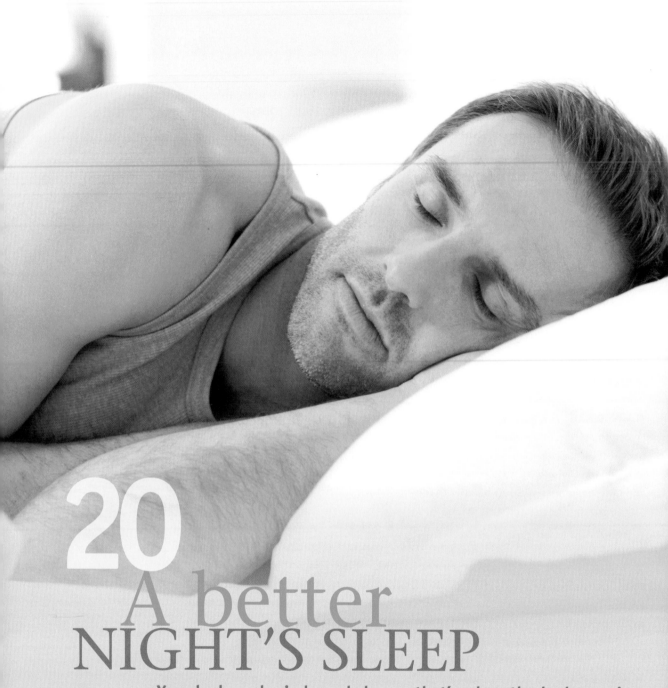

20
A better
NIGHT'S SLEEP

Your body and mind need sleep—that's when the body repairs itself and the mind sifts through the day's events, filing, and discarding as necessary. You know how much better you feel and function when you've slept well, so it should be no surprise that sleep plays a vital role in physical health, longevity, and emotional well-being.

Sleep your
WAY TO HEALTH

The stresses and strains of modern life, and our 24/7 lifestyles, are making it harder to get a good night's sleep. So it is no wonder that experts throughout the world are exploring old and new ways to help us get more and better-quality sleep and to use the power of sleep to benefit our health. Their key tips are shared on the following pages.

● **Drink cherry juice** If you regularly drink cherry juice, you could add up to 25 minutes a night to your sleep. Among volunteers studied by researchers at Northumbria University in the UK, those who drank 1oz (30ml) of Montmorency cherry juice twice a day for a week found that their daytime napping decreased and their nighttime sleep was prolonged. Further tests revealed that the juice stimulates the production of melatonin, the body's natural sleep-inducing chemical.

● **Sleep soundly to avoid colds** Try to have a full 7 to 8 hours sleep every night. Contrary to popular perception—and widespread claims that some successful public figures manage to be effective on only 3 or 4 hours sleep a night—it is not a smart move to skimp on sleep. Sleep deprivation will not only impair your judgement but also leave you vulnerable to disease. When a group of 153 healthy men and women were given nasal drops containing the common cold virus it was found that the less each of them slept the more likely they were to catch the cold.

● **Don't drive tired** Make sure you have had enough sleep before driving. Sleeping less than 5 hours a night can quadruple your risk of an accident. According to UK statistics, falling asleep is a factor in around

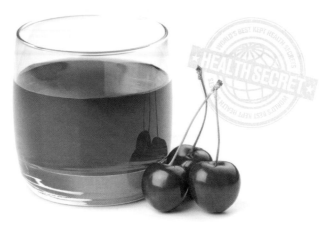

Drinking cherry juice triggers the production of melatonin, a natural chemical that encourages sleep.

20 percent of all accidents—most often caused by men aged 30 and under. Sufferers from sleep apnea are seven times more likely to have a crash, estimates the UK road safety charity Brake. You're much less able to coordinate your eye movements or control the steering wheel correctly when you're tired. If you have to drive, stop every 2 hours for a break or a nap. If you feel drowsy, stop immediately and rest before resuming your journey.

● **Don't decide when you're sleep deprived** Keep important money decisions for when you've had enough sleep. Lack of sleep can adversely affect the choices you might make at the gaming table or when buying and selling high-risk stocks and shares. Research has shown that sleepy players and investors often feel compelled to keep going rather than sensibly quitting when ahead. A study at Princeton University found sleep deprivation not only leads to excess production of the stress hormone corticosterone but also suppresses the action of cells in the hippocampus—the memory area. If you have to make important business decisions, make sure you're well rested.

● **Work with your body to fight infection** Use the power of sleep if you're ill or fighting an infection. When your body picks up an infection, such as the common cold virus, it begins working to produce a molecule called interleukin-1. This stimulates your lymphocytes, a type of white blood cell, to produce antibodies. The reason you feel sleepy when you have an

Getting good sleep helps you to master motor skills such as playing the piano.

HEALTH SECRET

infection is that interleukin-1 is also a sedative. So your immune system works to promote sleep, which will in turn help your immune system to do its job. If you're battling a cold or flu, don't fight drowsiness; your body will heal itself more quickly if you allow yourself to sleep.

● **Be a sober sleeper** Drink alcohol in moderation if you want a decent night's sleep. Because it is a sedative, alcohol helps you get to sleep but can interfere with the quality of your sleep throughout the night. It reduces the amount of rapid eye movement (REM) sleep—the sleep during which you dream—which has been identified by sleep experts as essential for mental acuity. And when dreams do occur, the influence of alcohol can turn them into disturbing nightmares. In addition, alcohol can make you wake up periodically, sweating heavily, and feeling so restless that you then stay awake for a long time before going back to sleep. To achieve top quality, brain-boosting sleep, stick to nonalcoholic beverages in the hours before bedtime.

● **Get more sleep for memory** Try to get a full night's sleep when studying for an exam or learning a new skill. Using MRI scans, researchers in the USA have discovered that during sleep some brain areas are more active than others. In students learning the piano, the cerebellum —the part of the brain involved with motor skills—was most active, but their limbic systems, which regulate anxiety and stress, were less active, resulting in better performance the following day. There is also evidence that the hippocampus, where memories are consolidated, is more active when you're asleep. So instead of doing extra revision or practice, sometimes it's better to put your head down and sleep.

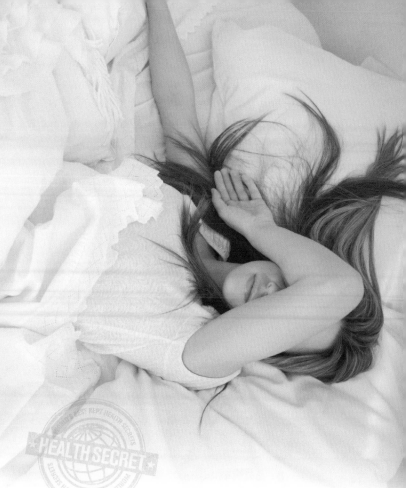

● **Slumber to stay slim** If you want to keep your weight in check, get plenty of sleep. In a 16-year US study, it was found that women who slept for 5 hours or less a night were 32 percent more likely to gain a significant amount of weight than those who slept for an average of 7 hours a night. The explanation for this is unclear, but it may be because those who sleep more are more likely to burn more energy during the day through fidgeting and other minor movements. It also seems that those who sleep less may produce more of the stress hormone cortisol, which stimulates hunger. Whatever the reason, getting enough sleep every night is a simple way to keep slim.

● **Let 'em sleep in** Young people need plenty of sleep, so make sure they get enough. Sleep promotes the release of the growth hormone essential to their development. When practical, they also need to sleep later in the mornings. This is because their hormonal body clock is on a different schedule than that of adults. In older people the release of the sleep-promoting hormone melatonin begins at around 10pm, but in teenagers it often doesn't start until after midnight, at about 1am. In the US, some schools have begun delaying the start of morning classes for this age group, with significant improvements in learning. It may be best to work with nature rather than try to fight it.

● **Sleep to steady your blood glucose** Lack of sleep over weeks and months can severely reduce the body's capacity to utilize insulin to process sugar, which can lead to symptoms of type 2 diabetes and, in some cases, increase the risk of developing the disease itself. In tests carried out on young adults deprived of sleep for six days, these adverse effects were

Teenagers really may need to sleep in—their hormonal body clocks often operate on a different schedule.

BELIEVE IT OR NOT!

Don't oversleep
As you get older, sleeping too much can be as harmful as sleeping too little. Sleep specialists in Spain found that older adults who sleep to excess increase their risk of Alzheimer's disease and other types of dementia. In their study of volunteers over 65, those who displayed dementia symptoms tended to sleep for 9 or more hours in every 24. By the time they are 65, most people get a maximum of 7 hours. Even if it doesn't cause dementia, sleeping too much can affect life expectancy. In a large American study, women who slept 9 to 11 hours a night were 3 percent more likely to have coronary heart disease than those who slept 8 hours.

quickly reversed following 12 hours of sleep, but for older people with chronic sleep loss the changes are not so easily countered. To reduce your risk of diabetes try to get 7 to 8 hours of sleep most nights.

● **Nap is a bright idea** If you feel like a daytime nap, it could be good for your creative juices. Research has shown that 30 percent of office workers have their best ideas when they're asleep rather than at their desks. Research has shown that our surreal dream sequences can sometimes produce real solutions to problems. People who work from home can easily try this technique for boosting creativity and a few forward-thinking employers have installed "napasiums" for sanctioned creative napping in the workplace.

● **Avoid cheese—if it gives you nightmares** The old wives' tale is true—eating cheese at night really can give you nightmares. Cheese contains the amino acid tyramine, which is involved in the production of adrenaline, a stress hormone. Excess levels of this hormone may in turn raise blood pressure, which is associated with nightmares. Other foods that contain tyramine and may disturb sleep include cured meats, fermented soy products, lima beans, and chocolate.

● **Learn to control your dreams** Lucid dreaming, a state of being awake within a dream and being able to direct its outcome, has been found to help people suffering from post-traumatic stress but can be helpful to anyone. You will benefit from the calming effects of being able to fly around your house, take yourself to a restful seashore, or imagine sitting in a beautiful garden. Try imagining a dream you

For further tips on lucid dreaming, see *Secrets of Dream Control,* page 286

want to resume as you fall asleep or training yourself to return to a dream as you are waking up.

● **Record your dreams** Keep a dream diary to help resolve problems that may be troubling you. Recording your dreams allows you to focus on difficulties, many of which may be long term or relate to your childhood. There is mounting evidence that if you have experienced divorce, bereavement, or separation, the nightmares that follow can actually help you come to terms with your loss. Dreams help you visualize what is going on in your life and let you find ways of dealing with problems by harnessing past experiences. To help you use your dreams:

★ **Keep** a notebook and pen beside the bed and write down your dreams as soon as you wake in the morning.

★ **Avoid** recording dreams in the middle of the night as this will interrupt your sleep.

★ **Record** the detail, including colors if they appear, and any feelings you had.

★ **Leave** space opposite each entry for any analysis you may wish to add.

★ **Review** the previous night's dreams before you go to bed.

● **Catch up on your sleep** Contrary to perceived wisdom, it is perfectly possible to make up a deficit of sleep according to a study at the University of Pennsylvania School of Medicine. Healthy sleepers who normally slept between 6.5 and 8.5 hours a night and who were neither shift workers nor long-haul travelers were only allowed 4 hours sleep for 5 nights in a row. Following tests, their alertness and ability to concentrate were found to be reduced. They were then allowed to sleep as long as they liked and were tested again, by which time their brain function had returned to normal.

When sleep ELUDES YOU

Having trouble sleeping is an age-old problem but fortunately medical science is constantly discovering new treatments for insomnia—and many old remedies are finding scientific backing. Here are some ideas that may help you sleep more soundly.

● **Listen to noise**—as long as it's white. White noise consists of every frequency audible to the human ear, which when played simultaneously creates a soothing hum or a sound like a gentle wind or the waves breaking on the seashore. This not only helps to drown out extraneous noise but fills the "space" in your brain that is otherwise taken up with anxious thoughts. It works for babies and small children, too. Consider investing in a white noise machine, download a white noise app for your smartphone, or simply listen to the sound produced by your radio when it's tuned between stations as you settle down for the night.

● **Keep cool** Cooling down your brain can apparently help you to sleep. Researchers at the University of Pittsburgh discovered that cooling the brain may help to induce sleep by slowing the activity of brain cells. Volunteers who spent the night wearing soft plastic caps through which cold water circulated had significantly improved sleep. Improve the quality of your sleep by keeping your bedroom cooler—no warmer than 65°F (18°C).

● **Rock yourself to sleep** The perfect way to get a baby to sleep works for adults, too. A Swiss experiment in which brain waves of volunteers taking naps were measured showed that it took 4 minutes for them to fall asleep while being rocked— a 30–40 percent improvement—and that they slept more deeply. The rocking stimulates receptors in the inner ear, which pass signals to the hypothalamus and cerebral cortex, rapidly synchronizing sleep-related brainwaves. So get yourself a rocking chair for an afternoon slumber.

The gentle sound of waves breaking on a shore is "white noise," which can help you drift off to sleep.

● **Identify your "sleep window"**
You'll have less trouble sleeping if you learn to recognize when your body rhythms are ready for sleep in the evenings and make that your bedtime. The brain functions in 90-minute cycles throughout the day and night, with periods of intense mental activity alternating with more relaxed times, during which our concentration lapses and we find it easier to fall asleep. Try to become aware of this pattern of waking activity so that you can pinpoint your "sleep window"—the best time to go to bed.

● **Sleep naturally** To help you sleep without the help of prescribed medicines, try one of these herbal preparations, all of which have a long history of treating insomnia effectively. Always check with your doctor if you are taking medication for another condition.

★ **Hops** Used by the ancient Chinese and early Europeans, dried hop flowers can be effective against insomnia when used as a pillow filling. They are often combined with valerian, a mixture shown in German trials to be as effective as benzodiazepine sleeping pills for remedying sleep disorders. The dried flowers can be made into an infusion using about a tablespoon (10g) in a liter of boiling water. Or add a liter of the infusion to warm bathwater for a sleep-inducing soak.

★ **Lavender** This favorite of the ancient Romans acts by helping to reduce stress. Make an infusion of 3–4 teaspoons (2–3g) of flowers with boiling water, and drink 1 cup (250 ml) of the cooled, strained liquid as a soothing nightcap. Or sprinkle 5 drops of lavender essential oil on your pillow or onto your chest before you go to bed.

★ **Magnolia** To help combat insomnia, particularly if the problem is anxiety related, try magnolia bark, a traditional Eastern remedy. Its sleep-inducing effect is thought to be due to the substances magnolol and honokiol, which lower the production of the stress hormone cortisol. Magnolia bark extract is available as capsules from health food stores.

★ **Passionflower** A cup of passionflower infusion, made with 3 teaspoons (2g) of the dried plant in a cup of boiling water, left for 15 minutes before straining, and taken before bed will help you get to sleep. The leaves and stems of this South American native, long used to treat insomnia and anxiety, contain substances called maltols, which have a sedative effect.

★ **Valerian** Preparations of the valerian root were recommended for insomnia by the ancient Greek physician Hippocrates and modern clinical studies in Brazil have proved that it can improve both the length and quality of sleep. Its key components are sedative compounds that calm muscle spasms, and others that block the transmission of signals in the brain.

● **Have some carbs** If you're trying to lose weight, find an alternative to a low-carbohydrate diet. These diets—the Atkins Diet, for example—tend to cause insomnia

Magnolia bark extract may help combat anxiety-related insomnia.

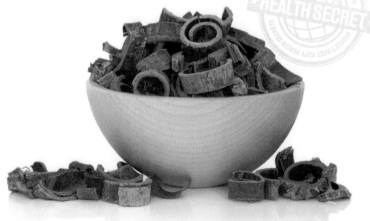

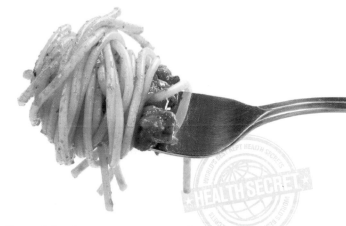

Spaghetti bolognese contains the right balance of nutrients to help you sleep better.

BODY POWER

Eat to sleep

It's worth considering the possibility that the foods you eat—or don't eat—may be the cause of your sleeping problem. Make sure you get enough of the following nutrients:

Tryptophan Stimulates the all-important production of melatonin. The time it takes you to fall asleep can be halved when your levels of this chemical are high. It is found in all high-protein foods, especially turkey, lean meat, eggs, and soybeans.

Vitamin B, particularly B_6, B_{12}, and niacin—lack of any of these is linked to insomnia. Eat whole grains, seafood, poultry, nuts, and lentils to ensure a good intake of these vitamins.

and nightmares. The main reason is that high-carbohydrate foods are rich in serotonin—a neurotransmitter that helps to promote sleep, among other effects. And a low-carbohydrate diet may reduce the levels of this brain chemical. To keep up your intake of serotonin and still lose weight, try stepping up your exercise regime.

● **Enjoy an early supper** Try not to eat after about 7pm. Going to bed with a full stomach is not only likely to cause indigestion but prevents the body from entering a state of relaxation because digestion is working at full tilt. According to the tenets of traditional Chinese medicine, the digestion is strongest in the morning and weakest in the final hours of the day—so putting it under strain is bound to disrupt sleep. Eat little and often throughout the day if you want a better night's sleep.

● **Eat spaghetti bolognese** This is an ideal supper dish for insomniacs—especially if you don't include a lot of meat. It provides the ideal balance of nutrients to raise the levels of tryptophan, a brain chemical that increases the secretion of the sleep-inducing hormone melatonin. Trytophan levels are raised most effectively by a meal that contains lots of carbohydrates and a small amount of protein. You can use this knowledge to make an ideal sleep-promoting late-night snack, such as a peanut butter sandwich.

● **Get your thyroid tested** Think about having a thyroid function test. Hyperthyroidism (sometimes called thyrotoxicosis), in which the gland is overactive, tends to "rev up" your body making your brain less able to know when to switch off and induce sleep. Even when sleep does happen, it is often fractured, and you may wake up a dozen times or more during the night, causing fatigue during the day. Additional symptoms of overactive thyroid include weight loss, anxiety, diarrhea, excessive sweating, and absent or light periods. See your doctor if you suspect this may be the cause of your sleep problem.

● **Clear your nose** Allergies caused by a reaction to dust mites or tree and grass pollens can indirectly affect your sleep by interfering with breathing. Dealing with nasal congestion can often bring about a dramatic improvement in sleep quality. Ask your doctor for advice on medication or other measures to control your symptoms.

For further tips on dealing with allergies that cause nasal congestion, see Chapter 3, *Breath of Life*

● **Have a milky bedtime drink** which contains both calcium and the amino acid tryptophan. Low calcium levels prevent the brain from achieving or maintaining the deepest levels of sleep, including REM (rapid eye movement) sleep, during which dreaming occurs. Tryptophan is essential for the manufacture of the sleep-inducing chemical melatonin. Magnesium, found in green leafy vegetables and legumes, is also needed for deep, uninterrupted sleep.

● **Cultivate friends** Try to keep connected to other people because feelings of loneliness can have a negative effect on sleep. In a study of adults in a close-knit community in South Dakota, researchers found that there was a strong connection between fragmented sleep and feeling lonely. Loneliness can be part of a negative cycle of thinking. If you break the cycle—for example, by finding ways to form new friendships—you hold the key to the resolution of your sleep problem. Don't hesitate to seek professional help, if you feel that your loneliness is linked to depression.

Having good friends combats loneliness, a key cause of insomnia.

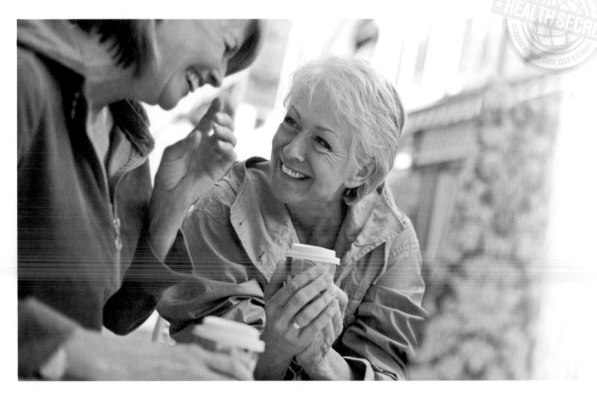

● **Don't exercise**—at least not just before bedtime. Getting enough exercise during the day is essential for good sleep, but be careful when you take it. Late afternoon to early evening is the best time of day for vigorous exercise. If you do an energetic workout any later, you may find it hard to relax adequately before you go to bed. But you can practice yoga and similar forms of gentle exercise during the evening without interfering with your ability to fall sleep.

● **Get on the couch** Psychotherapy can help you to sleep better. Short one-to-one cognitive behavior therapy (CBT) sessions have proved highly effective in curing insomnia, especially for those over 65. The therapy works by helping to reduce excessive arousal of the brain's "awake system," showing you how to replace negative thoughts such as "I'm so tired I'll never be able to function tomorrow" with positive ones such as "I've had other nights like this and I've still functioned well the next day." Ask your doctor about CBT therapists working in your area.

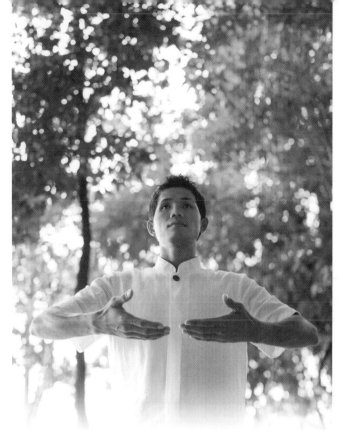

Regular tai chi practice can improve the quality and quantity of your sleep.

SURPRISINGLY EASY

Press it

Try acupressure before bed to induce sleep. According to French research, pressure applied to the Heart 7 point leads to a significant increase in both the length and quality of sleep. This pressure point is located on the palm side of your hand, on the wrist crease directly below your little finger. Locate the bony knob on the outside of your left wrist (little finger side) and Heart 7 is just next to this, in a small hollow. The best way to exert pressure throughout the night is with soft rubber acupressure cones, held on with a wrist band.

● **Move gently** Try movement therapies from the East, such as tai chi or yoga to relax your mind in preparation for sleep.

★ **Tai chi** When carried out for an hour a day for 24 weeks by a group of older people, tai chi—a kind of "moving meditation"—improved both the quality and quantity of sleep and reduced the time taken to nod off. The volunteers also experienced markedly improved mental abilities.

★ **Yoga** Before going to bed, relax in the Corpse Pose. Lie flat on your back with your arms by your sides and palms facing upward, and place your feet hip-width apart. Breathe deeply, close your eyes, then roll your head so that one ear and then the other touches the ground. Lie still and focus on your breathing for 10 minutes. You will find it hard not to fall asleep.

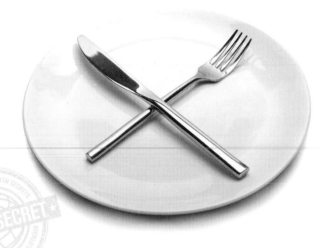

Fasting will help your body clock adjust to a new time zone.

● **See the light** If you're traveling between time zones, you can use light to reset your body clock and adjust melatonin production, which will help you to avoid jet lag. If traveling from west to east and while it is still dark, ideally at 4am, expose yourself to bright artificial light. If going in the other direction, do the same thing at 6am. It's also

helpful to alter your normal sleeping pattern to fit more closely with your schedule in the time zone to which you are traveling; reset your watch on takeoff; use the eye mask on the plane to synchronize with the darkness at your destination; on arrival, spend time outdoors in the light; and stay awake until it's bedtime.

● **Go without food** when traveling across several time zones. Experiments have shown that depriving the body of food for about 16 hours overrides its built-in circadian clock—the one that sets our approximate 24-hour cycle of sleep and wakefulness. But the clock is turned on again and rapidly reset as soon as food is consumed. If going hungry is not an option, try to time meals to fit with those of your destination.

● **Block it out** If you work at night, you may find it hard to sleep during daylight hours. To trick your body that it's nighttime, try using blackout curtains or blinds to block the light from your bedroom. Other good tips include:
★ **Wear sunglasses** on your way home to block out light and help stimulate melatonin production.
★ **Go to bed** as soon as you get home.
★ **Keep to your schedule** on days off and on weekends.
★ **Turn off the phone** so that your sleep is not disturbed.

● **Take a time pill** It is possible that one day you'll be able to pop a pill to treat jet lag. Researchers in the UK trying to find a cure for jet lag have discovered that an enzyme called casein kinase is essential to the fine tuning of our body clocks. Using this knowledge, they are working to develop a drug that will block the production of the enzyme to treat jet lag effectively.

BELIEVE IT OR NOT!

Pills may make sleeping problems worse

Sleeping pills can give temporary relief for insomnia. But American studies have shown that even the most recently introduced drugs for insomnia, such as zolpidem and zopiclone increase sleep time by an average of only 12 minutes, and may cause a range of side effects including sleepwalking and amnesia. What's more, many sleeping pills significantly reduce the amount of the deep, slow-wave non-REM sleep essential to waking up feeling refreshed. If you've been prescribed such medication for more than four weeks, you'll quickly build up tolerance and, when you stop, may find yourself suffering from "rebound insomnia." The message is to avoid sleeping pills or limit their use to the shortest time possible.

Hide your clock

Make sure that any timepieces in your bedroom are hidden away or covered up. This is because every time you wake in the night and look at the time you'll worry more about the amount of sleep you're losing and how little time there is left to get some sleep.

Take off your watch, hide your alarm clock, use duct tape to mask the time display on your radio, TV, or DVD player, and make sure your computer is turned off.

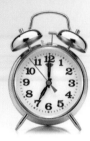

● **Cut back on zzzzs** Surprisingly, cutting down on how long you want to sleep might be the best way of curing your insomnia. Make a sleep log for a few weeks to determine how many hours, on average, you sleep each night. Then use this figure—say 5 hours—to set the time you will spend in bed. Each morning, record the proportion of that time you've actually been asleep and, once the figure passes 85 percent (in this case 3 hours 25 minutes), allow yourself another 15 minutes in bed. Then continue in this way until you're sleeping for at least 6 hours a night.

● **Don't just lie there** Instead of tossing and turning, get up if you haven't dropped off to sleep after 20 to 30 minutes of being in bed, and go and relax in a quiet, comfortable place, perhaps with a book and a cup of caffeine-free herb tea. When you begin to feel drowsy, go back to bed, but if you find you're lying awake for another 20 to 30 minutes, get up again. Repeat the routine until you fall asleep.

● **Avoid blue light** To boost the amount of melatonin your brain produces to induce sleep, pop on some amber goggles for a few hours before bedtime. This will help to prevent blue light—which inhibits melatonin production—from reaching your brain. As an alternative, look for light bulbs that do not contain blue light. Don't forget to turn off the computer and similar devices before you go to bed.

● **Get rid of the TV** Create a sleep-friendly environment by taking as much clutter out of your bedroom as possible. Electronic equipment such as TVs and computers, in particular, can hamper the process of falling asleep, possibly because of their associations with work or mental stimulation. Here are some more tips for making your bedroom into a place that is conducive to sleep:

★ **Install** light-blocking curtains or blinds.
★ **Paint** the walls in restful colors.
★ **Close** all cupboards and drawers.
★ **Adjust** the temperature to around 65°F (18°C) and have adequate ventilation.

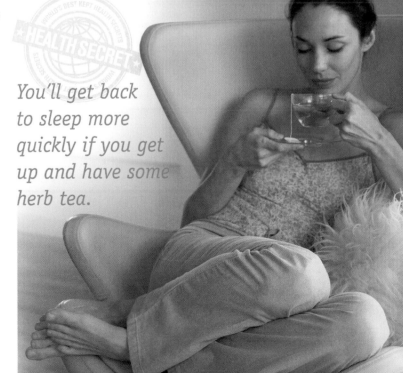

You'll get back to sleep more quickly if you get up and have some herb tea.

Secrets of
DREAM CONTROL

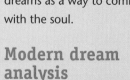

The often bizarre images that appear in the mind during sleep have fascinated people throughout the ages and remain the object of great curiosity. Yet despite continuing scientific investigation, there is still little consensus about the role dreams play in our mental and emotional health. Read on to discover ways in which you can learn to use your dreams to improve your well-being.

Dream caused by the Flight of a Bee around a Pomegranate One Second before Waking up was one of many disturbing images created by the surrealist artist Salvador Dali, who was influenced by Freud's work.

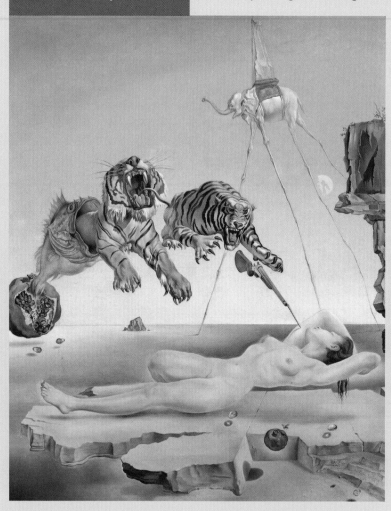

Throughout history, people of all cultures have sought to understand and interpret their dreams. The ancient Greeks and Romans believed they were direct messages from the gods or the dead and that they predicted the future. American Indians tried to encourage beneficial dreams by fasting, meditating, and choosing special places to sleep.

Shamans (medicine men and women or witchdoctors) in many cultures saw dreams as gateways to the spirit world, where they could learn the secrets of the dead. And Tibetan Buddhists have used dreams as a way to commune with the soul.

Modern dream analysis

Dream analysis entered the modern world with the work of Viennese psychiatrist and neurologist Sigmund Freud (1856–1939), who saw dreams as manifestations of our deepest desires and anxieties, which often related to childhood experiences repressed by the unconscious mind. His contemporary, Swiss psychiatrist and psychologist Carl Jung (1875–1961), believed that dreams accessed memories collected since time began, part of what he termed the "collective unconscious."

Twenty-first century psychologists are still divided over the purpose of dreams. Some believe they are no more than random bursts of nerve-cell activity in the brainstem. Others compare the brain to a computer in which dreams are responsible for filing away large amounts of mainly unnecessary data to make space for information we need to access from day to day. What is clear from many studies of people deprived of rapid eye movement (REM) sleep is that dreams are essential for mental well-being.

These color-coded scans show active (red) and inactive (blue) brain areas during non-REM sleep (left) and REM sleep (right).

Dream control

Most of us spend about a quarter of our sleeping time dreaming, whether we remember our dreams or not. This corresponds to the average length of time we spend in REM sleep. Monitoring of brain activity has shown that most dreaming occurs during this phase of sleep.

For most people, the memory of a dream fades rapidly upon waking. But others not only recall their dreams in great detail but are also aware while dreaming that they are dreaming—the experience has been described as waking up in a dream. These lucid dreamers can even learn to exert some control over the content of their dreams. Proponents of the benefits of lucid dreaming claim that the ability to control your dreams can enhance problem solving and creativity, and boost confidence, as well as provide great enjoyment. Research shows that lucid dreaming can also help control nightmares. You can now download an app or buy a facemask to give you aural or visual cues while you sleep, in an attempt to stimulate certain kinds of dream. Here are some tips on how to dream lucidly, based on the research of Stephen LaBerge and his colleagues at The Lucidity Institute:

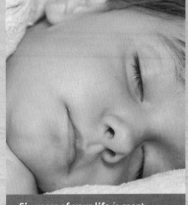

Six years of your life is spent dreaming, on average.

Mnemonic Induction of Lucid Dreams (MILD) Use this technique right after awakening from a dream, to help you re-enter the dream state and to stimulate lucid dreaming:
- **As soon as** you wake, recall the dream in as much detail as possible.
- **Tell yourself** while you fall back to sleep that you will remember that you're dreaming once you enter a dream.
- **Imagine** that you are back in an earlier dream (the one you just had

if you remember it) and that you recognize that you are dreaming. Look for something in the dream that indicates it is a dream. Repeat these steps until you fall asleep.

Wake up an hour early and do something to keep yourself alert for an hour, such as reading. Then do the MILD exercises for 10 minutes, before taking a nap for an hour—this is said to be one of the best ways to encourage lucid dreaming.

If you wake from a dreaming state (lucid or not), and you want to re-enter it, just lie still and wait; if this does not work, count yourself back to sleep in this way: "One, I'm dreaming; two, I'm dreaming," and so on.

If you achieve a lucid dreaming state, you may find that it seems to last for only a very short time and you emerge from it too early. A way to increase the apparent duration of the dream is to use a sensation trigger that will keep you rooted in it. Triggers suggested by researchers are spinning (so try to twirl around in the dream, like a dancer) and rubbing your hands together.

Special
SLEEP PROBLEMS

If you have a specific problem, such as snoring or obstructive sleep apnea syndrome (OSAS) that affects your sleeping, help is at hand. These surprisingly simple tips can make the difference for you (and your partner) between a sleep-deprived night and a full night's sleep.

● **Breathe moist air** Improve the quality of the air in your bedroom with a humidifier and you could find that your snoring problem, or that of your partner, disappears or noticeably reduces. Humid air works by helping to loosen the mucus in the respiratory system so that, rather than blocking the nose, the body is able to expel it more easily.

● **Exercise your tongue** Tone your tongue muscles to help stop yourself from snoring. Try fitting these exercises into your daily routine:

★ **Push** your tongue to the back of your front teeth and, as you do so, roll it around at the back of your mouth, using as much pressure as you can. Continue this exercise for 3 minutes.

★ **Repeat** each of the vowels (A, E, I, O, U) out loud for 3 minutes, stressing the tone of each one.

★ **Purse** your lips and try to keep them in position for 30 seconds.

★ **Contract** the muscles at the back of your throat for 30 seconds—this may produce a sound like a croaking frog.

● **Dilate your nostrils** Try putting on nasal strips at night to dilate your nostrils. If you snore because your nasal passages are blocked—due to an allergy such as hay fever, sinus infections, or unwanted growths such as polyps in the nose—nasal strips may help.

It's also possible to have surgery to keep the nasal passages open by inserting small rods into them. The surgical removal of troublesome polyps can be effective, too.

● **Watch your medications** Alcohol, and a variety of medications including antihistamines and sleeping pills, can cause relaxation of your tongue muscles leading to snoring. If your muscles are so relaxed and your tongue falls too far back in your mouth, a plastic mouth guard that pulls both it and the lower jaw forward can successfully reduce snoring.

● **Diet for quiet** Add exercise to your weight loss regimen to help tighten your neck muscles. Being overweight is a cause of OSAS—snoring plus frequent pauses in breathing. In a Greek study, a calorie-controlled diet combined with 30 minutes exercise a day proved effective, after six months, in producing both weight loss and less interruption of REM sleep from OSAS.

● **Mask the danger** OSAS is the most dangerous form of snoring. It also causes headaches and fatigue and is linked with high blood pressure, stroke, and type 2 diabetes. You can get relief with a continuous positive airway pressure (CPAP) device—a mask that fits over the nose connected to a bedside machine, which delivers a steady stream of pressurized air.

- **Search for the cause** It's particularly important to discover the cause of snoring in a child because it can lead to disturbed sleep and a reduced supply of oxygen to the brain, which can cause poor school performance and behavioral problems. Enlarged tonsils and adenoids, common in a small child, can cause snoring. Being overweight is also a risk factor because excess fat can constrict the throat and prevent the diaphragm from working properly. Seek your doctor's advice.

- **Cut down on caffeine** Found in coffee, tea, and cola, this stimulant slows down the body's absorption of iron, which is often deficient in people with restless leg syndrome. And caffeine is a well-known impediment to good sleep.

- **Keep a sleepwalker safe** Take every precaution if someone in your household is a sleepwalker. Keep them away from stairs—consider installing a stair gate. Lock windows and secure any potentially dangerous area in the house where a fall might occur. Affecting 1 in 10 children and 1 in 50 adults, sleepwalking can be brought on by sleep deprivation.

- **Give up the gum** If you grind your teeth at night, don't chew gum during the day—chewing clenches the jaw muscles, which can exacerbate the problem. If you find yourself clenching your teeth while you're awake, push the tip of your tongue between your teeth, as this can help train your jaw muscles to relax.

- **Try massage** To prevent restless legs at night, give your legs a good rub 2 or 3 hours before bedtime. It may also help to apply a hot or cold compress to your leg muscles—whichever works best.

- **Keep your legs calm with supplements** Try taking a daily supplement of 400mg magnesium combined with 800mg calcium if you suffer from restless leg syndrome. It may also be helpful to increase your intake of iron and folic acid, essential for the manufacture of oxygen-carrying blood cells and of myoglobin, the protein that stores oxygen in the muscles until it is needed. Achieve this by increasing the amount of leafy green vegetables, whole grains, and beans in your diet, plus red meat if you're not a vegetarian. Alternatively, take iron and folic acid as supplements.

For **further tips** on boosting your iron intake see Chapter 5, *Nutrition and Weight Control*

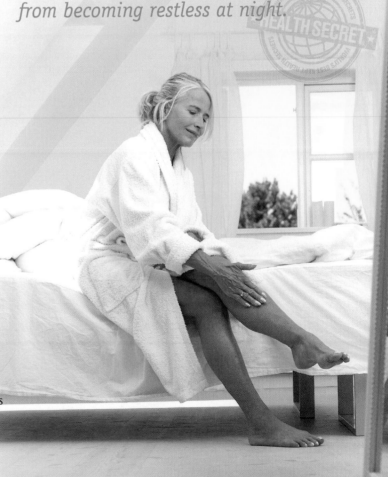

Massaging your legs can prevent them from becoming restless at night.

HEALTH SECRET

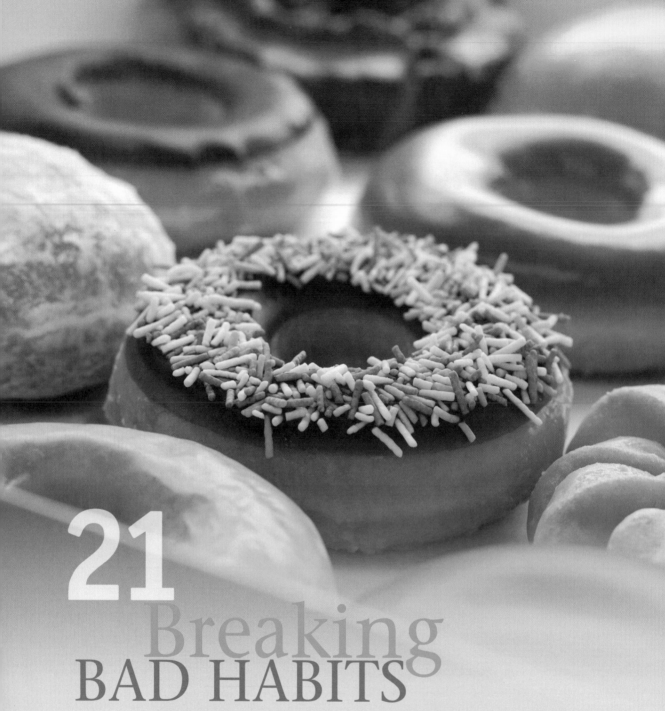

21
Breaking
BAD HABITS

It is so easy for health to be ruined when innocent pleasures turn into guilty addictions, or when daily routines are disrupted by irrational worries, obsessions, and phobias. But with the latest research in hand—plus some surprisingly effective traditional treatments—it's possible to get these bad habits under control, putting you back in the driver's seat.

Dealing with
CRAVINGS AND ADDICTIONS

We all know how damaging illegal drug abuse is to the body, but so is dependence on cigarettes and alcohol. Even food cravings, which we may think of as mere indulgence, can be detrimental to health. But there's a lot we can do to give ourselves a helping hand.

● **Walk away from bad habits** Just a brisk 15-minute walk can give you the help needed to kick your cravings. In research at the UK's Exeter University, chocoholics who were put on an exercise program reported a reduction in their desire for chocolate, both during and after exercise. And in studies of smokers, MRI scans revealed that exercise appeared to alter the activity of the reward centers in the smokers brains. It may be that the "feel good" endorphins produced during exercise have an effect, or that exercise causes more blood to flow to areas of the brain that are less involved with feelings of gratification.

● **Open up** Addicts do all they can to hide their problem for fear of being found out, from the shame they feel and because their lives are out of control. They may stash empty wine bottles away in cupboards, borrow money to cover gambling debts, or lie to mask their behavior. Admitting the problem to family or friends, a support group such as Alcoholics Anonymous, or a health professional who can recommend treatment such as psychotherapy, is a vital part of breaking the cycle of dependence.

● **Learn to say "no"** Cravings are always hard to resist. But help is at hand in the form of assertiveness training, in which you are coached to speak your mind calmly but forcefully. By practicing your arguments in advance and identifying problem scenarios and the way you handle them, you will gain the confidence to overcome difficulties and stick to your goals. As you become more optimistic and start to take control of your addiction, your thought patterns will change, giving you the power to say "no thank you." It's self-reinforcing: Every "no" will give you even greater strength to resist temptation the next time.

SURPRISINGLY EASY

Nail-biting photo finish
Help yourself to stop nail biting by taking snapshots of your bitten nails. Keep the photos on display to remind you how bad they look. Other tips:

● Choose just one nail to bite.

● Apply nail polish (colorless if necessary) to discourage biting.

● Buy one of the foul-tasting antibiting products on the market.

● Put strips of sticky tape over your nails.

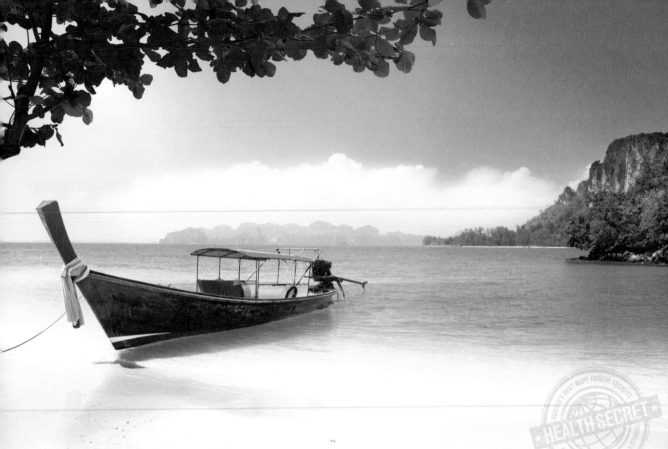

Refocusing your brain to visualize a rainbow or an idyllic scene instead of the food you crave could help you beat the addiction.

● **Get the knowledge** From the moment you decide to tackle a bad habit that risks becoming an addiction, finding out the facts can help to strengthen your willpower. It could be knowing that your lungs start repairing themselves and your blood pressure decreases within 20 minutes of your last cigarette, or that soon after you stop drinking, your damaged liver cells will start to repair themselves, or that you will have extra money in the bank to spend on treats for yourself and your family.

● **Change your vision** Researchers in Australia have found that cravings for treats such as chocolate, ice cream, and potato chips are linked to vivid "images" of these foods that form in the mind. Such mental imagery can occupy the brain so strongly

BELIEVE IT OR NOT!

Addictive genes

For addicts at a loss to understand their behavior, it may help to know that addiction may have a genetic cause— at least in part. Several genes are associated with dependence on alcohol, nicotine, cocaine, and other addictive substances. Studies show that the children of people addicted to drugs or alcohol have an 8 percent greater risk of becoming addicts themselves, while investigations of identical twins have revealed that addiction is 50 percent genetic and 50 percent due to poor coping skills—which means that it's always possible to take control and overcome an addiction.

that other brain functions, such as problem solving, suffer as a result. Researchers found that the cravings were significantly reduced when their subjects switched their mental imagery to a nonfood subject—for example, a rainbow or landscape—or watched a pattern of flickering black and white dots. There may soon be downloadable apps for people to view so that they can tackle their cravings quickly and effectively.

● **Don't go it alone** Addictions damage whole families, not just individuals. The partners of addicts may burden themselves with too many domestic responsibilities and chores and there may be conflict in the home. Some families live a life of denial and pretend that nothing is wrong, trapped in a vicious cycle of fear, hope, love, and guilt. Support groups such as Al-anon and Alateen offer help to the families of alcoholics, sympathizing with their embarrassment and pain and showing them what they need to do to break the cycle and heal both the addict and family relationships. Counseling of this kind, which may involve direct confrontation with the addict in the presence of a mediator, will help family members to move on with their lives, even if the addict refuses to take steps to address their problem.

● **Read the signals right** When a craving for alcohol sets in, it could be your brain sending a misleading message. What you perceive as an urge to drink alcohol may just be a sign that you're dehydrated. If so, a couple of glasses of water may make the desire go away. Alternatively, because alcohol supplies calories, it's possible that you're hungry. Eating a meal instead of pouring a drink is another effective way to stop the craving. When trying to give up alcohol, it's important that you always get

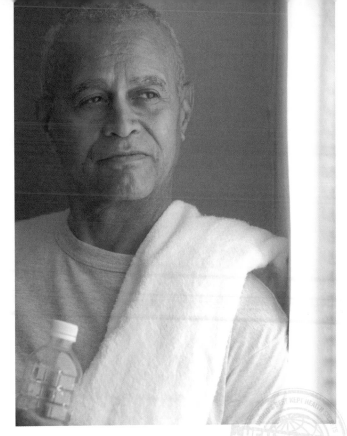

Alcohol cravings may actually be thirst or hunger; drinking water or eating can dampen the desire.

three meals a day—and keep yourself hydrated by drinking sufficient nonalcoholic fluids.

● **Be calm with balm** To calm the jitters that can set in when you give up smoking or drinking for good, try a herbal remedy such as lemon balm. Make a fragrant and soothing tea with a handful of chopped fresh leaves infused in boiling water. The plant is easy to grow in your garden or window box. Lemon balm also works well when combined with other plants, including hawthorn and passionflower.

● **Try milk thistle** This common herb, which grows in many parts of Europe and Asia, is renowned for its liver-healing properties. And the liver is one of the organs

SECRETS OF SUCCESS

Biofeedback
Addicts can learn to beat their dependency by looking at images of their brainwaves. Called biofeedback, this treatment uses a screen to display two sorts of waves: alpha waves (showing relaxation) and theta waves (reflecting calmness). Subjects are trained to de-stress by focusing on their breathing and heartbeat. By doing this, they not only soothe feelings of anxiety about getting their next drink or drug fix, but they can also see the effects of their mental state on the brainwaves displayed by the screen—which, in turn, helps to reinforce the effectiveness of their actions.

Angostura bitters, made from the root of the gentian plant, can ease the effects of too much alcohol.

most likely to be impaired by excessive alcohol consumption. Milk thistle has been shown to repair hepatocytes, a type of liver cell often damaged by alcohol. Take three cups of infusion a day (3 teaspoons of seeds to a cup of boiling water) or as tablets (one to two 200mg daily). Always check with your doctor before using a herbal remedy.

● **Take to water** If you want to be sure you don't drink too much, and to help avoid hangovers, drink water. Because alcohol is a diuretic that speeds water loss from body tissues, dehydration is one of the chief causes of hangovers. The best advice is to drink a glass of water before your first alcoholic drink. Then throughout the evening, alternate each alcoholic drink with a glass of water. Finally, drink a large glass of water before you go to bed.

● **Give it a rest** Even if you don't drink very much, you need to give your liver time to recover after consuming alcohol, so it's wise to refrain from drinking for two or

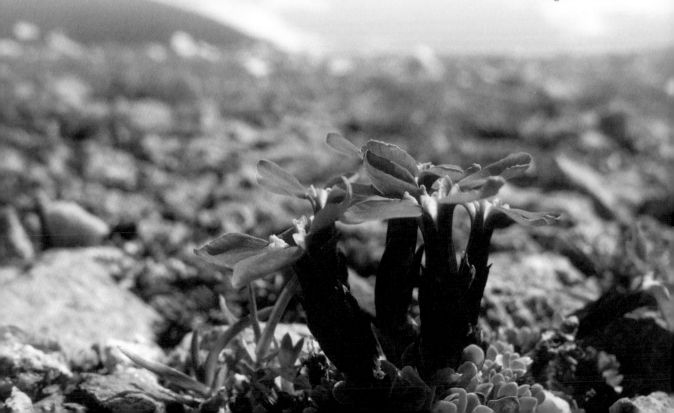

three days during the week. Regular drinking raises the risk of cirrhosis of the liver: One Japanese study has shown that drinkers who consumed their alcohol over five to seven days had higher death rates than those who drank it over one to four days.

● Get help from the liquor cabinet

Always try to avoid hangovers, but to ease a queasy stomach after a heavy night, add a few drops of Angostura bitters to a cup of boiling water. This cocktail ingredient, derived from gentian root, is a natural remedy for digestive problems. Tonic water is also an effective hangover cure. But it contains quinine, a bitter substance extracted from the bark of the South American cinchona tree, too much of which can disrupt heart rhythm, cause nervous tremors, and may damage the eyes. To avoid side effects, drink no more than one large glass of tonic water a day.

● Sweeten up

Because they contain fructose, which helps to speed up the breakdown of alcohol, both honey and fruit such as dates can help to prevent or cure hangovers. Honey in hot water is a time-honored hangover remedy.

● Make a meal of it

The best way to enjoy alcohol, and to minimize its effects, is to drink it with food. When food enters the stomach, the pyloric sphincter between the stomach and the duodenum closes to allow food to digest for as much as 8 hours. This helps to keep the alcohol confined in the stomach and slows the rate at which it is absorbed into the bloodstream.

● Postpone the pleasure

Use your emotional intelligence to break a bad habit. If you feel you need a drink of alcohol or a smoke, postpone the pleasure for a full hour.

You may then find that the urge disappears completely. Success in delaying gratification will also make you feel positive, optimistic, and good about yourself—all of which have been proven to be key factors in preventing and treating addictions of all kinds.

● Keep the choice wide

If you are prone to binge eating, the worst thing you can do is to follow a strict diet. The more foods you deny yourself, the less likely you are to solve the problem. While all foods are "legal," there are ways in which you can restrict the ones that trigger binges. One trick is to use a smaller plate, which limits you to smaller portions. Another is to eat "bad" foods in single servings out of the house; so rather than buying a big tub of ice cream, taking it home, and eating it all in front of the TV, buy a cone at your local ice cream parlor and savor every mouthful. As you gain control over your habit, introduce more and more healthy foods into your diet.

● Beat binge eating with breakfast

The old adage "breakfast is the most important meal of the day" holds true for those with a tendency to eat excessive amounts. Eating breakfast jump-starts the metabolism, so it can be a great help to binge eaters—especially if it's followed up with lunch and dinner. Skipping meals often leads to binge eating later in the day.

● Talk while you eat

As you eat, stay focused on the food. Eat as slowly as you can, with small bites, to give your stomach the chance to let you know when it's full, and put your knife and fork down between mouthfuls. Try to make mealtimes a relaxing time for conversation and discussion, which will also help slow your consumption and allow your natural appetite-regulating mechanisms to kick in.

● **Try psychological acupuncture** Also called emotional freedom technique (EFT), psychological acupuncture has proved effective in combating food cravings. The treatment involves tapping acupressure points while subjects concentrate on specific thoughts or emotions. At Griffith University, Australia, people receiving EFT found that food cravings, including those for sweet foods and salty snacks, were reduced after just four 2-hour sessions, and that the effects lasted for six months.

● **Hide the scale at first ...** Adding a few pounds to your weight when you give up smoking is an insignificant risk to health compared with the benefits to your heart and lungs and your reduced risk of cancer. Weight gain occurs because nicotine speeds up your digestion and metabolism, and reduces your appetite. And after quitting, you may use food to replace the oral stimulation of a cigarette and to help you

Eating mangoes can boost your serotonin levels, helping you to deal with the stress of giving up tobacco.

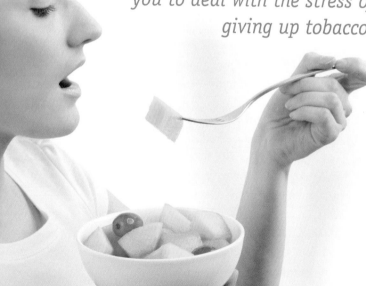

relax. In the short term, don't worry about what the scale says, just eat as healthy a range of foods as you can, including lots of whole grains, fruit, and vegetables.

● **... but keep a food diary** While you may want to snack more when you give up cigarettes, which does no harm in the short term, ultimately you will probably want to control your appetite and your weight. Writing down what you eat and when can help to identify the key times when you're substituting food for smoking. These are good moments to get out of the house and exercise, which will distract you from eating while helping to burn excess calories. It will also help get your heart and lungs back into tip-top condition.

● **Ban the desire with Zyban** A 21st-century drug, Zyban, which contains the antidepressant bupropion hydrochloride, was developed to help smokers. Tests at the University of Wisconsin showed Zyban to be twice as effective in helping smokers to quit as nicotine patches. The drug works to weaken the desire to smoke, possibly by affecting the neurotransmitters that are responsible for moderating mood.

● **Deprive yourself of funds** It seems obvious, but it's impossible to gamble if you don't have access to money. If you have a gambling addiction, empty your wallet, and cut up your credit and debit cards now. You may need to ask someone else to take control of your finances or get the bank to deal directly with all your payments. You'll also need to block online gambling sites on your computer. Remember that professional help is available via your doctor or the organization Gamblers Anonymous.

● **Stimulate your brain** One of the main problems in treating patients with addictions is restoring the ability of the brain to make its own opiates—the chemicals we know as endorphins. In the UK, Professor Karl Schmidt and Dr. Meg Paterson found that applying an extremely weak electric current to acupressure points at the back of the head stimulates the body to release endorphins. The treatment involves using a pocket-sized stimulator continuously for six to ten days. This can be effective within one or two weeks.

● **Have a mango** When you're struggling to give up smoking, your food choices can be critical. The pleasure rush from smoking a cigarette comes from the hormones dopamine and noradrenaline, and the feel-good hormone beta endorphin, whose release is triggered by nicotine. You can replace these substances with stress-relieving serotonin by getting plenty of exposure to bright light. Another way to increase serotonin levels is through diet. Serotonin-boosting foods include strawberries, oranges, mangoes, chickpeas, lentils, and hazelnuts. You should also eat foods that will encourage a steady, but slow release of dopamine, including yogurt, almonds, avocados, and legumes. Reducing the

BELIEVE IT OR NOT!

African plant may help addicts

Experts in New Zealand and Mexico are using the root of the iboga plant to help drug addicts, especially those dependent on opiates, kick the habit. The African plant has been used for thousands of years in ritual healing practices. But ibogaine, the alkaloid drug that is extracted from the plant, is controversial—not only because it is hallucinogenic and can cause a potentially lethal slowing of the heart, but also because it is illegal in many countries. The proponents of this drug believe that its effects on the brain are useful in helping people to resolve the behavioral problems that in many cases underlie their addiction.

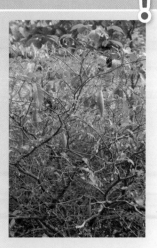

amount of animal protein in your diet will make these foods even more effective. And if you've just given up smoking, help your body to repair the cell damage caused by the habit by taking vitamin C supplements.

● **Eyedrop alert** A tell-tale sign that a young person is taking drugs is the frequent use of eyedrops to mask the red eyes and dilated or contracted pupils that result from illegal highs. Other signs may include:

★ **Skipping school** or college classes
★ **Money and valuables** disappearing from the home
★ **Refusing to tell** you about a new peer group and demanding more privacy.

If you suspect this problem, avoid an immediate confrontation. Seek help from your doctor or an organization such as Narcotics Anonymous.

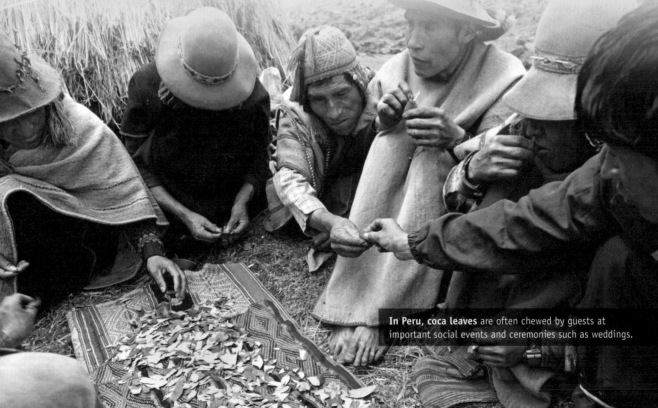

Secrets of
NATURE'S NARCOTICS

The potentially mind-altering effects of certain plants and fungi has long been recognized and harnessed by individuals and cultures around the world. And while they can be harmful and even lethal if misused, some of their powerful constituents have important medical applications, which continue to be developed for our benefit.

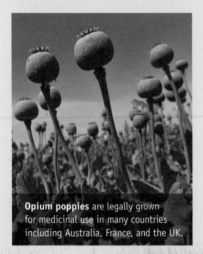

Opium poppies are legally grown for medicinal use in many countries including Australia, France, and the UK.

Despite, or perhaps because of the risks associated with their use, mind-altering plants and fungi have long fascinated humankind. Most of them contain compounds that are dangerous if taken in excess, but have also been used both as medicines and in religious rituals. Modern medical research is now beginning to understand the science that underlies these effects and is finding safer ways of using them.

Culture and history

For centuries, the people of South America have chewed coca leaves to quell hunger pangs and boost work stamina. They revered the plant as a gift from the gods. In 1860, German chemist Albert Niemann extracted cocaine from the leaves, initiating the use of the drug as a treatment for exhaustion and depression.

In Peru, coca leaves are often chewed by guests at important social events and ceremonies such as weddings.

The earliest evidence for the medicinal use of cannabis is in a Chinese manuscript from 2727 BC, which records it as a treatment for constipation, malaria, and rheumatism. And the ancient Persian texts of around 600 BC called bhang—dried cannabis—the "good narcotic." The seed pods of the opium poppy were used by the ancient Sumerians to make a pain-relieving medicine, and in ancient Egypt mothers gave opium to babies to induce sleep. Its recreational use came to the West in the 17th century, leading to the development of the modern narcotic painkillers morphine and codeine.

Studies of North African rock paintings from 9000 BC suggest that the effects of psilocybin—or "magic"—mushrooms were also known in ancient cultures. The Mayan and Aztec civilizations of Central and South America certainly used them to induce trances and to commune with the gods.

The Liberty Cap is one of the most potent species of magic mushroom.

Marijuana is made from the dried flowers and leaves of the cannabis plant.

Medical uses—now and in the future

While opiates have been used therapeutically in medicine for some centuries, scientists are still discovering the properties of other mind-altering plant-based drugs and revealing their potential to treat an array of diseases. A resultant medicine is then tested for safety and efficacy in clinical trials.

Coca cures Investigations at the Arizona Center for Integrative Medicine are focusing on the mix of alkaloids contained in the leaf and their use for treating conditions such as motion sickness, digestive complaints, and obesity. These substances must be taken by mouth, which minimizes any risk of addiction.

A change of view By the turn of the 21st century, the medicinal value of cannabis was becoming well known. In 2003, Canada became the first country to offer an extract of the plant for medical use in the form of the drug Sativex, which has since been licensed in several other countries, including the UK, where it can be prescribed to relieve some of the symptoms of multiple sclerosis. Research continues into the effectiveness of cannabis-derived drugs in relieving

the symptoms of other conditions associated with nerve damage, such as Parkinson's disease and spinal cord injuries. These drugs are also proving helpful in treating insomnia, anxiety, and loss of appetite.

Effective pain control With the invention of the hypodermic syringe, morphine became popular as an almost instant painkiller and was widely used in childbirth. Today, it is also available as tablets and liquid that can be taken orally and as skin patches. It works by inhibiting the action of pain receptors in the brain and is commonly used as an anesthetic during surgery and to treat the severe pain of serious injuries and many forms of cancer. Much current research focuses on developing drugs that act like opiates but without inducing tolerance and addiction. Such is the world shortage of opium that

the poppy is now being grown as a commercial crop in southern Britain and other European countries.

Help for depression? New research into the hallucinogenic drug psilocybin, which is obtained from psilocybin mushrooms, is exploring its use as an antidepressant. In studies at University College London, volunteers had psilocybin infused into their blood and the effects on their brains were monitored by MRI scans. The results showed that key of the areas of the brain affected by the drug are the posterior cingulated cortex, which is known to be involved in consciousness and self identity, and the medial prefrontal cortex, which is hyperactive in those suffering from depression. Work is now progressing on nonhallucinogenic versions of the drug.

Tackling fears, PHOBIAS AND OBSESSIONS

The stresses and demands of daily life make us all anxious from time to time. But when anxiety becomes extreme, when fears and worries appear to have no apparent or rational cause, or when we become so obsessive we cannot control our behavior, it's time to act.

● **Use computers to fight phobias**
About one in five people has a fear of flying, so great that it limits their holiday plans and can even put their careers at risk. Treatment has involved multiple visits to an airport with a therapist, but nowadays people are getting help from computer simulators. Subjects sit in an airline-style seat wearing a goggle-like device that fits over the head and eyes and transmits realistic images. The experience is so "real" that one participant in tests at the USA's Anxiety Disorders Center in Hartford, Connecticut, replied when asked to look out of the window: "No way. We're up too high." To be effective, the "flight" needs to last for about an hour, and it must be repeated occasionally. Similar technology is being used to help drivers face their fears, such as those resulting from traffic accidents.

● **Pop a pill before flying** If the prospect of flying sends you into a panic because you are sure the plane will crash or are afraid of heights, ask your doctor to prescribe a benzodiazepine tranquilizer. Drugs of this type can calm fears for just long enough to cope with flying. If you do take a tranquilizer, never mix it with alcohol, which will increase its side effects. These can include nausea, drowsiness, dizziness, slurred speech, and blurred vision. You may be advised to take a dose before flying, and to take an additional small dose if you feel anxious during the flight.

● **Seek SSRIs** Medication could be the answer for some agoraphobics. The lives of people who suffer from agoraphobia can be so limited that they become trapped in their

BELIEVE IT OR NOT!

Hard facts can calm fears
In successful "fear of flying" classes, aviophobics who are given the facts about how airplanes work and the safety of air travel compared with road or rail, and who have the opportunity to meet airline pilots and staff face to face, are much more able to conquer their fears. And when you do manage to get on the plane, simply closing your eyes and imagining that you're on a bus can really help, as there isn't a great deal of difference between air turbulence and driving on a bumpy road.

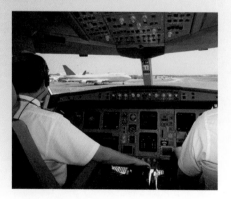

homes, unable to go out. Even when the condition is less severe, the fear of being in shopping centers, lines, elevators, and places from which they feel unable to escape, can still restrict people's lives. Of all the medications for treating agoraphobia, the most successful are antidepressants called selective serotonin re-uptake inhibitors, or SSRIs, which include the drug Prozac (fluoxetine). Ask your doctor about drug treatment if you suffer from agoraphobia.

● **Boost your levels** If your agoraphobia isn't severe or you don't want to embark on SSRI treatment (see above), you can boost your serotonin levels naturally. Get plenty of daylight, regular exercise, and eat a diet high in tryptophan, the amino acid from which serotonin is made. Try foods such as milk, yogurt, nuts, and seeds.

● **Stage your own recovery** Getting together with other sufferers to act out fears has proved extremely helpful for people who suffer from social phobias— that is, fear of situations in which you are convinced that you will be scrutinized, judged, or embarrassed in public. It can be fear of talking to strangers, speaking in public, or going to parties. By engaging in role play directed by a trained therapist, you'll be able to practice and prepare for the situations that frighten you, enabling you to overcome your paralysis and become more confident. There are support groups for most common phobias. Look on the Internet for one that is appropriate for you. Many such groups offer therapy of this kind.

● **Alter your reactions** Psychologists in Brazil have developed a novel method of treating arachnophobia—the fear of spiders. Many arachnophobes reject conventional treatments involving real spiders. The Brazilian approach gives each patient a CD of images with spider-like characteristics, varying from the vaulting in a Gothic cathedral to a camera on a tripod. Tests found that 42 percent of the arachnophobes who looked at the images twice a day for four weeks were able to touch a spider. After six months, more than 90 percent of the subjects were able to approach spiders without fear.

● **Desensitize yourself** It may seem contradictory, but imagining yourself in a situation that terrifies you can actually help you to confront fears that make you sweat,

Images that resemble spiders can help combat arachnophobia.

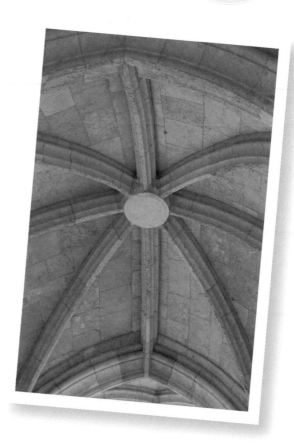

feel dizzy, or faint and give you palpitations and a pounding heartbeat. In this kind of therapy—which is particularly helpful for problems such as vertigo, claustrophobia, fear of water, the dark, or natural events such as storms and earthquakes—patients are encouraged to imagine the situations in which their fears arise. As they do this time and again, the situations begin to lose their anxiety-provoking ability, a process known as systematic desensitization.

● **See yourself confronting the fear**
Neurolinguistic programming (NLP) has recorded speedy success in alleviating fears and phobias. The treatment, carried out by a trained practitioner, takes place in several stages. First you have to imagine watching a black-and-white film of yourself confronting the situation or thing that frightens you— for example, being in a field with birds flying around your head, or holding a boa constrictor in your arms. In order to be able to view the film objectively, you are encouraged to feel yourself floating out of your body to a place where you are able to control the action, as if you were in the projection room of a movie theater. Once

Imagining yourself in a black-and-white film based on your fear can help you fight your phobia.

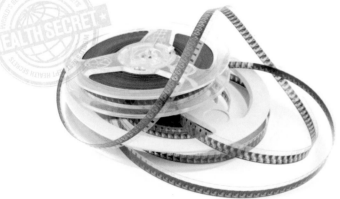

→

SURPRISINGLY EASY

Write it down
When you feel overcome by obsessive thoughts or feel spurred to carry out a compulsive action, write it down. Try to record exactly what you're thinking— however negative your thoughts may be, —even if it's the same thing over and over again. The more often you write down your thoughts, the more you'll find they'll lose their power over you.

you've "watched the film," and the birds, snakes, or other fearful objects have gone, you are then asked to visualize yourself stepping into the same scene in full color and re-enacting it from the beginning. The final stage is to imagine yourself meeting a flock of birds or picking up a snake; if the treatment has been successful, you'll find that your fear has dissipated.

● **Don't pass on your fears** Experts think that children of parents with anxiety disorders are at least seven times more likely to suffer problems than their peers. But this is not inevitable. In one US study, children who did not suffer from anxiety disorders and their parents who did have these problems were given a course of cognitive behavioral therapy (CBT). During eight weeks of treatment, the adults learned how to recognize what they were doing that might make their children anxious, such as being overprotective or worrying out loud. The children themselves learned such good coping skills that after a year not one of them had developed an anxiety disorder. In a similar group that did not receive CBT treatment, 30 percent of the children were diagnosed with anxiety issues severe enough to require therapy.

ARE MY HABITS A SIGN OF OCD?

Do you check several times that you've turned off the oven or always walk to the station on the same side of the street? Many of us have some compulsive habits; occasionally they get out of hand. This table describes the fears and actions typical of some of the most common forms of obsessive compulsive disorder (OCD). Talk to your doctor if your habits distress you or your family or begin to upset your daily life.

Your thoughts	Your actions
Fear of contamination from germs or dirt	● Repeatedly checking you body for signs of contamination ● Frequent washing ● Avoiding places or objects that you suspect may be a source of contamination
Fear of harmful consequences that may result from an oversight, such as leaving a door unlocked, a light burning, or the faucet running	● Repeatedly check locks, faucets, or switches ● Trying not to be the last person to leave the house ● Regularly seeking reassurance from others that everything is safe
Imagining that you may harm or cause distress to those you care for, such as hurting your child or betraying your partner	● Avoiding situations or objects that you fear may lead to harming, such as hiding sharp tools ● Focusing on a thought that seems to neutralize the risk
Fear of disorder or lack of symmetry and feeling anxious or distressed when objects are misaligned	● Constantly rearranging objects until they "feel right"
Fear of terrible consequences if you carry out tasks in the "wrong" order	● Re-doing actions that you feel may have been done "incorrectly"

● **Allow yourself a worry period** If you have obsessive compulsive disorder (OCD), a good way of overcoming your worries is to confine them to strictly timed 10-minute "worry periods," ideally first thing in the morning and in the early evening so that they don't interfere with your sleep. These sessions, which should take place in a specific location, are an ideal opportunity to record anxieties. If urges come into your head during the day, you can make a pact with yourself to postpone them until the worry period.

● **Know your value** The key to curing yourself of an obsessive compulsive disorder may lie in knowing yourself and using this knowledge to confront your fears. This is the basis of humanistic psychology, which asserts that everyone has an intrinsic worth and value and that to be mentally healthy, individuals must take personal responsibility for their actions. With the help of a therapist or analyst, the therapy concentrates on the present, not the past. It can work for you whether you're locked into a set of anxious thoughts, obsessed by fears or superstitions, or bound to rituals such as hand washing or double-checking.

● **See the funny side** Recognizing the absurdity of your obsessions can help you become more detached from your OCD. An award-winning American TV series featuring the OCD-suffering detective Adrian Monk, who cleans his hands every time he shakes hands with someone, has enabled sufferers to laugh at the problem, which affects one in 50 adults in the UK and USA.

● **Deal yourself a helping hand** The Q-sort test uses a deck of 100 cards to help people with OCD. On each card is written a

BODY POWER

Treat your body well—it's good for the mind

To keep anxiety to a minimum, it's important to keep your blood glucose levels as constant as possible during the day. When blood glucose drops or rises suddenly, anxiety kicks in. Begin the day with a good breakfast and throughout the day eat small, regular meals. Choose foods with a low GI (glycemic index) that release their energy more slowly, including whole grains, fruit, and vegetables. And avoid the sugar highs that come from eating cookies, cakes, and sweets.

personality trait, such as "very outgoing and social," "high self-esteem" or "organized and detail oriented." Participants are asked to sort the cards into nine piles on a scale from "not at all like me" to "very much like me," in categories that include "motivated," "educated," "lazy," and "easy to know." After

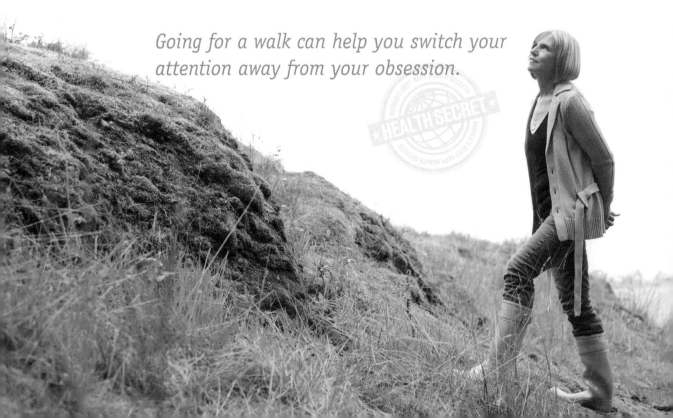

Going for a walk can help you switch your attention away from your obsession.

doing this, the cards are shuffled and you're asked to organize them again, but this time in a way that reflects your ideal self. Seeing the difference between the two will help you shift the focus of your thoughts so that you become more self-assured and positive, and less dependent on OCD behavior.

● **Take four steps** This simple plan can help you tackle your OCD.

★ **Re-label** If you're a hoarder, turn a compulsion on its head. Instead of thinking "I must hang on to these old newspapers, they may be useful one day," say "I don't really need them. It's my obsession that's telling me I can't let them go."

★ **Re-attribute** Admit that you have OCD and that it may be due to false brain messages. But distance yourself from it by telling yourself: "It's not me, it's the OCD."

★ **Re-focus** Do your best to distract yourself from your obsession. Instead of tidying or washing your hands, practice some yoga or meditation, or get out of the house and take a walk.

★ **Re-value** Downgrade your obsession by telling yourself it's not significant. You may not be able to make the thought disappear, but devaluing it can help you to ignore it.

● **Seek medication** If OCD is wrecking your life or making you depressed, ask your doctor about clomipramine, an antidepressant drug. It's one of the best medications for OCD, but it can take six to eight weeks before its full benefits are felt. Many OCD sufferers who take clomipramine agree that its side effects, such as dry mouth, fatigue, and weight gain, are outweighed by the relief provided from their obsessions.

● **Get support** Don't feel you have to cope with OCD on your own. Your family doctor can often provide valuable help and

advice, but talking to those who share your problem can be especially supportive. Visit the International OCD Foundation (www. iocdf.org) to find a local support group.

● **Deal with anxieties one by one**
By confronting things that make you anxious, you can diminish their effect. First make a list of the things you fear most. Tackle them one at a time, beginning with the least worrying. So, if you're least anxious about leaving the house without checking that the stove is off, begin with this. Instead of checking it several times, practice until you can look at it just once before you go out. Then go on to the next worry on the list. As you progress, monitor your anxiety levels—it's encouraging to see them drop.

INDEX

C

cabbage leaf compress 152

caffeine 85, 90, 203, 289
  see also chocolate; coffee;
    tea

calcium 21, 23, 55, 57, 80, 97, 98,
    119, 163, 164, 174, 177, 245,
    282, 289
  absorption 57
  non-dairy sources 23, 55–56, 59,
    163, 245

camellia nut oil 167

cancers
  chemotherapy 142, 172
  protection against 140–143
  protective foods 73, 95, 103, 118,
    140–143
  screening for 140, 195
  see also specific types of cancer

cannabis 299

canola oil 57, 70, 201, 227

capsaicin 272–273

capsaicin gel or cream 61

capsaicinoids 147

caraway seeds 84

carbohydrates 107–108
  FODMAPs 91
  low-carbohydrate diets 78, 245,
    280–281
  refined 86
  slow-release 201, 218
  unrefined 119

carcinogens 42

cardamom 89

cardiopulmonary resuscitation (CPR)
  27

carotenoids 34, 73, 75

carpal tunnel syndrome 206

carrots 69, 72, 136

casein kinase 284

castor oil 174

cataracts 73, 193

catechin 150

cerebellum 276

cervical cancer 195

chamomile 69, 151, 169

chasteberry 119, 124, 125

chatting 249

cheese 36, 76, 278

chemotherapy 142, 172

cherries 139

cherry juice 275

chewing gum 78, 84, 150, 224, 245,
  289

chewing sticks 157

chicken soup 34–35, 45

childbirth 128, 147

children
  anxiety disorders 302
  birth gaps 199
  brain development 199
  exercise 25, 200–201
  food refusal 75
  heart health 25
  myopia 257–258
  snoring 289
  television viewing 199

chiles 61, 78, 89, 136, 272–273

chocolate 39, 47, 142, 215, 238
  addiction 291

cholecystitis 86

cholesterol
  blood test 195
  and gallstones 85, 86, 87
  HDL cholesterol 21, 23, 29, 30,
    31, 71, 77–78, 227, 243
  LDL cholesterol 18, 21, 29, 30, 39,
    77–78, 126–127, 227, 243
  lowering 18, 20, 21, 22, 23, 29,
    30, 31, 35, 87, 108, 129
  oxidation 20, 39
  testing 30–31

choline 227

cholinesterase 237

chronic obstructive pulmonary
  disease (COPD) 41, 42, 51

chronic venous insufficency (CVI) 39

cider vinegar 84

cinnamon 89, 157

circadian clock 284

cirrhosis 295

citrus fruits 29, 86, 98, 134, 140,
  147, 229–230
  see also specific fruits

clams 75

claustrophobia 302

cleavers 100

clomipramine 305

clot-busting drugs 38

cloves 151, 152

cluster headaches 204

coal tar 170

cobalamin 243

coca leaves 298, 299

cocaine 298

coconut oil 77–78

celiac disease 93

coenzyme Q10 125

coffee 121, 160, 203
  decaffeinated 244
  and dementia risk reduction 233
  and depression 222–223

cognitive behavioral therapy (CBT)
  16, 283, 302

cognitive decline 229
  see also memory problems

cognitive fluency 228

cola 57, 97

cold remedies 47

cold sores 154, 155

colds see coughs and colds

collagen 163, 164, 166

colon cancer 94, 129, 141

colonic irrigation 92

colorectal cancer 95

color therapy 217, 219

compliments 215

compression stockings 33

computer simulators 300

computer, working at a 13, 66, 259,
  260

conjugated linoleic acid 21, 86

Conn's syndrome 36

W

X, Y

Z